Allergy Products Directory 1995-1996

Controlling Your Environment

by Carol Rudoff, MA, President, American Allergy Association

Edited by Joann Blessing-Moore, MD
Clinical Assistant Professor, Stanford University Medical Center

Important information. Please read.

This publication is designed to provide general information regarding services and products only. It is violable with the understanding that Allergy Publications, Inc. Is not engaged in rendering any medical or other advice in use or selection. If any medical or other professional assistance is required, the services of a competent physician should be sought.

Throughout this book, trademarked names are used. If a trademark notation was omitted, it was not done to infringe. We use the names only in an editorial fashion, and to the benefit of the trademark owner, with no intention of infringement of the trademark.

Mention of a product or service or facility by name does not constitute or imply an endorsement or recommendation. No product or procedure or location or facility or approach is safe or appropriate for everyone and purchases of products for personal or other use should be discussed with your doctor.

Acceptance of advertisements for publication does not imply endorsement of the products advertised.

This publication and the information contained in these listings was compiled as carefully as possible. Allergy Publications, Inc. cannot guarantee the correctness of all the information contained herein and cannot accept responsibility for omission or errors. The Directory is provided as is.

Offers from previous directories are now replaced by this new publication.

Library of Congress Catalog Card Number: 95-75930
Allergy Products Directory: ISBN 0-944569-02-1
Controlling Your Environment: ISBN 0-944569-03-X

Acknowledgments

Joann Blessing-Moore, MD

Clinical Assistant Professor

Stanford University Medical Center

Department of Allergy

Private Practice, Allergy and Pediatric Pulmonary

Disease

for reviewing the articles and listings in this directory

Gabriel Groner, PhD

Insight Solutions, Palo Alto, CA

for understanding the complex structure

of this directory and constructing an intelligent

program to create it

"This directory is really impressive. It puts practical information and tips into the hands of people who need them most. Great for people with asthma and allergies, their families, and the people who care for them."

Asthma and Allergy Foundation of America

"Allergy Products Directory" provides easy access to the incredible network of allergy products throughout the United States. This much needed directory has proved to be a tremendous value to the many people that are in search of more information."

Allergy and Asthma Network
Mothers of Asthmatics, Inc.

TABLE OF CONTENTS

Controlling Your Environment

Table of Contents

Controlling Your Environment

Table of Contents

Controlling Your Environment

Table of Contents

Controlling Your Environment

Table of Contents

HOW TO USE THIS DIRECTORY

INTRODUCTION TO *ALLERGY PRODUCTS DIRECTORY*

Allergy Products Directory lists a wide variety of resources and products that can help individuals and families with their allergy problems.

These resources and products are also of help to the doctors, nurses, respiratory therapists, social workers, and dietitians who counsel and treat such individuals and their families.

There are 3897 listings from more than one thousand companies, publishers, and organizations, plus instructive articles, how-to articles, and informative articles that will orient you to the listings.

WHAT'S NEW IN THIS EDITION?

ON LINE ADDRESSES

On-line resources are a new addition to the Directory. You'll find databases, on-line services, discussion groups, bulletin boards, CD-ROM's, and computer programs for the patient and for the professional.

E-MAIL ADDRESSES

Also new is the addition of e-mail addresses when available.

FAX NUMBERS

Fax numbers have been listed when available.

SPANISH LANGUAGE INFORMATION

These publications and education programs have been listed separately for easy referencing.

NUMBER OF CATEGORIES

The number of categories has been greatly increased for greater specificity and clarity.

EXPANSION OF ARTICLES

Articles have been re-written, updated, expanded, and corrected in accordance with new medical information, new standards, and new approaches.

Controlling Your Environment

How to Use This Directory

INCREASE IN NUMBER OF COMPANIES AND LISTINGS

There are many more listings and many more companies listed and these companies and products are cross referenced wherever appropriate.

HOW IS *ALLERGY PRODUCTS DIRECTORY* ARRANGED?

To improve accessibility, the Directory is divided into four Directories, each covering a major topic.

Controlling Your Environment

Here you'll find in-depth articles on assessing and selecting air filters and other products which humidify, dehumidify, heat, and condition your home. Environmental irritants are discussed with suggestions on handling or avoiding them.

The problems with dust and mold in bedroom environments are carefully reviewed with specific suggestions for improvement. Stinging and biting insects are described and steps to take if you are stung are covered in depth along with places to avoid and other precautions. Traveling with allergies has always been difficult. This article discusses how travel affects those with pollen allergy, food allergy, dust and mold allergy, and allergy to environmental smoke.

Listings include filters, dust and pollen controls, mold and mildew aids, specialty stores with mail order catalogues and special services, and titles of books on allergy for adults, children, and professionals.

Allergy/Asthma Finding Help

This volume covers a wide range of help resources with far-ranging capabilities in many areas from organizations to resource centers, telephone information lines, special libraries, newsletters, hospital departments, directories, clearinghouses, emergency preparation and help, patient education programs.

You'll find on line databases, on line services, discussion groups, bulletin boards, CD-ROMs, and computer programs for professionals and for individuals.

Various insurance options are explained and along with standards to evaluate individual and group policies. The

Controlling Your Environment
How to Use This Directory

myriad of medical initials, HMO's, IPA's, SFH's, FFS's, PPO's, HBH's, SFH's and EPO's, are demystified.

Asthma Resources Directory

Today, asthma control involves medication, environmental control, patient education, and measurement of lung function. Medication management evolves during the on-going relationship between you and your doctor. Environmental control is addressed in *Controlling Your Environment.* The last two aspects of management are addressed in this volume.

Asthma triggers, irritant-free pest control, environmental irritants, pulmonary function, and respiratory tools are major explanatory articles. *Talking to Your Doctor* helps you prepare and organize your thoughts and gives you check lists of information your doctor will want to know, and physical signs you should be aware of in order to make decisions about emergency needs, and information the emergency room will need to know.

The article on camps and asthma camps provides you with ideas on evaluating camps and assuring a safe camping experience for your child. You'll also have check lists to assess facilities and programs and information on making your child's experience a productive and meaningful one. The list of specialty camps is arranged by state.

Protecting Your Skin

Offered are two major articles: *Allergic and Irritant Contact Dermatitis* discusses medications, contacts, types of exposures (with special attention to nickel and latex), temperature, foods, even contact lenses solutions and eyeglass frames. Intimate use products and sunscreens are described and *Cosmetics.*

Listings include personal care items (from cosmetics to deodorants) to household products such as cleaning aids and repair products, even shoes and diapers, and specialty stores with mail order catalogues.

Food Allergy Resources (available in 1996)

This volume presents orgaizations, resource centers, hot lines, and health lines that are in-depth sources of information along with libraries and on line help through publications and recipe books round out this major source of help.

WHAT KIND OF INFORMATION IS PROVIDED IN A LISTING?

You will find the name of the product, book, program, or resource listed first, an explanation or description, and the companies or publishers or organizations that have that product or resource available. Selection should be made after discussion with your doctor because individual needs and environments vary and should be considered.

The addresses and telephone numbers of companies are supplied with each listing. All cross-referencing is done for you by listing all products, resources, and buying information in each appropriate chapter.

ANTICIPATED AREA CODE CHANGES

In 1995, several area codes changed. Certain sections of area code 206 in Washington state changed to 360; from July 9 you must use the new code. In Alabama certain sections of 205 became 334; from July 16 you must use the new code. In Arizona, Phoenix remained 602 while the rest of the state is 520; from July 23 you must use the new code. In Virginia, area code 703 split to create 540; from July 15 you must use the new code.

HOW DO I FIND WHAT I NEED?

Listings are alphabetized on a word-by-word basis. A listing for *Allergy* will be placed before *AllergyRite.* Companies that use a first name or initial and last name as in *L.L. Bean Co.* are alphabetized on a letter-by-letter basis since this is how the company is known. Names that begin with a number are listed first in order.

Each volume is divided into topic chapters and within those chapters are subheadings of products or services. For example, the section on emergencies is divided into preparing for emergencyes, help during emergencies, emergency communication devices, and travel emergencies.

Under each of those subsections you will find the product name, a description, and the providing company's address, telephone, and fax numbers. Telephone only services will list the service title, a description of the service, and the telephone number.

services will list the service title, a description of the service, and the telephone number.

The *Table of Contents* is comprehensive with a list of major headings as well as subheadings. Each chapter begins with its chapter title. Running heads on each page indicate the chapter. The index enables you to go quickly to the specific reference you wish.

POSTAL TWO-LETTER ABBREVIATIONS

We have used the postal service two-letter abbreviations for states, possessions, and Canadian provinces as follows:

Alabama	AL	Ohio	OH
Alaska	AK	Oklahoma	OK
Arizona	AZ	Oregon	OR
Arkansas	AR	Pennsylvania	PA
California	CA	Rhode Island	RI
Colorado	CO	South Carolina	SC
Connecticut	CT	South Dakota	SD
Delaware	DE	Tennessee	TN
Florida	FL	Texas	TX
Georgia	GA	Utah	UT
Hawaii	HI	Vermont	VT
Idaho	ID	Virginia	VA
Illinois	IL	Washington	WA
Indiana	IN	West Virginia	WV
Iowa	IA	Wisconsin	WI
Kansas	KS	Wyoming	WY
Kentucky	KY	District of Columbia	DC
Louisiana	LA	Guam	GU
Maine	ME	Puerto Rico	PR
Maryland	MD	Virgin Islands	VI
Massachusetts	MA		
Michigan	MI		
Minnesota	MN	CANADA	
Mississippi	MS		
Missouri	MO	Alberta	AB
Montana	MT	British Columbia	BC
Nebraska	NE	Manitoba	MB
Nevada	NV	New Brunswick	NB
New Hampshire	NH	Newfoundland	NF
New Jersey	NJ	Nova Scotia	NS
New Mexico	NM	Prince Edward Island	PE
New York	NY	Quebec	PQ
North Carolina	NC	Saskatchewan	SK
North Dakota	ND	NW Territories	NT
		Yukon Territory	YK

YOUR HOME ENVIRONMENT

Perennial rhinitis and asthma are very common respiratory complaints. Rhinitis symptoms include runny and stuffy nose, itching eyes, sore throat, sneezing, coughing, and, perhaps, sinusitis. Asthma symptoms include wheezing, coughing, difficulty breathing (especially at night), and difficulty breathing from exercise, strong odors, or cold air or allergic causes.

Controlling the indoor environment is very important since we spend the vast majority of our time indoors and a very large part of that indoor time in our bedrooms

Sometimes eczema, a skin allergy that results in a rash that itches and is red, develops from exposure to preservatives in products, oils, and resins, or plant products.

Controlling the indoor environment is very important since we spend the vast majority of our time indoors (at home, shopping, at recreational and entertainment events, or at work) and a very large part of that indoor time in our bedrooms.

HOUSE DUST MITES

House dust is a mixture of house dust mite protein, the dander from your pets, cockroaches, molds, outdoor pollen, and spores. Dust mites (*Dermatophagoides pteronyssinus*) are so small they can only be seen through a microscope. They are arachnids (in the same family as spiders) and live in mattresses, bedding, carpets, upholstery, clothing, and anything with fabric, especially nubby and textured fabrics, even stuffed toys.

One female dust mite can lay up to 50 eggs every three weeks!

Dusts fall on and cling to heavily upholstered and overstuffed furniture and flocked wallpapers. They live on human skin scales and so live anywhere that we live.

It is the waste products and body parts of the mites to which most people react. Since one female mite can lay up to 50 eggs every three weeks, your bed alone can be host to untold numbers. These are persistent and numerous adversaries.

Controlling Your Environment

Home Environment

Avoid carpeting where possible. Vacuuming stirs up and scatters dust. Mites have sticky pads on their feet that cling strongly to surfaces, so vacuuming is generally not effective at removing live mites, but does remove the feces and body parts that can be inhaled. When you walk on the carpet, mite waste matter floats up and can be inhaled and cause allergic symptoms. Therefore, you should vacuum thoroughly and often even though you are not getting rid of the mites themselves, you are removing mite feces and body parts.

Mites have sticky pads on their feet that cling strongly to surfaces, so vacuuming is generally not effective at removing live mites, but does remove the feces and body parts that can be inhaled.

When you make the bed or air it out or change sheets, you are disturbing mite waste matter and may experience symptoms. Washing in hot water is effective in keeping mite populations down.

You will want to strive for a clean, uncluttered look. Only keep display items that you really love. Don't try to fill every square inch of space. Consider displaying in glass-door cabinets. Hardwood and tile flooring have a beautiful look and can be damp mopped. Make it easy for yourself to keep your rooms clean.

PREPARING AND MAINTAINING THE BEDROOM

If you have a family history of this type of allergy problem, it is a good idea to prepare and maintain the bedroom before your child is born. It is still a good idea even if a child has no symptoms. According to Dr. Joann Blessing-Moore, there are good data to indicate that such precautions can delay the onset of allergies.

You will want to concentrate on keeping your bedroom or the bedrooms of your allergic children as dust free as you can because so many hours are spent in the bedroom. This can be done by isolating the bedroom as much as possible from the air circulation pattern of the house. Keep the doors and windows closed at all times. Install a window air conditioner if you don't have central air conditioning. Keep pets out. Remember, most doctors prefer you find your pet another home.

Controlling Your Environment

Home Environment

Do not pull up carpeting with your allergic child home.

Reactions can be severe.

With care and planning, you may find that symptoms can diminish considerably in this room and that it can be used during the day for other activities as well as for moments of relief.

If you or your child have severe problems, adapt the Japanese way of leaving your shoes outside the bedroom so as not to track in outdoor grime.

If at all possible, empty the bedroom and remove the carpeting. **Do not pull up and remove the carpeting with your allergic child at home. Reactions can be severe.** If you have hardwood floors, just clean them and enjoy their beauty. Otherwise, if you can, select vinyl or linoleum. They are easier to keep clean and will not harbor dust mites.

Everything that goes into a bedroom should be needed and easily washable, including, rugs, drapes, bedspread, blankets, or comforters.

Clean the walls, the floor, and ceiling; the windows, window sills, and molding; the closet, the light fixtures, and door molding. Clean the radiator. You can cover forced hot-air heating vents with a double layer of cheesecloth to trap larger particles, but cheesecloth will not trap pollen. Cheesecloth should be replaced at least weekly. More often is better. You may also use replaceable fiber glass or plastic filters. Replace them monthly.

Everything that goes into a bedroom should be needed and should be easily washable, including, rugs, drapes, bedspread, blankets, or comforters. The bedroom should be completely cleaned once a week, including mopping the floor and cleaning the walls and window sills.

Toys should be washable and preferably made of wood, plastic, or metal; if favorite stuffed toys remain, they must be hot water washable and dryable in the drier. Keep them in the dryer for at least 45 minutes. Store stuffed toys each night, preferably in a plastic bag. Do not leave them on a shelf.

The bedroom should be completely cleaned once a week, including mopping the floor and cleaning the walls and window sills.

The good news here is that Abstract #440 at the American Academy of Allergy meeting, March 12-17, 1993

Controlling Your Environment

Home Environment

indicated that velour blanket squares put into a dryer for at least 45 minutes was effective in lowering mite population from an average of 547 mites in an 8-inch square to 8 mites in an 8-inch square. This means that a favorite stuffed toy or blankets which cannot take extensive washings *may* be effectively treated in the dryer only. Talk to your doctor.

The following article is an in-depth look at what you can do to make your child's bedroom or your own bedroom as comfortable and as allergen-free as possible. Specific aspects of the bedroom environment are explored with specific action suggestions. (Products mentioned are found in our listings.)

RUG

As it is the largest potential collector of dust in the bedroom, make every effort to remove the carpet and its underlying pad which can also support mold. **Remember: Do not pull up the carpeting with your allergic child at home. Reactions can be severe.**

When installing new carpeting in other areas of the house, use a low-emitting adhesive if adhesives are needed. Try to be outside during installation and stay away for a while after installation. Open doors and windows during installation. If you have fans or an air conditioner, use them for a couple of days after installation.

Vacuuming does not lower your live dust mite population because live mites cling to the carpet fibers.

Vacuuming does not lower your live dust mite population. Live mites cling to the carpet fibers. Vacuuming will decrease mite feces and body parts which can be stirred up and inhaled when walking.

✔ Vacuum while your allergic child is at school

✔ If you are allergic to dust and must do the vacuuming, be sure to wear a mask with an appropriate level of protection while you vacuum

✔ Don't take your mask off as soon as you finish because your vacuuming will have stirred up all sorts of problem-causing particles that can float around for at least 15 minutes

✔ Investigate a central vacuum system that is vented outdoors or investigate a vacuum with high efficiency filters.

✔ Another possible solution is to use disposable plastic drop cloths found at paint stores. Tape them over your old

Controlling Your Environment

Home Environment

rug. If you leave your shoes outside the door, your plastic rug may last a week or two.

✔ A spray that keep the dust mite population down are also available

FLOOR

When you remove old carpeting in an older home, you may discover hardwood floors beneath. These are easier to keep clean than carpets.

> **WARNING: Do not pull up the carpeting with your allergic child or anyone with a severe reaction in the house. The reaction can be severe. Stay away from the house for as long as possible.**

If you have tile, it is not only attractive, it makes a good playing floor and spills from crafts projects, snacks, and accidents wipe up easily. If you use a throw rug, it should be lintless cotton that you can easily wash each week. If your floor is in poor condition, cover it with linoleum or vinyl and use molding to seal spaces between the baseboard and the floor. Mop weekly and twice a month, damp mop with a disinfectant solution that fights mold. One part chlorine bleach to 10 parts water is a good disinfectant.

BED

Since we spend the most hours in bed, do not place your bed in line with the air vent because dust and molds can be blown into the room through the vent by the heating and cooling systems.

Avoid bunk beds.

The upper bed is more difficult to clean and dust can fall on the lower bed.

Avoid bunk beds. The upper bed is more difficult to clean and dust can fall on the lower bed. If you must use bunk beds, remember to cover the mattresses and pillows on both beds and do not keep stuffed animals on the upper bunk. Do not use the upper bunk for storage of any kind.

Your mattress should be synthetic. The bed should be of metal or wood. First, thoroughly clean the bed frame and springs. Try to vacuum the bed frame at least monthly, preferably, more often. Thoroughly vacuum and dust the bedsprings.

Controlling Your Environment

Home Environment

MATTRESS ENCASINGS

Since dust mites flourish in your mattress, a cover or case made of plastic or vinyl (not cotton) with a zipper should enclose it. Cover the full length of the zipper with wide masking tape. You can use a washable, cotton mattress pad under the sheet. Be sure to also cover the box spring.

PILLOWS

Your pillows should be a non-allergenic, washable synthetic like dacron or polyester. Look for a "hypoallergenic" label and wash your pillow weekly in hot water and dry in a hot dryer. Encase it inside a plastic or vinyl cover and cover the zipper with wide masking tape.

Feather pillows can't be washed and are allergens in their own right. They also contain dust mites and mold. Even if you encase a feather pillow, the dust-proof cover will only protect you from dust mites, not from feather allergens.

Even if you encase a feather pillow, the dust-proof cover will only protect you from dust mites not from feather allergens.

If you use foam rubber pillows, they must be replaced every few months or at least annually because they disintegrate and because molds can grow on them.

SHEETS AND PILLOWCASES

Cotton is preferred. When you change the sheets, vacuum the encasings that are on the pillows, mattress, and box springs and sponge them clean.

BLANKETS AND BEDSPREADS

Blankets should be synthetic or cotton and washed weekly. Avoid woolen blankets and down comforters. The bedspread should also be cotton or a washable synthetic, and both should have a smooth finish. Be sure to wash with hot water and dry bedding in a dryer if available. Heat kills mites.

CEILING AND WALLS

If possible, the walls and ceiling should be smooth, without a finish and without a wallpaper that collects dust.

Controlling Your Environment

Home Environment

After washing thoroughly with a mild water and bleach combination of one part chlorine bleach to 10 parts water, ceilings and walls may be painted or papered with a washable wallpaper. Be sure to use mildew-resistant adhesive. Vacuum the ceiling and walls monthly.

WINDOWS AND WINDOW TREATMENT

In humid climtes, and when pollen and mold are problems, keep the windows closed. The windows should fit tightly. Use weather stripping. Install a window air conditioner if you don't have central air conditioning.

Sheets make colorful, washable, and easily replaceable curtains.

Venetian blinds and shutters collect dust and are not easily cleaned. Bright, colorful curtains that can easily be taken down weekly and laundered are best. Sheets make colorful, washable curtains. They work well and can be colorful accessories in a child's room and sophisticated color accents in an adult room

Window shades provide privacy and light control. They can be laminated with fabrics that match bedspreads and are available in contrasting or harmonizing colors. Shades will need to be wiped with a mild disinfectant solution that prevents mold. Be sure to wipe both sides of the shade. If you live in a high humidity area, you may find you need to use this mold preventive weekly.

FURNITURE

Furniture should have simple lines and not be ornate with grooves that catch dust. A desk chair should be a washable vinyl or plastic. Heavily upholstered furniture

Avoid ornate furniture with grooves that catch dust.

and pillows can be champion collectors of dust and don't belong in the bedroom. Padding should be a foam plastic. Remember that kapok and feathers can produce allergens and foam rubber supports mold. Twice a month wipe the vinyl with a disinfectant solution that fights mold like one part chlorine bleach to 10 parts water.

Controlling Your Environment

Home Environment

BOOKS

Books and bibelots are dust collectors and support mold growth. Either store them in another room or put them, and any magazines, inside a cabinet with doors.

PICTURES

If you are willing to clean and dust them each week, you can hang pictures. Pennants can contain hair and should taken down from bedrooms walls.

DOOR

Try to keep the bedroom door closed all the time.

CLOSETS

Closets are a part of the room. Think of the bedroom closet as a room in your bedroom and treat it exactly as you do the bedroom. Bedroom closets are also dust collectors that can spew dust into the bedroom air whenever you fling open the door.

Don't store anything in the closet.

Keep only clothes currently in use.

Don't store items in the closet, especially books. Keep only clothes currently in use in the closet. If you must store clothing in the closet, store it in plastic bags without mothballs or camphor. Keep shoes on a shoe rack that you can easily remove from the closet so that you can clean the floors and corners. When you clean the bedroom, clean the closet, the closet floor, and then close its door.

AIR CLEANER

These are discussed in-depth later in *Controlling Your Environment*. Air cleaners cannot take the place of environmental controls in your home and if you use them, they should be used along with the methods discussed above and not instead of.

HUMIDITY

Dust mites do not survive at humidity levels less than 20%. The more humid the air in your home is, the more

Controlling Your Environment

Home Environment

dust mites you will have, so try to keep the humidity level in your home low. Thirty-five to 45% humidity may be a good compromise, although some sources prefer lower. As a rule of thumb, if the outdoor temperature is 40°, inside humidity should be 45%; if outdoor temperature is 0 degrees, inside humidity should be 25%.

Keeping the room temperature below 70°
and room humidity below 50% helps to control dust mites.

Keeping the room temperature below 70° and room humidity below 50% helps to control dust mites. During showering or cooking, use an exhaust fan.

Air conditioners can help keep your mite population down by removing excess humidity from the atmosphere. An electric blanket or sheet on 'low' during the day keeps the dust mite population in your bed low also.

PETS

Pets should not be allowed in the bedroom and should be kept out of the house. Many doctors prefer that their patients not keep pets at all. It takes many, many months for dander to dissipate from your home.

HEATING/COOLING SYSTEMS AND DUCTWORK

Try to make the bedroom independent of the household's heating and cooling systems. You can then use separate heating units, air conditioners, and air filters to control dust and mold and keep the room much cleaner with less effort.

If you have a forced air heating system, use a special dust filter on the furnace and install an air purifier. Furnaces and cooling systems trap dust and dirt. In order for them to function efficiently, their filters must either be cleaned or changed frequently. Filters and purifiers are discussed elsewhere in *Allergy Products Directory*.

If you have a forced air heating system,
use a special dust filter on the furnace and install an air purifier.

Furnaces and cooling systems trap dust and dirt.

In the fall, before starting your heating system, clean or vacuum the registers thoroughly. In the summer, before

Controlling Your Environment

Home Environment

starting your cooling system, clean or vacuum the registers thoroughly; otherwise, months of accumulated dust and molds can be spewed into your home.

Electric heat is the cleanest. Avoid fans and blowers in favor of radiation or convection heating units.

Air conditioners and dehumidifiers seem to help keep mite population low by removing excess water (humidity) from the atmosphere. These units must be kept scrupulously clean and free of mold and bacteria growth. (See *Living with the Air in Your Home* in this Directory.)

Help us to help you. Mention *Allergy Products Directory.*

LIVING AREAS

In theory, you would like to handle other main living areas as though they were bedrooms. Remove moldy carpet pads and carpets, take down draperies, remove stuffed furniture and pillows, pack away accessories, and keep only those special items that you are willing to keep scrupulously clean.

As a practical matter, cast a careful eye over your living areas. If you have a family room, you probably spend a fair amount of time there and so do your children. It may be the kind of room you would tackle next. If the carpeting is old, consider replacing it with tile that can handle spills and scuffing when your children play. Tile is also easily mopped.

Tackle your family room next.

You and your family spend a great deal of time in it.

For other living areas (dining room or dining area, living room, den, sunroom) consider how you can replace aging carpets, drapes, stuffed furniture, pillows. Save your budget for replacing major items like carpeting. Can you use area rugs? Is there a wood floor under the old carpet? Is there a tile flooring that will give your home a new look?

MOLD CONTROL - INDOOR MOLDS

Mildew is a fungus that grows as a surface mold on just about anything. Mildew spores are in the air waiting for a welcoming environment: warm and moist.

Where there are warmth, moisture (humidity) and darkness, there are molds. You can smell them. They have

Controlling Your Environment

Home Environment

a musty odor which experience has taught us to associate with mildew. You can sometimes see where mildew has discolored a material.

Wherever you find warmth, moisture, and darkness, you'll find mold.

To eliminate molds, you must eliminate the conditions that encourage them. Ventilating rooms and closets and lighting them keeps them dry and inhibits mold formation. Lowering the humidity level to below 40 percent contributes to an environment that does not encourage mold.

MILDEW ON WALLS

If your walls are mildewed, don't paint over them. The mildew will grow through the new paint. Instead, wash the wall. Try one of the following:

One ounce of bleach in three quarts of water. Let the mixture dry on the wall surface for 20 minutes, then rinse thoroughly with fresh water. Let the wall dry before painting.

Add one quart liquid chlorine bleach to three quarts of warm water. Stir in one-third cup powdered laundry detergent. Apply with a sponge or nylon brush. Leave on long enough for the black stains to turn white, but don't let it dry. Rinse thoroughly and then let dry. (U.S. Dept. of Agriculture)

> **WARNING — Do not mix bleach with ammonia. The combination can release a poisonous gas**

Ask at the paint store about paint additives that may help control mildewing. Some exterior paints may be formulated with such additives in them.

BASEMENT

To control dampness in basements, use an electric heater or dehumidifier or, if possible, leave screened windows opened. Keep an incandescent light burning. Humidity levels should be maintained between 30 and 50%. Repair and water proof concrete or cinder block walls.

Ask a building contractor about plastic shields under cement flooring and for closet walls. Do not use a basement as a living area unless it does not leak, is dry and mold-free and has sufficient ventilation. Avoid carpets as they can become moldy rapidly.

Controlling Your Environment

Home Environment

BATHROOMS

In your bathrooms, window sills, shower stalls, shower curtains, and tile grout encourage mold growth. Scrub this growth with a brush dipped in a liquid bleach solution or commercially available mold-preventive. (See *Fighting Mold.*) Use paint in your bathroom rather than wallpaper and give mold less of a hiding place.

Use paint in your bathroom rather than wallpaper and give mold less of a hiding place.

Replace shower curtains that are mildewed. Carpeting in the bathroom develops mold rapidly and should be avoided. If the room doesn't have a vent fan, install one or keep the window opened. After the family's bathing and showering is done, leave the bathroom door opened and the vent fan going until the humidity level is down.

CLOSETS

Damp closets can be helped by installing fans, louvered doors, opening windows, burning an incandescent light, or using a small dehumidifier.

KITCHEN

Cooking raises the level of moisture in the air, supporting mold growth, while use of cleaning chemicals, storage of cleaning chemicals and leftover products, placement of household plants (See below.), and pest

Cooking raises the level of moisture in the air, supporting mold growth.

Use the exhaust fan when cooking and cleaning.

control procedures mean following careful steps to keep the kitchen clear of indoor pollutants. Use the exhaust fan when cooking and cleaning. Do not use the oven to heat the room. Discard old or unused chemical products. Read the chapter on non-irritating pest control.

If your laundry equipment is in the area, be sure the clothes dryer vents outdoors. Turn on ventilating fans while using laundry equipment.

Controlling Your Environment

Home Environment

REFRIGERATOR

Molds or mildew grow on the gasket around the inside of the refrigerator door. Inside the refrigerator, you'll find mold on spoiled fruit or old cheese. Keep refrigerators clean and

throw out spoiled food. Do not try to cut away mold that you can see and save the rest of the food. The mold has penetrated rest of the food and none of it should be eaten.

More recent thought is that larger foods with the mold cut away leaving a broad, clean border may be safe to eat. Smaller foods like grapes should be thrown away if mold is on them. Consider the cost and replaceability of the item and err on the side of caution.

Protect yourself by wearing a mask with an appropriate level of protection or have someone else clean the dusty coils of the refrigerator. You'll save money on the cost of running the appliance.

TRASH COMPACTOR

Don't neglect regular cleaning of your trash compactor. It will encourage mold, especially in warmer weather, when you may notice a distinctly unpleasant odor. Let the container air in full sunlight or wash thoroughly with soap and let dry completely.

PLANTS

Molds also grow on the surface of clay pots, dead leaves, and on the soil of your house plants. Depending upon your degree of sensitivity, you may need to scrub the clay pots, keep your plants free of dead leaves, and put charcoal on the soil, or you may try growing cactus, or you may have to give your plants away. Also consider that any water spillage on carpeting and padding will support mold growth.

ATTIC MILDEW

Attics need ventilation (roof fan or louvers) as well as a vapor barrier. Activities like showering, bathing, cooking, or laundering, produce a great deal of moisture that is absorbed into the air of your home. Your home needs sufficient ventilation for water vapor to escape.

Your home needs sufficient ventilation for water vapor to escape.

Older homes, probably built without vapor barriers, are vulnerable to moisture in the air, and condensation.

Controlling Your Environment

Home Environment

Unfortunately, the newer homes of today are more energy-efficient and tightly sealed. There are usually not as many air exchanges per hour as older, more leaky houses are likely to have. When windows must be kept closed because of pollen and molds, ventilation becomes inadequate to handle the excess moisture that daily activities produce.

Older homes, more likely built without vapor barriers, are vulnerable to moisture in the air. When moist, warm, indoor air touches cold surfaces inside the wall, it causes condensation.

A vapor barrier (plastic sheeting or foil) on the warm side of the wall keeps heated, moist indoor air from meeting cold surfaces inside the wall and causing condensation. This condensation makes insulation less effective and can result in peeling exterior paint.

Crawl spaces should be ventilated and covered with plastic sheeting to prevent mold spores in the moist ground from entering your house. Be on the alert for the musty odor that indicates mildew caused by water seepage.

APPLIANCES

Appliances that release combustion pollutlants are space heaters, gas ranges, ovens, furnaces, gas water heaters, gas clothes dryers, charcoal grills, wood or coal-burning stoves, and fireplaces. Combustion pollutants are particles or gases that result from burning fuels like gas, kerosene, wood, or coal. Combustion also releases water vapor that can cause high humidity, encouraging house dust mites, molds, and bacteria.

OTHER SOURCES OF MOLD

Other sources of mold in your home are kapok, foam pillows, wallpaper, dirty upholstery, old carpet padding, and wet wallpaper, foam pillows, dirty upholstery, and wet swimsuits and towels that have been thrown down on the floor rather than hung up to dry.

Don't forget to clean your home's gutters and downspouts and keep roofing in good repair, especially on the shady side of the house.

Wet swimsuits and towels that have been thrown on the floor rather than hung up to dry are prime sources of mold.

Controlling Your Environment

Home Environment

Remember that dehumidifiers, cold mist vaporizers, humidifiers, and air conditioners must be kept clean because molds and bacteria will grow in their water

reservoirs. Fix water leaks promptly to avoid mold formation.

If you are building a home, there are techniques that may be employed to cut down on moisture, especially in basements. Be sure to talk to your architect or builder about placing sheet plastic barriers, especially for cement flooring, to act as moisture barriers.

DON'T FORGET YOUR CAR

Like your heating furnace, when you first turn on your car's air conditioner for the summer, it will throw out a spume of dust. Have the conditioner and the vents cleaned before you use the system. Remove the condensation water to keep the system free of mold.

Keep the floor mats clean and dry them in the sun. Don't allow children to eat or drink in the car and be very careful yourself. Spills on upholstery can support mold growth.

MOLD CONTROL — OUTDOOR MOLDS

Grass and leaves have a great deal of mold growth. When you rake, you scatter the mold and their spores become airborne. If you are allergic and you must care for your garden, wear a mask with an appropriate level of protection, and take your medication before gardening.

Do be sure your allergic children remain indoors while you are raking or mowing. Mold-allergic children shouldn't bounce on your leaf piles or walk through fallen leaves because that also disturbs the mold spores.

Mold-allergic children shouldn't bounce on your leaf piles or walk through fallen leaves because that disturbs the mold spores.

Keep your yard clean and don't use compost piles. Cut grass, barns, and wooded areas are sources of mold. Your compost heap is a major source of mold from decaying leaves and grass. Try to keep the garden clear of debris and dying plants. Areas with hay stacks and barns or granaries and farms are important mold sources.

Garbage containers are mold sources as well and should be kept clean along with the area around them. Some

Controlling Your Environment

Home Environment

sources recommend that borax be poured inside the cans to fight mold.

Garbage containers are mold sources and should be kept clean along with the area around them

---

Being outdoors on dry windy days, especially in rural areas, should be avoided. If farming or gardening activity is on-going, and children are very sensitive, they should stay in a clean-air room with the doors and windows closed.

Outdoor molds easily enter your home environment. Keep your windows closed and use a window air conditioner. If you can afford only one air conditioner, put it in the bedroom.

ANIMAL EXPOSURE

DANDER AS A CARRIER OF GLANDULAR SECRETIONS

Although your pet's dander or skin flakes are an allergic component of house dust, they are also an allergen by themselves. Dander is a long-lasting problem. It can remain in a home that has not had a pet for months, even years.

Some individuals are more sensitive to animal dander than others. Completely eliminating the animal from the home may be the only solution. For some, keeping the pets outdoors may be sufficient. However, children may actually spend more time outdoors with their pets because they are lonely for them.

GLANDULAR SECRETIONS

Dander carries glandular secretions that are on the skinflakes, the hair, or in saliva. Proteins from glandular secretion are carried on your pet's dander. When your pet licks itself, glandular secretions are spread over its fur.

Cat glandular secretion is such a strong allergen that you may have difficulty being with a friend who owns a cat. Your friend's clothing may have cat dander on it and you can react to the glandular secretion proteins carried by dander on the clothing.

Cat glandular secretion is such a strong allergen, that you may have difficulty being with a friend who owns a cat.

Fel d I, a protein in cat skin, can be washed away. Some recent studies seem to indicate that *if* the cat is washed once a week for 10 minutes and *if* it spends most of its time

Controlling Your Environment

Home Environment

outdoors, *if* the carpeting in the home is eliminated, and *if* air filters are used and *if* a thorough house cleaning schedule initiated, *then* —*some* time may be able to be spent with the cat.

These are severe measures for a possible occurrence, especially considering the pollen and moldy leaves that cling to your cat's fur. Also consider how you plan to bathe a cat once a week for 10 minutes. Further, these measures do not account for cat saliva, another strong allergen.

SALIVA AS A CARRIER

Pet saliva is an allergen. If you are very sensitive, your skin may turn red and itch where your pet licks you. Cat saliva deposited on cat hair during grooming aerosolizes and is found in the air, on your furniture and on your clothing. Saliva is also a carrier of gland secretion, picked up as cats lick themselves.

URINE

Sand boxes may become contaminted with cat urine and feces even when you don't own a cat. Be sure to keep sand boxes covered. As cats urinate, the urine becomes contaminated by the secretions that are on the skinflakes and the hair. Cat boxes are also sources of allergen from urine.

FLEAS

The majority of the fleas that your pet has been supporting remain in your home in the carpeting, in the cracks of the floor, or on furniture. Without your pet, it takes time and lots of it before that population actually declines.

Fleas can remain in their pupa stage for up to one year.

Keep this in mind when moving into a home where a pet once lived.

Fleas can remain in their pupa stage for up to one year. Keep this in mind when moving into a home where a pet once lived. (Bio-Integral Resource Center has a booklet, *Least-Toxic Pest Management for Fleas* PO Box 7414, Berkeley, CA 94704)

Controlling Your Environment

Home Environment

TRANSPORT

When your pet comes indoors, it brings moldy leaves clinging to its fur along with pollen it has picked up while romping. This increases the allergic load in the household. Even allowing a pet indoors for a short time is questionable because your forced air heating system can spread dander throughout the house. Once a pet is in a house, the allergen can remain in the environment for months; therefore, many doctors prefer that pets be given to other homes.

AVOIDANCE

Even when the decision to give a pet away is carried out, contacts with animal dander are difficult to avoid. Direct exposures can occur at a friend's home, a baby sitter's home, the park, a dog straying onto school property.

Dander travels on people's clothing and your child can be exposed to pet owners at school, at the supermarket, at a department store, on the street, at a friend's home (even when the friend does not own a dog), almost anywhere. Other family members may be in situations where there are animals and bring dander home on their clothing.

HELP US TO HELP YOU

When writing to the companies and organizations listed here, be sure to use the initials (APD) as part of the address and tell them you saw them listed in *Allergy Products Directory.*

If you call, be sure to tell them you found them in *Allergy Products Directory.*

This is important to you because:

- Lets the company know that its listings have helped you.

- Encourages the company to keep *Allergy Products Directory* informed of its new products so that we can keep you informed.

- Enables us to keep our listings accurate and up-to-date for you on the latest products, services, and innovations.

- Enables us to keep the Directory price low for you.

Thank you for your help.

DUST AND POLLEN CONTROL AIDS

MITE-PROOF MATTRESS ENCASEMENTS

All-Vinyl Boxspring/Mattress Encasing

Zippered vinyl encasing; most sizes
Available from:
Skin & Allergy Shop,™The
310 E. Broadway (APD)
Louisville, KY 40202
800-366-6483
In KY 502-585-4824
Fax 502-589-3429

Aller-Shield® Encasings

Vinyl coated knitted, mildew-resistant nylon mattress, box spring, and pillow covers; cleanable in washing machine and dryer; cotton-free, cotton lint-free, napless; seams back-tacked, edges bound, zippers rust-free and opens on three sides of mattress or box spring; most sizes
Available from:
Environtrol® Corporation
PO Box 31313 (APD)
St. Louis, MO 63131
800-423-1982
In St. Louis 314-966-6886

Aller-Shield® Encasings

Embossed, 6-gauge vinyl coated mattress, box spring, and pillow covers; cleanable in washing machine and dryer; cotton-free, cotton lint-free, napless; seams back-tacked, edges bound, zippers rust-free and opens on three sizes of mattress or box spring; water-proof, flame retardant; zippers rust-free and opens on three sizes of mattress or box spring; most sizes
Available from:
Environtrol® Corporation
PO Box 31313 (APD)
St. Louis, MO 63131
800-423-1982

In St. Louis 314-966-6886

Aller-Tech Vinyl Box Spring Protector

6-gauge vinyl; zipper encasement; fire retardant; most sizes
Available from:
Allergy Asthma Technology
4151 N. Kedzie (APD)
PO Box 18398 (APD)
Chicago, IL 60618
800-621-5545
312-465-8020
Fax 312-465-7619
and:
Priorities®
70 Walnut St. (APD)
Wellesley, MA 02181
800-553-5398

Aller-Tech® Bedding Protector

Vinyl or vinyl with nylon covers for mattress, box springs, and pillows; zipper; washable; most sizes
Available from:
Allergy Asthma Technology
4151 N. Kedzie (APD)
PO Box 18398 (APD)
Chicago, IL 60618
800-621-5545
312-465-8020
Fax 312-465-7619

Aller-Tech® Breathable Mattress/Box Spring Protector

Cotton protector with "breathable" vapor transmissible membrane; barrier layer non-permeable to allergens; fire retardant; zipper; mattress in many sizes; box spring in many sizes; greater depth for heavily padded mattresses
Available from:
Allergy Asthma Technology
4151 N. Kedzie (APD)
PO Box 18398 (APD)
Chicago, IL 60618
800-621-5545

312-465-8020
Fax 312-465-7619

Aller-Tech® Breathable Pillow Protector

Cotton protector with "breathable" vapor transmissible membrane; barrier layer non-permeable to allergens; fire retardant; zipper; standard, queen, king
Available from:
Allergy Asthma Technology
4151 N. Kedzie (APD)
PO Box 18398 (APD)
Chicago, IL 60618
800-621-5545
312-465-8020
Fax 312-465-7619

Aller-Tech® Mattress/Box Spring Protector

Nylon lined with vinyl by a dipping process; fire retardant; machine wash; zipper; mattresses in many sizes; box springs in many sizes; greater depth for heavily padded mattresses
Available from:
Allergy Asthma Technology
4151 N. Kedzie (APD)
PO Box 18398 (APD)
Chicago, IL 60618
800-621-5545
312-465-8020
Fax 312-465-7619

Aller-Tech® Pillow Protector

Nylon lined with vinyl by a dipping process; fire retardant; zipper; machine wash; standard, queen, king
Available from:
Allergy Asthma Technology
4151 N. Kedzie (APD)
PO Box 18398 (APD)
Chicago, IL 60618
800-621-5545
312-465-8020
Fax 312-465-7619

Aller-Tech® Vinyl Boxspring/Mattress Encasing

Zippered, "non-allergenic" 6-gauge vinyl encasing; most sizes
Available from:
A-Plus Allergy Equipment & Supply
8325 Regis Way (APD)
Los Angeles, CA 90045-2646
Orders 800-86-ALLER (862-5537)
310-337-7468
Fax 310-337-1971
and:
Absolute Environmental's Allergy Store
2615 S. University Dr. (APD)
Davie, FL 33328
Nationwide 800-771-ACHOO (2246)
In FL 800-329-3773
Broward 305-472-3773
Fax 305-474-0133
and:
Allergy Asthma Technology
4151 N. Kedzie (APD)
PO Box 18398 (APD)
Chicago, IL 60618
800-621-5545
312-465-8020
Fax 312-465-7619
and:
Allergy Relief Products
9 Renata Ct. (APD)
Dundas, ON L9H 6X1
Canada
905-628-5324 ?416
Fax 416-628-1734
and:
American Allergy Supply
PO Box 722022 (APD)
Houston, TX 77272-2022
800-321-1096
713-995-6110
and:
National Allergy Supply, Inc.
4400 Georgia Hwy. 120 (APD)
PO Box 1658 (APD)
Duluth, GA 30136
800-522-1448
In Atlanta 404-623-8077
Fax 404-623-5568

Controlling Your Environment

Dust and Pollen Control

Allergen Tight™ Mattress/Boxspring Encasing

Zippered covers for mattresses, boxsprings; unbleached cotton cloth with rubberized backing
Available from:
Allergy Relief Distributors
Div. of E.C.Environmental Control, Inc.
177 Telegraph Rd. #365 (APD)
Bellingham, WA 98226
206-734-1646
Fax 206-734-3696
Canadian office in Vancouver, BC

Allergen Tight™ Mattress/Boxspring Encasing

Zippered covers for mattresses, boxsprings; vinyl
Available from:
Allergy Relief Distributors
Div. of E.C.Environmental Control, Inc.
177 Telegraph Rd. #365 (APD)
Bellingham, WA 98226
206-734-1646
Fax 206-734-3696
Canadian office in Vancouver, BC

Allergen Tight™ Pillow Encasing

Zippered covers for pillows; unbleached cotton cloth with rubberized backing
Available from:
Allergy Relief Distributors
Div. of E.C.Environmental Control, Inc.
177 Telegraph Rd. #365 (APD)
Bellingham, WA 98226
206-734-1646
Fax 206-734-3696
Canadian office in Vancouver, BC

Allergen Tight™ Pillow Encasing

Zippered covers for pillows; vinyl
Available from:
Allergy Relief Distributors
Div. of E.C.Environmental Control, Inc.
177 Telegraph Rd. #365 (APD)
Bellingham, WA 98226
206-734-1646
Fax 206-734-3696
Canadian office in Vancouver, BC

Allergy Control™ Covers

Washable and dryable covers have an allergen barrier; non-vinyl; allows water vapor transmission. Economy model is tricot for box springs and mattress; original model is cotton-polyester for pillow, mattress, box springs, water beds; custom sizes; ultra model is 3-ply material for pillow and mattress.
Available from:
Allergy Control Products, Inc.
96 Danbury Rd. (APD)
PO Box 793 (APD)
Ridgefield, CT 06877
800-422-DUST (3878)
203-438-9580
Fax 203-431-8963

Cloth/Vinyl Encasing

Poly cotton fabric thermally bonded to 6-gauge vinyl; washable; fully zippered; glue-free
Available from:
Absolute Environmental's Allergy Store
2615 S. University Dr. (APD)
Davie, FL 33328
Nationwide 800-771-ACHOO (2246)
In FL 800-329-3773
Broward 305-472-3773
Fax 305-474-0133

Comfortech™ Comforter Cover

Comforter encasing or inner liner under decorative duvet cover of miteproof Comfortech™ membrane; zipper; blue, beige, white, rose; twin, queen, king
Available from:
National Allergy Supply, Inc.
4400 Georgia Hwy. 120 (APD)
PO Box 1658 (APD)
Duluth, GA 30136
800-522-1448
In Atlanta 404-623-8077
Fax 404-623-5568

Controlling Your Environment

Dust and Pollen Control

Cotton/Poly Mattress Protector

Vinyl-backed, cotton/polyester blend protector; 5-gauge vinyl; zipper encasement; fire-retardant; most sizes
Available from:
Priorities®
70 Walnut St. (APD)
Wellesley, MA 02181
800-553-5398

Cotton/Poly Pillow Protector

Vinyl-backed, cotton/polyester blend protector; 5-gauge vinyl; zipper encasement; fire-retardant; standard, queen, king
Available from:
Priorities®
70 Walnut St. (APD)
Wellesley, MA 02181
800-553-5398

DERPI Dustop Encasing

Polyethylene base encasing with covered zipper, including tape for dust-free seal; case can be shaken to clean or remove tape to wash separately in warm water, air dry, replace tape; pillow cases, single, double, king size mattress encasings, single, double, king size duvet covers; special sizes available for cots, futons, cushions, bunkbeds
Available from:
Allergy Relief Products, Ltd.
39 Spring Crescent (APD)
Southampton SO2 1FZ
England
44-0703-586709
Fax 44-0703-676226

Dust Proof Mattress Encasing

Cotton/polyester; zipper; most sizes; custom sizes
Available from:
Allergy Clean Environments
501 Station Ave. (APD)
Haddon Heights, NJ 08035
800-882-4110
In NJ 609-546-1101
Fax 609-546-1466

URL:
http:\\WWW.infomall.com\allergy.html

Envirocase®

Cotton and Supplex® nylon with Miteguard® barrier finish; flame retardant, water proof, machine washable; mattress (many sizes), box springs, pillow (standard, queen, king) encasings
Available from:
Skin & Allergy Shop,™ The
310 E. Broadway (APD)
Louisville, KY 40202
800-366-6483
In KY 502-585-4824
Fax 502-589-3429

Intervent™

Breathable fabric is a barrier to house dust mite. Called expanded polytetrafluoroethylene membrane, it is integrated into mattress construction and provides outer covering for pillows; fabric can be wiped with damp cloth. It functions as a highly efficient filter down to 0.001 micron
Available in England from
Slumberland Plc
Medicare Division
Salmon Fields
Oldham OL2 6SB
England
Telephone 061 628 5293
Intervent is also available as an interliner for mattresses, pillows, and duvets. It is called expanded polytetrafluoroethylene membrane
Available in England through
Freephone 0800 515730
Expected availability in the U.S. 1995,1996
Available from:
W.L. Gore & Associates, Inc.
297 Blue Ball Rd. (APD)
Elkton, MD 21921
800-431-4673
Canada 800-523-4673
Orders Canada only 800-636-4777

Controlling Your Environment

Dust and Pollen Control

and
W.L. Gore & Associates (UK) Ltd.
Church Gate, Church Street W.
Woking, Surrey GU2 1DJ
England

Linen/Non-Vinyl Encasing
Linen (polycotton) covered with a non-vinyl, mite-proof membrane; mattress and pillow encasing; all sizes; custom sizes
Available from:
Absolute Environmental's Allergy Store
2615 S. University Dr. (APD)
Davie, FL 33328
Nationwide 800-771-ACHOO (2246)
In FL 800-329-3773
Broward 305-472-3773
Fax 305-474-0133

Mite Proof Duvet Cover
Breathable fabric bonded to mite-proof inside barrier; seams reinforced with cotton binding; tricot knit or cotton polyester, zipper; most sizes
Available from:
Allergy Relief Products
9 Renata Ct. (APD)
Dundas, ON L9H 6X1
Canada
905-628-5324 ?416
Fax 416-628-1734

Mite Proof Mattress Encasing
Breathable fabric bonded to mite-proof inside barrier; seams reinforced with cotton binding; tricot knit, cotton polyester, or stretchable polyester knit; zipper; most sizes
Available from:
Allergy Relief Products
9 Renata Ct. (APD)
Dundas, ON L9H 6X1
Canada
905-628-5324 ?416
Fax 416-628-1734
and:
American Allergy Supply
PO Box 722022 (APD)
Houston, TX 77272-2022

800-321-1096
713-995-6110
and:
National Allergy Supply, Inc.
4400 Georgia Hwy. 120 (APD)
PO Box 1658 (APD)
Duluth, GA 30136
800-522-1448
In Atlanta 404-623-8077
Fax 404-623-5568

Mite Proof Pillow Encasing
Breathable fabric bonded to mite-proof inside barrier; seams reinforced with cotton binding; tricot knit, cotton polyester, or stretchable polyester knit; zipper; standard, queen, king
Available from:
Allergy Relief Products
9 Renata Ct. (APD)
Dundas, ON L9H 6X1
Canada
905-628-5324 ?416
Fax 416-628-1734
and:
American Allergy Supply
PO Box 722022 (APD)
Houston, TX 77272-2022
800-321-1096
713-995-6110
and:
National Allergy Supply, Inc.
4400 Georgia Hwy. 120 (APD)
PO Box 1658 (APD)
Duluth, GA 30136
800-522-1448
In Atlanta 404-623-8077
Fax 404-623-5568

Mite-N-Case® Pillow Cover
Cotton terry pillow cover, vinyl backing; reinforced seams; zipper; standard, queen, king
Available from:
Aller-Guard,® Inc.
Southgate Office Park

Controlling Your Environment

Dust and Pollen Control

1645 S.W. 41st St. (APD)
Topeka, KS 66609-1250
800-234-0816
913-267-9333
Fax 913-267-0072

Mite-N-Case® Pillow/Mattress Cover

Poly cotton pillow, vinyl backing; reinforced seams; zipper; standard, queen, king; and mattress cover, vinyl backing; zipper; most
Available from:
Aller-Guard,® Inc.
Southgate Office Park
1645 S.W. 41st St. (APD)
Topeka, KS 66609-1250
800-234-0816
913-267-9333
Fax 913-267-0072

Mite-N-Case® Pillow/Mattress Cover

Tricot pillow, vinyl backing; reinforced seams; zipper; standard, queen, king; and mattress cover, vinyl backing; zipper; most sizes
Available from:
Aller-Guard,® Inc.
Southgate Office Park
1645 S.W. 41st St. (APD)
Topeka, KS 66609-1250
800-234-0816
913-267-9333
Fax 913-267-0072

Mite-N-Case® Mattress/Box Spring

All-vinyl mattress or box spring cover; heavy gauge; zipper; most sizes
Available from:
Aller-Guard,® Inc.
Southgate Office Park
1645 S.W. 41st St. (APD)
Topeka, KS 66609-1250
800-234-0816
913-267-9333
Fax 913-267-0072

Mite-N-Case® Box Spring Cover

All vinyl, box spring cover; 6-gauge vinyl; zipper; most sizes
Available from:
Aller-Guard,® Inc.
Southgate Office Park
1645 S.W. 41st St. (APD)
Topeka, KS 66609-1250
800-234-0816
913-267-9333
Fax 913-267-0072

Pillow/Mattress Encasing

Knitted nylon fabric coated on one side with vinyl; waterproof; washable
Available from:
Allergy Alternative
440 Godfrey Dr. (APD)
Windsor, CA 95492
800-838-1514

Provin™ Protector

Vinyl box spring protector; heat-sealed; reinforced seams; zipper; available; most sizes
Available from:
Allergy Control Products, Inc.
96 Danbury Rd. (APD)
PO Box 793 (APD)
Ridgefield, CT 06877
800-422-DUST (3878)
203-438-9580
Fax 203-431-8963

Stretchlite® Knit Encasement

Knit fabric covered with a non-vinyl mite-proof membrane; mattress and pillow encasing; all sizes; custom sizes
Available from:
Absolute Environmental's Allergy Store
2615 S. University Dr. (APD)
Davie, FL 33328
Nationwide 800-771-ACHOO (2246)
In FL 800-329-3773
Broward 305-472-3773
Fax 305-474-0133

Controlling Your Environment

Dust and Pollen Control

Tricot Mattress Encasing

Tricot cloth bonded (no glue) to vinyl encasing; zipper; machine washable in hot water, dry on low; most sizes; some custom sizes
Available from:
A-Plus Allergy Equipment & Supply
8325 Regis Way (APD)
Los Angeles, CA 90045-2646
Orders 800-86-ALLER (862-5537)
310-337-7468
Fax 310-337-1971
and:
Allergy Clean Environments
501 Station Ave. (APD)
Haddon Heights, NJ 08035
800-882-4110
In NJ 609-546-1101
Fax 609-546-1466
URL:
http:\\WWW.infomall.com\allergy.html

Tricot Pillow Encasing

Nylon tricot cloth bonded (no glue) to vinyl encasing; zipper; machine washable in warm water, dry on low; standard, queen, king
Available from:
A-Plus Allergy Equipment & Supply
8325 Regis Way (APD)
Los Angeles, CA 90045-2646
Orders 800-86-ALLER (862-5537)
310-337-7468
Fax 310-337-1971
and:
Allergy Clean Environments
501 Station Ave. (APD)
Haddon Heights, NJ 08035
800-882-4110
In NJ 609-546-1101
Fax 609-546-1466
URL:
http:\\WWW.infomall.com\allergy.html

Vinyl Barrier Cover

Zippered, rubberized vinyl covers for mattress and boxspring; many sizes; pillow;
Available from:
Allergy Shop, Ltd.

3420 Cardston Crescent N.W. (APD)
Calgary, AB T2L 0S6
Canada
403-289-9052

Vinyl Mattress Cover

Dust-proof encasings with 50/50 cotton-polyester laminated to 5-gauge vinyl; zipper encasement; most sizes
Available from:
Allergy Relief Shop,™ Inc.
3371 Whittle Springs Rd. (APD)
Knoxville, TN 37917
Orders 800-626-2810
Questions 615-522-2795

Vinyl Mattress Protector

Cotton terry knit, 5-gauge vinyl-backed protector; zipper encasement; fire retardant; most sizes
Available from:
Priorities®
70 Walnut St. (APD)
Wellesley, MA 02181
800-553-5398

Vinyl Mattress/Boxspring Encasing

"Non-allergenic" covers made of waterproof, stainproof, and dustproof vinyl; 6-gauge; rust-proof zippers; electronically sealed and bartacked seams; clean with cloth or sponge; most sizes
Available from:
Absolute Environmental's Allergy Store
2615 S. University Dr. (APD)
Davie, FL 33328
Nationwide 800-771-ACHOO (2246)
In FL 800-329-3773
Broward 305-472-3773
Fax 305-474-0133
and:
Allergy Supply Co.
11994 Star Court (APD)
Herndon, VA 22071
800-323-6744
Metropolitan DC 703-391-2011
Fax 703-391-2014
BBS 703-521-0638

Controlling Your Environment
Dust and Pollen Control

and:
Allergy-Asthma Shopper™
PO Box 239 (APD)
Fate, TX 75132
800-447-1100
Fax 903-883-4513

Vinyl Pillow Encasing
"Non-allergenic," vinyl covers; rust-proof zippers; electronically sealed seams; standard, queen, king
Available from:
Allergy Supply Co.
11994 Star Court (APD)
Herndon, VA 22071
800-323-6744
Metropolitan DC 703-391-2011
Fax 703-391-2014
BBS 703-521-0638
and:

Vinyl Pillow Protector
Cotton terry knit, 5-gauge vinyl-backed protector; zipper encasement; fire retardant; standard, queen, king
Available from:
Priorities®
70 Walnut St. (APD)
Wellesley, MA 02181
800-553-5398

Vinyl-Coated Cotton Knit Pillow Cover
Terry knit pillow covers, cotton thermally bonded to vinyl; washable; standard, queen, king
Available from:
Absolute Environmental's Allergy Store
2615 S. University Dr. (APD)
Davie, FL 33328
Nationwide 800-771-ACHOO (2246)
In FL 800-329-3773
Broward 305-472-3773
Fax 305-474-0133
and:
Allergy Supply Co.
11994 Star Court (APD)
Herndon, VA 22071
800-323-6744
Metropolitan DC 703-391-2011

Fax 703-391-2014
BBS 703-521-0638
and:
Allergy-Asthma Shopper™
PO Box 239 (APD)
Fate, TX 75132
800-447-1100
Fax 903-883-4513
and:
Skin & Allergy Shop,™The
310 E. Broadway (APD)
Louisville, KY 40202
800-366-6483
In KY 502-585-4824
Fax 502-589-3429

Vinyl-Coated Terry Cloth Mattress Encasing
Terry cloth thermally bonded to vinyl; no glue; washable; zippered; washable
Available from:
Absolute Environmental's Allergy Store
2615 S. University Dr. (APD)
Davie, FL 33328
Nationwide 800-771-ACHOO (2246)
In FL 800-329-3773
Broward 305-472-3773
Fax 305-474-0133
and:
Skin & Allergy Shop,™The
310 E. Broadway (APD)
Louisville, KY 40202
800-366-6483
In KY 502-585-4824
Fax 502-589-3429

Vinyl-Knit Mattress Cover
Fire retardant covers; machine wash and dry; rust-proof zippers; twin, full, queen, king
Available from:
Allergy Supply Co.
11994 Star Court (APD)
Herndon, VA 22071
800-323-6744
Metropolitan DC 703-391-2011
Fax 703-391-2014
BBS 703-521-0638

Controlling Your Environment

Dust and Pollen Control

Vinyl-Knit Pillow Cover
Fire retardant covers; machine wash and dry; rust-proof zippers; standard, queen, king
Available from:
Allergy Supply Co.
11994 Star Court (APD)
Herndon, VA 22071
800-323-6744
Metropolitan DC 703-391-2011
Fax 703-391-2014
BBS 703-521-0638

HEPA VACUUM CLEANERS

3M Service Vacuum Cleaner
Designed to clean toner from photocopying machines and general clean up; 10 micron toner/dirt filter; optional fine particle filter, .3 to .5 micron for laser toner and dust/dirt filter; grounded, case with self-storing hose, crevice nozzle, tubular nozzle, dusting brush, adaptor; 9 lbs.
Available from:
Jensen® Tools, Inc.
7815 S. 46th St. (APD)
Phoenix, AZ 85044-5399
800-426-1194
In AZ 602-968-6231
Fax 800-366-9662

Allergy Vacuum
Captures dust, pollen, mold, dander; disposable paper bag, pre-filter, impact filter, HEPA filter, 99% effective at 0.3 micron; vacuum does not operate if HEPA filter is removed; casters, hose, cord, tool kit
Available from:
Hako® Minuteman ®, Inc.
111 S. Rohlwing Road (APD)
Addison, IL 60101
708-627-6900
Fax 708-627-1130

Allervac
Four-filter system with filter bag; prefilter efficient to 3 micron; HEPA filter 99.97% efficient to 0.3 micron; microfilter catches dust and particles generated by motor; casters; telescopic wand, floor tool for hardwood floors, corner tool, upholstery tool
Available from:
Euroclean
905 W. Irving Park (APD)
Itasca, IL 60143
800-545-HEPA (4372)
Fax 708-773-2859
and:
Priorities®
70 Walnut St. (APD)
Wellesley, MA 02181
800-553-5398

Drum Kit 600
HEPA filter and vacuum head fits standard 55-gal. drum; handles wet and dry clean-ups; industrial waste
Available from:
Euroclean
905 W. Irving Park (APD)
Itasca, IL 60143
800-545-HEPA (4372)
Fax 708-773-2859

Fantom® Two Cyclone Vacuum
HEPA filter (99.97% at 0.3 micron); HEPA replacement indicator; filters output air; no collection bags; blockage warning whistle; 10 ft. cleaning wand, attachments
Available from:
Allergy Asthma Technology
4151 N. Kedzie (APD)
PO Box 18398 (APD)
Chicago, IL 60618
800-621-5545
312-465-8020
Fax 312-465-7619
and:
Allergy-Asthma Shopper™
PO Box 239 (APD)
Fate, TX 75132
800-447-1100
Fax 903-883-4513

Controlling Your Environment

Dust and Pollen Control

Hako Minuteman HEPA

Disposable paperbag, polyester filter bag 99% efficient at 1.5 micron; impaction filter 95% efficient at 0.3 micron; and HEPA filter; 1.2 hp motor; 4-gal., polyethylene tank; 99 CFM; tool kit and caddy, 40' cord; other attachments; home use
Available from:
A-Plus Allergy Equipment & Supply
8325 Regis Way (APD)
Los Angeles, CA 90045-2646
Orders 800-86-ALLER (862-5537)
310-337-7468
Fax 310-337-1971

Hako Minuteman ULPA

Disposable paperbag, cloth filter bag and ULPA (ultra low particulate air) filter; 1.2 hp motor; 4-gal. tank; 99 CFM; optional swivel casters and other attachments; industrial, commercial, institutional use
Available from:
Hako® Minuteman ®, Inc.
111 S. Rohlwing Road (APD)
Addison, IL 60101
708-627-6900
Fax 708-627-1130

HEPA VAC 100

HEPA filter removes 99.97% of dust and dirt particles 0.3 micron and larger; multilayered disposable paper bag (2-1/2 gal. capacity), pre-filter; 2-stage motor; on/off switch; 1.125 horsepower motor; 70 cu. ft./min. airflow; 14 lbs.
Available from:
Pure Air Systems, Inc.
425 Duffey St. (APD)
PO Box 418 (APD)
Plainfield, IN 46168
800-869-8025
317-839-9135
Fax 317-839-8567

Hoover Office Machine Vacuum

Removes toner powder from photocopying machines; double-layer filter bags, .3 micron, prevent particle re-entry into air; shoulder straps, dusting brush, crevice tool, crevice tool brush, snorkel, dusting brush; 8.3 lbs.
Available from:
Jensen® Tools, Inc.
7815 S. 46th St. (APD)
Phoenix, AZ 85044-5399
800-426-1194
In AZ 602-968-6231
Fax 800-366-9662

Lindhaus™ DP-5 Upright Vacuum

Traps dust, pollen, bacteria, spores; natural fiber paper bag traps dust; high efficiency bag liner traps dirt and fine dust; washable, urethane inlet filter protects motor; motor filter cleans air through the motor; 2 Filtrete ™ microfilters rated 99.7% efficient trap micro particle emissions; ball bearing motors, ball bearing power brush; vacuum host port for tools
Available from:
National Allergy Supply, Inc.
4400 Georgia Hwy. 120 (APD)
PO Box 1658 (APD)
Duluth, GA 30136
800-522-1448
In Atlanta 404-623-8077
Fax 404-623-5568

Miele Vacuum Cleaner 280i

Dust collected in double layer bag; filter traps particles to 0.5 micron; prevents escape of allergens from its exhaust; 7.5 qt. capacity bag with protective closeable flap; on/off flip switches and cord rewind; electronic suction power control; optional power brush
Available from:
Allergy Control Products, Inc.
96 Danbury Rd. (APD)
PO Box 793 (APD)
Ridgefield, CT 06877
800-422-DUST (3878)
203-438-9580
Fax 203-431-8963
and:

Controlling Your Environment

Dust and Pollen Control

Allergy Relief Products
9 Renata Ct. (APD)
Dundas, ON L9H 6X1
Canada
905-628-5324 ?416
Fax 416-628-1734

Mite Hunter SCP92

Recycles heated air from motor inside dust bag after vacuuming to kill dust mites; built-in thermostat turns off automatically; micron filter and high-density outlet filter to prevent mites and fine dust particles from escaping
Available from:
Sanyo Fisher (USA) Corp.
21314 Lassen St. (APD)
Chatsworth, CA 91311-2329
818-998-7322
Consumer Help Desk Ext. 496
and
Central Reg. 708-297-0269 Ext. 534
Eastern Reg. 201-641-2333 Ext. 461

Mite Hunter SCP93

Recycles heated air from motor inside dust bag after vacuuming to kill dust mites; built-in thermostat turns off automatically, indicator panel shows function on; micron filter and high-density outlet filter to prevent mites and fine dust particles from escaping
Available from:
Sanyo Fisher (USA) Corp.
21314 Lassen St. (APD)
Chatsworth, CA 91311-2329
818-998-7322
Consumer Help Desk Ext. 496
and
Central Reg. 708-297-0269 Ext. 534
Eastern Reg. 201-641-2333 Ext. 461
and:
Solutions®
PO Box 6878 (APD)
Portland, OR 97228
800-342-9988
Fax 503-643-1973

Nilfisk GB Series Vacuum

Central system vacuums for hospitals and industrial use; HEPA models 733, 833, 933, 1033 vary in power and area of effectiveness; selection on the basis of hose lengths, sizes of piping, and purpose determined upon consultation with representative
Available from:
Nilfisk Ltd.
Nilfisk of America, Inc.
300 Technology Dr. (APD)
Malvern, PA 19355
800-NILFISK (645-3475)
In PA 610-647-6420
and
396 Watline Ave. (APD)
Mississauga, ON L4Z 1X2
Canada

Nilfisk Gore-Tex® 3-Stage Filtered Vacuum GS-90

Gore-Tex® microfilter membrane material has teflon-like coating for HEPA-like filter effect; retains 99.995% of particles down to 0.33 micron; replaceable; plastic container; cannister for home use; Nilfisk recommends that a replaceable microstatic exhaust diffuser be used as a final filter for carbon dust from the motor
Available from:
Allergy Clean Environments
501 Station Ave. (APD)
Haddon Heights, NJ 08035
800-882-4110
In NJ 609-546-1101
Fax 609-546-1466
URL:
http:\\WWW.infomall.com\allergy.html
and:
Allergy-Asthma Shopper™
PO Box 239 (APD)
Fate, TX 75132
800-447-1100
Fax 903-883-4513
and:
American Allergy Supply

Controlling Your Environment

Dust and Pollen Control

PO Box 722022 (APD)
Houston, TX 77272-2022
800-321-1096
713-995-6110
and:
Flowright Int'l Products
1495 N.W. Gilman Blvd. #4 (APD)
Issaquah, WA 98027
206-392-8357
and:
Nilfisk Ltd.
Nilfisk of America, Inc.
300 Technology Dr. (APD)
Malvern, PA 19355
800-NILFISK (645-3475)
In PA 610-647-6420
and
396 Watline Ave. (APD)
Mississauga, ON L4Z 1X2
Canada

Nilfisk Gore-Tex® Filtered Vacuum GS-80

Gore-Tex® microfilter; microstatic exhaust filter; HEPA filter removes 99.97% of dust and dirt particles 0.3 micron and larger; aluminum container; upholstery nozzle, drapery insert; crevice toools
Available from:
Allergy-Asthma Shopper™
PO Box 239 (APD)
Fate, TX 75132
800-447-1100
Fax 903-883-4513
and:
Flowright Int'l Products
1495 N.W. Gilman Blvd. #4 (APD)
Issaquah, WA 98027
206-392-8357

Nilfisk HEPA Vacuum GS-80

Felt microfilter; HEPA removes 99.97% of dust and dirt particles 0.3 micron and larger; aluminum container; upholstery nozzle, drapery insert; crevice toools
Available from:
Allergy Shop, Ltd.
3420 Cardston Crescent N.W. (APD)

Calgary, AB T2L 0S6
Canada
403-289-9052
and:
Flowright Int'l Products
1495 N.W. Gilman Blvd. #4 (APD)
Issaquah, WA 98027
206-392-8357

Nilfisk HEPA/ULPA 4-Stage Vacuum GS-90

Filters for dust and allergens. 2-ply cellulose (paper) bag collects dust. Permanent, cleanable main filter of napped cotton retains 99.5% of particles to 4 micron. Replaceable microfilter made of wool-rayon felt retains 99.5% of particles to 2 micron; this filter is used with a HEPA or ULPA filter. Replaceable HEPA (tightly woven glass fiber paper) filter traps (DOP test) 99.99% of particles down to 0.3 micron in exhaust dust. Replaceable ULPA (very tightly woven glass fiber paper) filter available; 2.25 gal. disposable bag; cannister; plastic container; attachments available
Available from:
Absolute Environmental's Allergy Store
2615 S. University Dr. (APD)
Davie, FL 33328
Nationwide 800-771-ACHOO (2246)
In FL 800-329-3773
Broward 305-472-3773
Fax 305-474-0133
and:
Air Doctors, Inc.
3632 Meadow Ln. (APD)
Jackson, MS 39212
PO Box 7147 (APD)
Jackson, MS 39282-7147
601-371-8928
Fax 601-373-2623
and:
Allergy Asthma Technology
4151 N. Kedzie (APD)
PO Box 18398 (APD)
Chicago, IL 60618
800-621-5545
312-465-8020

Controlling Your Environment

Dust and Pollen Control

Fax 312-465-7619
and:
Allergy Clean Environments
501 Station Ave. (APD)
Haddon Heights, NJ 08035
800-882-4110
In NJ 609-546-1101
Fax 609-546-1466
URL:
http:\\WWW.infomall.com\allergy.html
and:
Allergy Control Products, Inc.
96 Danbury Rd. (APD)
PO Box 793 (APD)
Ridgefield, CT 06877
800-422-DUST (3878)
203-438-9580
Fax 203-431-8963
and:
Allergy Shop, Ltd.
3420 Cardston Crescent N.W. (APD)
Calgary, AB T2L 0S6
Canada
403-289-9052
and:
Allergy Supply Co.
11994 Star Court (APD)
Herndon, VA 22071
800-323-6744
Metropolitan DC 703-391-2011
Fax 703-391-2014
BBS 703-521-0638
and:
Allergy-Asthma Shopper™
PO Box 239 (APD)
Fate, TX 75132
800-447-1100
Fax 903-883-4513
and:
American Allergy Supply
PO Box 722022 (APD)
Houston, TX 77272-2022
800-321-1096
713-995-6110
and:
Environtrol® Corporation
PO Box 31313 (APD)
St. Louis, MO 63131
800-423-1982
In St. Louis 314-966-6886

and:
Flowright Int'l Products
1495 N.W. Gilman Blvd. #4 (APD)
Issaquah, WA 98027
206-392-8357
and:
National Allergy Supply, Inc.
4400 Georgia Hwy. 120 (APD)
PO Box 1658 (APD)
Duluth, GA 30136
800-522-1448
In Atlanta 404-623-8077
Fax 404-623-5568
and:
Nilfisk Ltd.
Nilfisk of America, Inc.
300 Technology Dr. (APD)
Malvern, PA 19355
800-NILFISK (645-3475)
In PA 610-647-6420
and
396 Watline Ave. (APD)
Mississauga, ON L4Z 1X2
Canada
and
Skin & Allergy Shop,™The
310 E. Broadway (APD)
Louisville, KY 40202
800-366-6483
In KY 502-585-4824
Fax 502-589-3429

Princess III Bagless Home Cleaning System

Filters air to 3 micron; filters dirt, dust, pollen, pollutants; 25-foot cord, 10-foot hose; accessories; 2-1/2 gal. dirt container is up-ended to empty; optional filter is 99% efficient to 0.3 micron
Available from:
Allergy Supply Co.
11994 Star Court (APD)
Herndon, VA 22071
800-323-6744
Metropolitan DC 703-391-2011
Fax 703-391-2014
BBS 703-521-0638

Controlling Your Environment

Dust and Pollen Control

Royal Vacuum Cleaner 4600

Retains dust, pollen to 0.5 particle size; metal tank; all attachments; uses Micro-Fresh™ bags
Available from:
Allergy Clean Environments
501 Station Ave. (APD)
Haddon Heights, NJ 08035
800-882-4110
In NJ 609-546-1101
Fax 609-546-1466
URL:
http:\\WWW.infomall.com\allergy.html
and
Royal Appliance Mfg. Co.
650 Alpha Dr. (APD)
Cleveland, OH 44143-2172
800-321-1134 Ex 533
216-449-6150
Fax 216-449-7806

Scooter™ Multi-Purpose Mini-Vacuum Kit

Compact vacuum to clean dust on computer and typewriter keyboards; cleans work surfaces, projector and camera lenses; batteries
Available from:
Jensen® Tools, Inc.
7815 S. 46th St. (APD)
Phoenix, AZ 85044-5399
800-426-1194
In AZ 602-968-6231
Fax 800-366-9662

Thermax AF®

Dust and odor filter; washable urethane foam filter; disposable electrostatically charged filter; traps allergens, contaminants in a water filtration system; waterlift 89 inches; air intake 80.9 CFM
Available from:
Allergy Relief Shop,™ Inc.
3371 Whittle Springs Rd. (APD)
Knoxville, TN 37917
Orders 800-626-2810
Questions 615-522-2795

Toner Vacuum Cleaner

Cleans pollutants that clog computers, copiers, printers, disk drives; triple filtration system with toner filter and fiberglass filter; accessories; 7 lbs
Available from:
Jensen® Tools, Inc.
7815 S. 46th St. (APD)
Phoenix, AZ 85044-5399
800-426-1194
In AZ 602-968-6231
Fax 800-366-9662

Ultra Clean Allergy Vacuum

HEPA filter traps particles 0.3 micron in size; 8-quart collection capacity; 6-foot hose, wand, combination bare floor/carpet tool, other tools; 17" wide x 22" high; optional electric power head
Available from:
Fortress Industries, Inc.
12451 US 27 (APD)
DeWitt, MI 48820
800-526-2569
517-669-8861
Fax 517-669-8836

UZ 774

Wet or dry hazardous materials without electrical supply; 15 gal. capacity; HEPA filter; 55 lbs.
Available from:
Euroclean
905 W. Irving Park (APD)
Itasca, IL 60143
800-545-HEPA (4372)
Fax 708-773-2859

UZ 775 Industrial

Wet or dry hazardous materials without electrical supply; optional HEPA filter; 17.5 gal. capacity; 106 lbs
Available from:
Euroclean
905 W. Irving Park (APD)
Itasca, IL 60143
800-545-HEPA (4372)
Fax 708-773-2859

Controlling Your Environment

Dust and Pollen Control

UZ 877 HEPA Industrial

Wet or dry applications; 11 gal. capacity; reusable microfilter; HEPA filter; 37 lbs.
Available from:
Euroclean
905 W. Irving Park (APD)
Itasca, IL 60143
800-545-HEPA (4372)
Fax 708-773-2859

UZ 878 HEPA Industrial

Wet or dry applications; 15 gal. capacity; reusable microfilter; HEPA filter; 55 lbs.
Available from:
Euroclean
905 W. Irving Park (APD)
Itasca, IL 60143
800-545-HEPA (4372)
Fax 708-773-2859

UZ 930 HEPA Industrial

Hazardous dust and dirt removal; HEPA filter; 4-gal capacity; optional back-pack harness; 17.5 lbs.
Available from:
Euroclean
905 W. Irving Park (APD)
Itasca, IL 60143
800-545-HEPA (4372)
Fax 708-773-2859

UZ 932 HEPA Home Use

HEPA filter for dust, allergens, and harmful bacteria; 1.25 horsepower motor; 2-1/2 gal. capacity; 14 lbs.
Available from:
Euroclean
905 W. Irving Park (APD)
Itasca, IL 60143
800-545-HEPA (4372)
Fax 708-773-2859

UZ 948 Industrial

For hazardous material pick up; wet or dry applications; asbestos; multi-filter HEPA cartridge; 130 lbs.
Available from:
Euroclean
905 W. Irving Park (APD)
Itasca, IL 60143
800-545-HEPA (4372)
Fax 708-773-2859

UZ 964 Ergoclean Home Use

3-stage filter system with microfilter traps pollen, bacteria, allergens; with belt for hip-use; 7.4 lbs.
Available from:
Euroclean
905 W. Irving Park (APD)
Itasca, IL 60143
800-545-HEPA (4372)
Fax 708-773-2859

Vita-Vac™

Charcoal/HEPA-type filter efficient to 0.3 micron; traps dust, pollen; filter bag which inhibits mold growth inside cellulose bag which traps dust
Available from:
N.E.E.D.S.
527 Charles Ave. 12A (APD)
Syracuse, NY 13209
800-634-1380
Fax 800-295-NEED (6333)
and:
Vita-Mix® Corp.
8615 Usher Rd. (APD)
Cleveland, OH 44138-2199
800-VITAMIX (848-2649)

MASKS

3M Dust/Pollen Filter Mask - Non-Toxic Particles

Filters dusts, and pollen; indoors/outdoors; reusable; replaceable; not a respirator
Available from:
3M Company
PO Box 33275 (APD)
St. Paul, MN 55133-3275
3M Center Bldg.(APD)
St. Paul, MN 55144-1000
Medical information 800-328-0255
Medical information local 612-736-4930

Controlling Your Environment

Dust and Pollen Control

Customer service 800-423-5197
Outside CA 800-423-5146
In CA 818-341-1300
and:
Allergy Asthma Technology
4151 N. Kedzie (APD)
PO Box 18398 (APD)
Chicago, IL 60618
800-621-5545
312-465-8020
Fax 312-465-7619
and:
Allergy Control Products, Inc.
96 Danbury Rd. (APD)
PO Box 793 (APD)
Ridgefield, CT 06877
800-422-DUST (3878)
203-438-9580
Fax 203-431-8963
and:
Allergy Relief Shop,™ Inc.
3371 Whittle Springs Rd. (APD)
Knoxville, TN 37917
Orders 800-626-2810
Questions 615-522-2795
and:
Allergy Supply Co.
11994 Star Court (APD)
Herndon, VA 22071
800-323-6744
Metropolitan DC 703-391-2011
Fax 703-391-2014
BBS 703-521-0638
and:
Environtrol® Corporation
PO Box 31313 (APD)
St. Louis, MO 63131
800-423-1982
In St. Louis 314-966-6886
and:
Gempler's
211 Blue Mounds Rd. (APD)
PO Box 270 (APD)
Mt. Horeb, WI 53572
800-382-8473
Fax 800-551-1128
and:
National Allergy Supply, Inc.
4400 Georgia Hwy. 120 (APD)
PO Box 1658 (APD)

Duluth, GA 30136
800-522-1448
In Atlanta 404-623-8077
Fax 404-623-5568

3M Face Mask

Filters dust, mold, airborne particles; sealing ring; adjustable nose bridge; double straps; exhale valve flap; not compatible with eye glasses.
Available from:
3M Company
PO Box 33275 (APD)
St. Paul, MN 55133-3275
3M Center Bldg.(APD)
St. Paul, MN 55144-1000
Medical information 800-328-0255
Medical information local 612-736-4930
Customer service 800-423-5197
Outside CA 800-423-5146
In CA 818-341-1300

3M Non-Toxic Particle Mask 8500

Protects against dusts from alfalfa, pollen, animal dander, sawdust, calcium carbonate, gypsum, and limestone; does not protect from toxic particulates or spray paint
Available from:
Industrial Safety Co.
1390 Neubrecht Rd. (APD)
Lima, OH 45801-3196
Orders 800-537-9721
Customer Service 419-227-6030
Fax 419-228-5034
and:
Interex Safety & Industrial Supplies
176 Newington Rd. (APD)
W. Hartford, CT 06110
800-225-5910
Fax 800-334-2594
and:
Masuen™ Co.
490 Fillmore Ave. (APD)
Tonawanda, NY 14150
800-831-0894
In IL 312-956-1255
Fax 800-222-1934

Controlling Your Environment

Dust and Pollen Control

Air Clear®

Velux fabric outside catches pollen; foam inner layer; acetate inner layer; hand wash, air dry; small, medium, large
Available from:
Airgard, Inc.
12601 Pleasant Grove #10 (APD)
Syracuse, IN 46567
219-457-5237

Aseptex-Plus Molded Face Mask

3M mask fluid resistant; fiberglass-free; high filtration efficency of 99%; various colors
Available from:
IDE Interstate Dental Supply Catalog
1500 New Horizons Blvd. (APD)
Amityville, NY 11701-1130
800-666-8100
Fax 516-957-1678

AWO1 Airwear Mask

Mask of "hypoallergenic" neoprene with activated charcoal filter
Available from:
RESPRO Products
Boboli Imports, Inc.
11203-63 St. (APD)
Edmonton, AB T5W 4E5
Canada
403-448-0393
Fax 403-448-9044

AWO2 Foam Mask

Mask with replaceable, activated charcoal filter
Available from:
RESPRO Products
Boboli Imports, Inc.
11203-63 St. (APD)
Edmonton, AB T5W 4E5
Canada
403-448-0393
Fax 403-448-9044

Care-flo Air Cap CF 20

Not a mask, but a plastic hat with high, rounded bill or front brim attached to a clear plastic face plate that covers the face to chin level; under the bill is a blower and a filter that traps 99% of particles greater than one micron (pollen is between 10 and 100 micron); a belt-worn battery holds 3 C cells for forty hours of blower power; blower moves filtered air down the face, behind the face plate
Available from:
Neoterik Health Technologies, Inc.
Neoterik Center, Box 128 (APD)
Woodsboro, MD 21798
301-845-2777
Fax 301-845-2213

HEPA Mask

Two replaceable HEPA filters for particulates; two replaceable charcoal filters for gases and chemical fumes; mask is made of silicon; compatable with eye glasses
Available from:
Allergy Asthma Technology
4151 N. Kedzie (APD)
PO Box 18398 (APD)
Chicago, IL 60618
800-621-5545
312-465-8020
Fax 312-465-7619
and:
Pro-Tech Respirators, Inc.
107 E. Alexander St. (APD)
Buchanan, MI 49107
616-695-9663

HEPA Tech™

Uvex® foam sealed mask; disposable; three sizes; NIOSH approved
Available from:
Direct Safety Co.
7815 S. 46th St. (APD)
Phoenix, AZ 85044-5399
PO Box 50050 (APD)
Phoenix, AZ 85076-0050
800-528-7405
In AZ 602-968-7009
Fax 800-366-9662

Controlling Your Environment

Dust and Pollen Control

Ideal Molded Face Mask

Adjustable nose band with elastic band; two sizes
Available from:
IDE Interstate Dental Supply Catalog
1500 New Horizons Blvd. (APD)
Amityville, NY 11701-1130
800-666-8100
Fax 516-957-1678

Maxi-mask®

Disposable dust and pollen face mask
Available from:
Priorities®
70 Walnut St. (APD)
Wellesley, MA 02181
800-553-5398

Moldex® Disposable Mask 1100

Protects from dusts and non-toxic particles; contour design; compatible with eyeglass use
Available from:
Allied Glove & Safety Products Corp.
4711 W. Armitage Ave. (APD)
Chicago, IL 60639
800-621-3861
312-804-1800
Fax 312-804-1810
and:
Direct Safety Co.
7815 S. 46th St. (APD)
Phoenix, AZ 85044-5399
PO Box 50050 (APD)
Phoenix, AZ 85076-0050
800-528-7405
In AZ 602-968-7009
Fax 800-366-9662
and:
Industrial Safety Co.
1390 Neubrecht Rd. (APD)
Lima, OH 45801-3196
Orders 800-537-9721
Customer Service 419-227-6030
Fax 419-228-5034
and:
Interex Safety & Industrial Supplies
176 Newington Rd. (APD)
W. Hartford, CT 06110

800-225-5910
Fax 800-334-2594

Net Particulate Mask Model 0401

Viledon/Microdon filtration media; for dust and mist; 90% efficient at 0.1 micron; nose contour; adhesive and additive-free
Available from:
Allergy Relief Shop,™ Inc.
3371 Whittle Springs Rd. (APD)
Knoxville, TN 37917
Orders 800-626-2810
Questions 615-522-2795

No-Fog Face Mask

3M mask directs moist breath away from eyewear; does not rest against mouth; fluid resistant inner layer; available in tie-on and surgical tie-on
Available from:
IDE Interstate Dental Supply Catalog
1500 New Horizons Blvd. (APD)
Amityville, NY 11701-1130
800-666-8100
Fax 516-957-1678

Pleated Mask

Ear loop bands; green and pink
Available from:
IDE Interstate Dental Supply Catalog
1500 New Horizons Blvd. (APD)
Amityville, NY 11701-1130
800-666-8100
Fax 516-957-1678

Pura-Mask® Disposable

Protects against dust, pollen, bacteria; self-adjusting molded nose contour; nose bridge seats glasses and goggles; "non-allergenic fiber"
Available from:
Consolidated Plastics Co., Inc.
8181 Darrow Rd. (APD)
Twinsburg, OH 44087
800-362-1000
216-425-3900
Fax 216-425-3333

Controlling Your Environment

Dust and Pollen Control

Respro™ Anti-Pollution Mask

Replaceable charcoal filter for bicyclists; traps ozone, nitrogen oxides
Available from
Boboli Imports
9936-77 Ave. (APD)
Edmonton, AB T6E 1M5
Canada

Respro™ Face Mask

Neoprene mask with elecrostatically charged filter; velcro closure; low inhalation resistance and two valves; can be worn with glasses; replaceable filter
Available from:
Allergy Control Products, Inc.
96 Danbury Rd. (APD)
PO Box 793 (APD)
Ridgefield, CT 06877
800-422-DUST (3878)
203-438-9580
Fax 203-431-8963

Sportsta Mask

"Hypoallergenic" neoprene with replaceable filter effective to 0.3 micron
Available from:
RESPRO Products
Boboli Imports, Inc.
11203-63 St. (APD)
Edmonton, AB T5W 4E5
Canada
403-448-0393
Fax 403-448-9044

Travenol/Baxter "Fog-Free"

Designed to keep eyewear fog-free
Available from:
IDE Interstate Dental Supply Catalog
1500 New Horizons Blvd. (APD)
Amityville, NY 11701-1130
800-666-8100
Fax 516-957-1678

Travenol/Baxter Molded Mask

Mask stands away from face
Available from:
IDE Interstate Dental Supply Catalog
1500 New Horizons Blvd. (APD)

Amityville, NY 11701-1130
800-666-8100
Fax 516-957-1678

Travenol/Baxter Procedure Mask

Ear loops; yellow
Available from:
IDE Interstate Dental Supply Catalog
1500 New Horizons Blvd. (APD)
Amityville, NY 11701-1130
800-666-8100
Fax 516-957-1678

Willson 6000 Series

Silicone half-mask with dual dust/mist pre-filter pads for moldy grain, silage, pollen, field dusts; replacement cartridges to match contaminant
Available from:
Gempler's
211 Blue Mounds Rd. (APD)
PO Box 270 (APD)
Mt. Horeb, WI 53572
800-382-8473
Fax 800-551-1128

COTTON MASKS

May be helpful for some

Cotton Face Mask with Carbon

Washable mask with ties and patch of refillable carbon
Available from:
N.E.E.D.S.
527 Charles Ave. 12A (APD)
Syracuse, NY 13209
800-634-1380
Fax 800-295-NEED (6333)

Cotton Mask with Charcoal

Fitted cotton mask with charcoal for particulate protection and odor adsorption
Available from:
Allergy-Asthma Shopper™
PO Box 239 (APD)
Fate, TX 75132

Controlling Your Environment
Dust and Pollen Control

800-447-1100
Fax 903-883-4513

Cotton Mask

Fitted all cotton mask traps particulates
Available from:
Allergy-Asthma Shopper™
PO Box 239 (APD)
Fate, TX 75132
800-447-1100
Fax 903-883-4513

Hand-Held Mini-Mask

All cotton mask with charcoal insert fits in pocket for unplanned needs
Available from:
Allergy-Asthma Shopper™
PO Box 239 (APD)
Fate, TX 75132
800-447-1100
Fax 903-883-4513

Reusable Cotton Mask

Cotton face mask, 300 thread count, with replaceable charcoal filter from coconut shell carbon; blocks dust, fumes, odors
Available from:
Allergy Resources
Mail: PO Box 888 (APD)
UPS: 264 Brookridge Ave. (APD)
Palmer Lake, CO 80133
Orders 800-USE-FLAX (873-3529)
Company plans to move; use 800 #

RESPIRATORS

3M Dust/Mist Respirator 8710

Protects against cotton and textile dusts, silica, dry fertilizer, livestock barns, haying, grinding feeds; upper and lower straps; do not use for harmful vapors
Available from:
Allergy Alternative
440 Godfrey Dr. (APD)
Windsor, CA 95492

800-838-1514
and:
Allergy-Asthma Shopper™
PO Box 239 (APD)
Fate, TX 75132
800-447-1100
Fax 903-883-4513
and:
Consolidated Plastics Co., Inc.
8181 Darrow Rd. (APD)
Twinsburg, OH 44087
800-362-1000
216-425-3900
Fax 216-425-3333
and:
Gempler's
211 Blue Mounds Rd. (APD)
PO Box 270 (APD)
Mt. Horeb, WI 53572
800-382-8473
Fax 800-551-1128
and:
Industrial Safety Co.
1390 Neubrecht Rd. (APD)
Lima, OH 45801-3196
Orders 800-537-9721
Customer Service 419-227-6030
Fax 419-228-5034
and:
Interex Safety & Industrial Supplies
176 Newington Rd. (APD)
W. Hartford, CT 06110
800-225-5910
Fax 800-334-2594

3M Dust/Mist Respirator 8715

Protects against cotton and textile dusts, silica; adjustable nose clip for reliable seal; nose cushion reduces fogging of eyeglasses; withstands humidity
Available from:
Conney Safety Products
3203 Latham Dr. (APD)
PO Box 44190 (APD)
Madison, WI 53744-4190
800-356-9100
Fax 800-845-9095
and:
Industrial Safety Co.

Controlling Your Environment

Dust and Pollen Control

1390 Neubrecht Rd. (APD)
Lima, OH 45801-3196
Orders 800-537-9721
Customer Service 419-227-6030
Fax 419-228-5034
and:
Interex Safety & Industrial Supplies
176 Newington Rd. (APD)
W. Hartford, CT 06110
800-225-5910
Fax 800-334-2594

3M Dust/Mist Respirator 9913

Protection against dusts and mists with permissible exposure level not less than .05 mg/m3 SUPERSCRIPT; carbon media for nuisance odors, gases, vapors, paint spray
Available from:
Allergy-Asthma Shopper™
PO Box 239 (APD)
Fate, TX 75132
800-447-1100
Fax 903-883-4513
and:
Allied Glove & Safety Products Corp.
4711 W. Armitage Ave. (APD)
Chicago, IL 60639
800-621-3861
312-804-1800
Fax 312-804-1810
and:
Consolidated Plastics Co., Inc.
8181 Darrow Rd. (APD)
Twinsburg, OH 44087
800-362-1000
216-425-3900
Fax 216-425-3333
and:
E.L. Foust Co., Inc.
PO Box 105 (APD)
Elmhurst, IL 60126
800-225-9549
708-834-4952
Fax 708-834-5341
and:
Interex Safety & Industrial Supplies
176 Newington Rd. (APD)
W. Hartford, CT 06110
800-225-5910

Fax 800-334-2594
and:
N.E.E.D.S.
527 Charles Ave. 12A (APD)
Syracuse, NY 13209
800-634-1380
Fax 800-295-NEED (6333)

3M High Efficiency Respirator 9970

Industrial use respirator; manufacturing dusts, fumes, mists, soot, metal and wood shavings, agricultural molds, pollen and smoke; filters to 1 micron; adjustable contoured nose clip, foam face seal ring, exhalation valve; medium and large
Available from:
3M Company
PO Box 33275 (APD)
St. Paul, MN 55133-3275
3M Center Bldg.(APD)
St. Paul, MN 55144-1000
Medical information 800-328-0255
Medical information local 612-736-4930
Customer service 800-423-5197
Outside CA 800-423-5146
In CA 818-341-1300
and:
Absolute Environmental's Allergy Store
2615 S. University Dr. (APD)
Davie, FL 33328
Nationwide 800-771-ACHOO (2246)
In FL 800-329-3773
Broward 305-472-3773
Fax 305-474-0133
and:
Allergy Asthma Technology
4151 N. Kedzie (APD)
PO Box 18398 (APD)
Chicago, IL 60618
800-621-5545
312-465-8020
Fax 312-465-7619
and:
Allergy Clean Environments
501 Station Ave. (APD)
Haddon Heights, NJ 08035

Controlling Your Environment

Dust and Pollen Control

800-882-4110
In NJ 609-546-1101
Fax 609-546-1466
URL:
http:\\WWW.infomall.com\allergy.html
and:
Allergy Clean Environments
501 Station Ave. (APD)
Haddon Heights, NJ 08035
800-882-4110
In NJ 609-546-1101
Fax 609-546-1466
URL:
http:\\WWW.infomall.com\allergy.html
and:
Allergy Control Products, Inc.
96 Danbury Rd. (APD)
PO Box 793 (APD)
Ridgefield, CT 06877
800-422-DUST (3878)
203-438-9580
Fax 203-431-8963
and:
Allergy Relief Products
9 Renata Ct. (APD)
Dundas, ON L9H 6X1
Canada
905-628-5324 ?416
Fax 416-628-1734
and:
Allergy-Asthma Shopper™
PO Box 239 (APD)
Fate, TX 75132
800-447-1100
Fax 903-883-4513
and:
National Allergy Supply, Inc.
4400 Georgia Hwy. 120 (APD)
PO Box 1658 (APD)
Duluth, GA 30136
800-522-1448
In Atlanta 404-623-8077
Fax 404-623-5568

3M Nuisance Odor Respirator

Dust and mist respirator with activated charcoal to remove odors and organic vapors; grain dust, hay dust, pollen, and livestock dander
Available from:

Gempler's
211 Blue Mounds Rd. (APD)
PO Box 270 (APD)
Mt. Horeb, WI 53572
800-382-8473
Fax 800-551-1128

3M Toxic Dust/Fume Respirator

Protects from grain and hay dusts, welding fumes; charcoal layer removes nuisance levels of livestock odors; exhalation valve
Available from:
Gempler's
211 Blue Mounds Rd. (APD)
PO Box 270 (APD)
Mt. Horeb, WI 53572
800-382-8473
Fax 800-551-1128

Chemisorb Respirators

Protects from organic vapors, odors, dust, smoke; activated charcoal filters from coconut-shell carbon or BS-6016 respirator with activated charcoal and particle filter
Available from
Safpac Pty, Ltd.
62 Lynch Crescent (APD)
Brighton, Vic., 3186
Australia
03-592-8269

Fresh-Aire Respirator

Replaceable cartridge traps particulates and gases, including pollen, spores, and 1.0 ppm ozone and 0.2 ppm sulfur dioxide (smog components); facepiece is soft PVC
Available from:
Environtrol® Corporation
PO Box 31313 (APD)
St. Louis, MO 63131
800-423-1982
In St. Louis 314-966-6886

Gerson Dust/Mist Respirator 1710

Formable nosepiece; foam inner seal; protects against dusts and mists
Available from:

Controlling Your Environment

Dust and Pollen Control

Conney Safety Products
3203 Latham Dr. (APD)
PO Box 44190 (APD)
Madison, WI 53744-4190
800-356-9100
Fax 800-845-9095

Gerson Dust/Mist Respirator 1725

Protects against dusts and mists; exhalation valve for humidity; Conney notes non-irritating inner lining
Available from:
Conney Safety Products
3203 Latham Dr. (APD)
PO Box 44190 (APD)
Madison, WI 53744-4190
800-356-9100
Fax 800-845-9095

Moldex® Dust/Mist Respirator 2200

Polymesh shell molds to facial contours; protects from dusts and mists; rubber straps; disposable. Flame retardants are added to decrease flammability so discuss this with your doctor.
Available from:
Allied Glove & Safety Products Corp.
4711 W. Armitage Ave. (APD)
Chicago, IL 60639
800-621-3861
312-804-1800
Fax 312-804-1810
and:
Conney Safety Products
3203 Latham Dr. (APD)
PO Box 44190 (APD)
Madison, WI 53744-4190
800-356-9100
Fax 800-845-9095
and:
Direct Safety Co.
7815 S. 46th St. (APD)
Phoenix, AZ 85044-5399
PO Box 50050 (APD)
Phoenix, AZ 85076-0050
800-528-7405
In AZ 602-968-7009
Fax 800-366-9662

and:
Gempler's
211 Blue Mounds Rd. (APD)
PO Box 270 (APD)
Mt. Horeb, WI 53572
800-382-8473
Fax 800-551-1128
and:
Industrial Safety Co.
1390 Neubrecht Rd. (APD)
Lima, OH 45801-3196
Orders 800-537-9721
Customer Service 419-227-6030
Fax 419-228-5034

Moldex® Dust/Mist Respirator 2300

Exhale valve controls over-heating; molded nose area compatible with eyeglass use; cotton inside, plastic exterior; disposable
Available from:
Conney Safety Products
3203 Latham Dr. (APD)
PO Box 44190 (APD)
Madison, WI 53744-4190
800-356-9100
Fax 800-845-9095
and:
Gempler's
211 Blue Mounds Rd. (APD)
PO Box 270 (APD)
Mt. Horeb, WI 53572
800-382-8473
Fax 800-551-1128
and:
Industrial Safety Co.
1390 Neubrecht Rd. (APD)
Lima, OH 45801-3196
Orders 800-537-9721
Customer Service 419-227-6030
Fax 419-228-5034
and:
Skin & Allergy Shop,™ The
310 E. Broadway (APD)
Louisville, KY 40202
800-366-6483
In KY 502-585-4824
Fax 502-589-3429

Controlling Your Environment
Dust and Pollen Control

Moldex® Dust/Mist Respirator 2400

Charcoal layer inside mask removes nuisance odors; polymesh outershell; one-way exhale valve
Available from:
Gempler's
211 Blue Mounds Rd. (APD)
PO Box 270 (APD)
Mt. Horeb, WI 53572
800-382-8473
Fax 800-551-1128

North Disposable Respirator

Protects against dusts and fumes; coaxial inhalation and exhalation valve controls over-heating
Available from:
Industrial Safety Co.
1390 Neubrecht Rd. (APD)
Lima, OH 45801-3196
Orders 800-537-9721
Customer Service 419-227-6030
Fax 419-228-5034

Respirator CF 60

Airflow box with battery, blower, and filter attaches to belt; plastic tube leads up to user's hat or sun visor and blows filtered air across eyes and nose
Available from:
Neoterik Health Technologies, Inc.
Neoterik Center, Box 128 (APD)
Woodsboro, MD 21798
301-845-2777
Fax 301-845-2213

Technirama TK2

Respirator with anti-fogging nose-cup, speaking diaphragm, neoprene/rubber barrier; replaceable HEPA filter cartridge; silicone rubber facepiece optional
Available from:
Neoterik Health Technologies, Inc.
Neoterik Center, Box 128 (APD)
Woodsboro, MD 21798
301-845-2777
Fax 301-845-2213

Willson® Freedom 2000™ 1HA-0278

Respirator in three sizes; nose bridge compatible with eyeglass use; for dusts and mists; disposable
Available from:
Industrial Safety Co.
1390 Neubrecht Rd. (APD)
Lima, OH 45801-3196
Orders 800-537-9721
Customer Service 419-227-6030
Fax 419-228-5034
and:
Interex Safety & Industrial Supplies
176 Newington Rd. (APD)
W. Hartford, CT 06110
800-225-5910
Fax 800-334-2594

Willson® Freedom 2000™ 1HA-0302

Respirator in three sizes; nose bridge compatible with eyeglass use; for dusts and mists; HEPA, dusts, mists, fumes
Available from:
Interex Safety & Industrial Supplies
176 Newington Rd. (APD)
W. Hartford, CT 06110
800-225-5910
Fax 800-334-2594

HELMETS

Kasco Industrial Air Purifiers

This series of purifiers has passed safety impact and penetration tests; unless you work in a situation where you need this extra protection (and if you do, information is available from the company), other Kasco products are less expensive
Available from:
St. George Co., Ltd.
20 Consolidated Dr. (APD)
PO Box 430 (APD)
Paris, ON N3L 3T5
Canada
519-442-2046

Controlling Your Environment

Dust and Pollen Control

Fax 519-442-7191
U.S. 800-461-4299

Kasco K8OE-T5A

Helmet for industrial use; belt battery and fan-motor; HEPA filter removes 99.7% of particulate matter; 2 lbs.
Available from:
St. George Co., Ltd.
20 Consolidated Dr. (APD)
PO Box 430 (APD)
Paris, ON N3L 3T5
Canada
519-442-2046
Fax 519-442-7191
U.S. 800-461-4299

Kasco K8OE-T8A

Helmet for industrial use; 2 HEPA filters remove 99.7% of particulate matter; transformer/-charger; 2 lbs.
Available from:
St. George Co., Ltd.
20 Consolidated Dr. (APD)
PO Box 430 (APD)
Paris, ON N3L 3T5
Canada
519-442-2046
Fax 519-442-7191
U.S. 800-461-4299

Kasco K8OS-T1 Air Purifier

Helmet for agricultural spraying; runs off tractor battery, independent belt powerpack; pesticide filter (organic vapor/HEPA combination); 1 lb. 12 oz.
Available from:
St. George Co., Ltd.
20 Consolidated Dr. (APD)
PO Box 430 (APD)
Paris, ON N3L 3T5
Canada
519-442-2046
Fax 519-442-7191
U.S. 800-461-4299

Kasco K8OS-T4 Air Purifier

Helmet for agricultural spraying; runs off tractor battery; 3 pesticide

filters (organic vapor/HEPA combination); 1 lb. 12 oz.
Available from:
St. George Co., Ltd.
20 Consolidated Dr. (APD)
PO Box 430 (APD)
Paris, ON N3L 3T5
Canada
519-442-2046
Fax 519-442-7191
U.S. 800-461-4299

Kasco K8OS-T5 Air Purifier

Helmet for agricultural spraying; 6-volt, belt battery; pesticide filter; (organic vapor/HEPA combination)
Available from:
St. George Co., Ltd.
20 Consolidated Dr. (APD)
PO Box 430 (APD)
Paris, ON N3L 3T5
Canada
519-442-2046
Fax 519-442-7191
U.S. 800-461-4299

Kasco K8OS-T5N

Helmet for agricultural spraying; 6-volt, belt battery; 3 pesticide filters
Available from:
St. George Co., Ltd.
20 Consolidated Dr. (APD)
PO Box 430 (APD)
Paris, ON N3L 3T5
Canada
519-442-2046
Fax 519-442-7191
U.S. 800-461-4299

Kasco K8OS-T8N

Helmet for dust-filled environments; helmet contains batteries, fan-motor, 2 pesticide filters (organic vapor/HEPA combination); 1 lb. 12 oz.
Available from:
St. George Co., Ltd.
20 Consolidated Dr. (APD)
PO Box 430 (APD)
Paris, ON N3L 3T5

Canada
519-442-2046
Fax 519-442-7191
U.S. 800-461-4299

Kasco PROF 88 Air Purifier

Helmet for agricultural spraying; helmet contains batteries, twin fan motor unit, 2 pesticide filters; can recharge from tractor battery; 4.5 lbs.
Available from:
St. George Co., Ltd.
20 Consolidated Dr. (APD)
PO Box 430 (APD)
Paris, ON N3L 3T5
Canada
519-442-2046
Fax 519-442-7191
U.S. 800-461-4299

KOMPAT 12

Helmet for dust-filled environments; runs off tractor battery; helmet contains fan-motor and filter effective to 5 micron (ragweed); 2 lbs.
Available from:
St. George Co., Ltd.
20 Consolidated Dr. (APD)
PO Box 430 (APD)
Paris, ON N3L 3T5
Canada
519-442-2046
Fax 519-442-7191
U.S. 800-461-4299

KOMPAT 6

Helmet for dust-filled environments; helmet contains batteries, fan-motor, filter effective to 5 micron (ragweed); 3 lbs.
Available from:
St. George Co., Ltd.
20 Consolidated Dr. (APD)
PO Box 430 (APD)
Paris, ON N3L 3T5
Canada
519-442-2046
Fax 519-442-7191
U.S. 800-461-4299

HOUSEKEEPING AIDS
CLEANING AIDS

Acarex Dust Mite Test Kit

Indicates dust mite levels in carpeting, draperies, bedding, and upolstered furniture by taking a sample of dust from your vacuum cleaner, mixing it with packet, and comparing results with a chart
Available from:
Allergy Asthma Technology
4151 N. Kedzie (APD)
PO Box 18398 (APD)
Chicago, IL 60618
800-621-5545
312-465-8020
Fax 312-465-7619

Acarosan® Dust Mite Eliminator

Benzyl benzoate solution destroys dust mites; removes allery-containing excrement; powder brushes into carpet, vacuums out. Contains benzyl benzoate. May not be available in California. Discuss with your doctor the application of this product after use of water or an active cleaning substance. (Ref. J. Allergy Clin Immunol. 2/92 pg. 637)
Available from:
Absolute Environmental's Allergy Store
2615 S. University Dr. (APD)
Davie, FL 33328
Nationwide 800-771-ACHOO (2246)
In FL 800-329-3773
Broward 305-472-3773
Fax 305-474-0133
and:
Air Doctors, Inc.
3632 Meadow Ln. (APD)
Jackson, MS 39212
PO Box 7147 (APD)
Jackson, MS 39282-7147
601-371-8928
Fax 601-373-2623
and:
Allergy Asthma Technology
4151 N. Kedzie (APD)

Controlling Your Environment

Dust and Pollen Control

PO Box 18398 (APD)
Chicago, IL 60618
800-621-5545
312-465-8020
Fax 312-465-7619
and:
Allergy Clean Environments
501 Station Ave. (APD)
Haddon Heights, NJ 08035
800-882-4110
In NJ 609-546-1101
Fax 609-546-1466
URL:
http:\\WWW.infomall.com\allergy.html
and:
Allergy Control Products, Inc.
96 Danbury Rd. (APD)
PO Box 793 (APD)
Ridgefield, CT 06877
800-422-DUST (3878)
203-438-9580
Fax 203-431-8963
and:
Allergy Solutions
4909 W. Park Blvd. #169 (APD)
Plano, TX 75093
800-380-SNEEZ (7633)
214-612-4188
Fax 214-985-5573
and:
Allergy Supply Co.
11994 Star Court (APD)
Herndon, VA 22071
800-323-6744
Metropolitan DC 703-391-2011
Fax 703-391-2014
BBS 703-521-0638
and:
Allergy-Asthma Shopper™
PO Box 239 (APD)
Fate, TX 75132
800-447-1100
Fax 903-883-4513
and:
American Allergy Supply
PO Box 722022 (APD)
Houston, TX 77272-2022
800-321-1096
713-995-6110
and:

Skin & Allergy Shop,™The
310 E. Broadway (APD)
Louisville, KY 40202
800-366-6483
In KY 502-585-4824
Fax 502-589-3429

Aeroallergen Assessments

Detects presence of D. pteronyssinus, D. farinae, cat, cockroach, and a mold spore count from your dust sample
Available from:
Allergy Clean Environments
501 Station Ave. (APD)
Haddon Heights, NJ 08035
800-882-4110
In NJ 609-546-1101
Fax 609-546-1466
URL:
http:\\WWW.infomall.com\allergy.html

ALK Indoor Allergen Analysis

Test measures cat and mite allergen levels in dust samples from living or working environments; repeat measurements monitor effectiveness
800-326-9181 Ext. 222

Aller Search ADS™ Spray

Denatures mite, cat, pollen, mold, and feather allergen protein; use on carpets or upholstered furniture; contains 3% tannic acid
Available from:
Absolute Environmental's Allergy Store
2615 S. University Dr. (APD)
Davie, FL 33328
Nationwide 800-771-ACHOO (2246)
In FL 800-329-3773
Broward 305-472-3773
Fax 305-474-0133
and:
Allergy Control Products, Inc.
96 Danbury Rd. (APD)
PO Box 793 (APD)
Ridgefield, CT 06877
800-422-DUST (3878)
203-438-9580
Fax 203-431-8963

and:
American Allergy Supply
PO Box 722022 (APD)
Houston, TX 77272-2022
800-321-1096
713-995-6110
and:
Priorities®
70 Walnut St. (APD)
Wellesley, MA 02181
800-553-5398

Aller-Vac™

Disposable vacuum cleaner bag made of DuPont HYSURF™ replaces standard bags to trap pollen, spores, dust mite allergens, bactaeria, cat dander; 97% efficient to 1 micron; available for some models of standard vacuums: Eureka, Hoover, Electrolux, Regina, Sears, Panasonic, Dirt Devil
Available from:
Allergy Solutions
4909 W. Park Blvd. #169 (APD)
Plano, TX 75093
800-380-SNEEZ (7633)
214-612-4188
Fax 214-985-5573
and:
National Allergy Supply, Inc.
4400 Georgia Hwy. 120 (APD)
PO Box 1658 (APD)
Duluth, GA 30136
800-522-1448
In Atlanta 404-623-8077
Fax 404-623-5568
and:
West Coast Shoe Co.
52828 N.W. Shoe Factory Ln. (APD)
PO Box 607 (APD)
Scappoose, OR 97056-0607
800-326-2711
503-543-7114
Fax 503-543-7110

Allergex® Dust Immobilizer

Inhibits the release of dust from upholstery, draperies, bedding, and blankets; liquid concentrate or aerosol for draperies, carpets, and fabrics;

used on pets to reduce free dander; aerosol and concentrate for dipping, sponging, or spraying. Avoid contact with skin; avoid breathing vapor or mist
Available from:
A-Plus Allergy Equipment & Supply
8325 Regis Way (APD)
Los Angeles, CA 90045-2646
Orders 800-86-ALLER (862-5537)
310-337-7468
Fax 310-337-1971
and:
Absolute Environmental's Allergy Store
2615 S. University Dr. (APD)
Davie, FL 33328
Nationwide 800-771-ACHOO (2246)
In FL 800-329-3773
Broward 305-472-3773
Fax 305-474-0133
and:
Allergy Alternative
440 Godfrey Dr. (APD)
Windsor, CA 95492
800-838-1514
and:
Allergy-Asthma Shopper™
PO Box 239 (APD)
Fate, TX 75132
800-447-1100
Fax 903-883-4513
and:
Allergy Asthma Technology
4151 N. Kedzie (APD)
PO Box 18398 (APD)
Chicago, IL 60618
800-621-5545
312-465-8020
Fax 312-465-7619
and:
Allergy Solutions
4909 W. Park Blvd. #169 (APD)
Plano, TX 75093
800-380-SNEEZ (7633)
214-612-4188
Fax 214-985-5573
and:
Allergy Shop, Ltd.
3420 Cardston Crescent N.W. (APD)
Calgary, AB T2L 0S6

Controlling Your Environment

Dust and Pollen Control

Canada
403-289-9052
and:
American Allergy Supply
PO Box 722022 (APD)
Houston, TX 77272-2022
800-321-1096
713-995-6110
and:
National Allergy Supply, Inc.
4400 Georgia Hwy. 120 (APD)
PO Box 1658 (APD)
Duluth, GA 30136
800-522-1448
In Atlanta 404-623-8077
Fax 404-623-5568
and:
Priorities®
70 Walnut St. (APD)
Wellesley, MA 02181
800-553-5398
and:
Skin & Allergy Shop,™ The
310 E. Broadway (APD)
Louisville, KY 40202
800-366-6483
In KY 502-585-4824
Fax 502-589-3429

Allergy Control™ Solution

Inactivates allergy-causing substances in dust, including dust mite particles and animal dander; for carpets and upholstered furniture; spray solution dries within three hours, lasts 2 to 3 months
Available from:
Allergy Control Products, Inc.
96 Danbury Rd. (APD)
PO Box 793 (APD)
Ridgefield, CT 06877
800-422-DUST (3878)
203-438-9580
Fax 203-431-8963
and:
Allergy Relief Products
9 Renata Ct. (APD)
Dundas, ON L9H 6X1
Canada
905-628-5324 ?416

Fax 416-628-1734
and:
Priorities®
70 Walnut St. (APD)
Wellesley, MA 02181
800-553-5398

Allersearch .ADS™

Non toxic, 3% tannic acid spray renders house dust mite droppings non-allergenic; use on carpets and upholstery every 2 months if humidity is over 50%; read instructions and spot test area to be treated; avoid white or near-white fabrics
Available from:
Aller-Guard,® Inc.
Southgate Office Park
1645 S.W. 41st St. (APD)
Topeka, KS 66609-1250
800-234-0816
913-267-9333
Fax 913-267-0072
and:
Allergy Asthma Technology
4151 N. Kedzie (APD)
PO Box 18398 (APD)
Chicago, IL 60618
800-621-5545
312-465-8020
Fax 312-465-7619
and:
Allergy Clean Environments
501 Station Ave. (APD)
Haddon Heights, NJ 08035
800-882-4110
In NJ 609-546-1101
Fax 609-546-1466
URL:
http:\\WWW.infomall.com\allergy.html
and:
National Allergy Supply, Inc.
4400 Georgia Hwy. 120 (APD)
PO Box 1658 (APD)
Duluth, GA 30136
800-522-1448
In Atlanta 404-623-8077
Fax 404-623-5568

Controlling Your Environment
Dust and Pollen Control

Allersearch X-Mite™ All-in-One

Controls dust mites, mite allergen, and animal dander; can be used on carpets and some fabrics; moist powder based on tannic acid; covers 115 sq. ft. of carpet
Available from:
American Allergy Supply
PO Box 722022 (APD)
Houston, TX 77272-2022
800-321-1096
713-995-6110
and:
National Allergy Supply, Inc.
4400 Georgia Hwy. 120 (APD)
PO Box 1658 (APD)
Duluth, GA 30136
800-522-1448
In Atlanta 404-623-8077
Fax 404-623-5568

Capture® Carpet Care

Dry carpet cleaner; moisture-free use does not support mold growth; includes spot cleaner and brush
Available from:
Allergy Asthma Technology
4151 N. Kedzie (APD)
PO Box 18398 (APD)
Chicago, IL 60618
800-621-5545
312-465-8020
Fax 312-465-7619
and:
Allergy Control Products, Inc.
96 Danbury Rd. (APD)
PO Box 793 (APD)
Ridgefield, CT 06877
800-422-DUST (3878)
203-438-9580
Fax 203-431-8963

DMC Dust Mite Anti-Microbial Treatment

Disinfectant and fungicide; can be sprayed on carpets, bedding, and upholstered furniture or used in warm water laundry
Available from:
Allergy-Asthma Shopper™

PO Box 239 (APD)
Fate, TX 75132
800-447-1100
Fax 903-883-4513

DRI-APP™

Applicator for cleaning powders
Available from:
Allergy Control Products, Inc.
96 Danbury Rd. (APD)
PO Box 793 (APD)
Ridgefield, CT 06877
800-422-DUST (3878)
203-438-9580
Fax 203-431-8963

Dust Analysis Test

Separate tests for your house dust; collector and insructions; test for dust mite allergen, cockroach, cat allergen, mold spore count
Available from:
Allergy-Asthma Shopper™
PO Box 239 (APD)
Fate, TX 75132
800-447-1100
Fax 903-883-4513

Dust Bunny® Cloth

Electrostatically charged fibers attract and hold dust; washable; residue-free; use a mop cover for walls and floors
Available from:
Allergy-Asthma Shopper™
PO Box 239 (APD)
Fate, TX 75132
800-447-1100
Fax 903-883-4513

Dust Cloth

Cloth treated to attract and hold dust; greaseless; lint-free; odor-free; washable; 14"x18"
Available from:
Allergy Control Products, Inc.
96 Danbury Rd. (APD)
PO Box 793 (APD)
Ridgefield, CT 06877
800-422-DUST (3878)

Controlling Your Environment

Dust and Pollen Control

203-438-9580
Fax 203-431-8963

Dust Grabber™

Fabric with permanent electrostatic surface charge; washable; odor-free, chemical-free; does not feel tacky; leaves no film; 14x14 cloth stretchable, can be clipped to mop head
Available from:
National Allergy Supply, Inc.
4400 Georgia Hwy. 120 (APD)
PO Box 1658 (APD)
Duluth, GA 30136
800-522-1448
In Atlanta 404-623-8077
Fax 404-623-5568

Greer Indoor Allergen Spray

Neutralizes house dust allergens from mites, animals, insects; spray onto upholstery and rugs
Available from:
Skin & Allergy Shop,™The
310 E. Broadway (APD)
Louisville, KY 40202
800-366-6483
In KY 502-585-4824
Fax 502-589-3429

Johns Hopkins Dust Mite Test Kit

Indictes dust mite allergen, cat allergen, cockroach allergen levels, mold spores in your home
Available from:
Allergy-Asthma Shopper™
PO Box 239 (APD)
Fate, TX 75132
800-447-1100
Fax 903-883-4513

Micro-Clean™ Vacuum Bags

Multi-layer bags reduce allergen escape; made with treated anti-bacterial paper; available for some models of Hoover®, Eureka®, Electrolux®, Panasonic®, Sanyo®, Oreck®, Regina®, Singer®, Sharp®, and Kenmore®

Available from:
Allergy Asthma Technology
4151 N. Kedzie (APD)
PO Box 18398 (APD)
Chicago, IL 60618
800-621-5545
312-465-8020
Fax 312-465-7619
and:
Allergy Control Products, Inc.
96 Danbury Rd. (APD)
PO Box 793 (APD)
Ridgefield, CT 06877
800-422-DUST (3878)
203-438-9580
Fax 203-431-8963
and:
American Allergy Supply
PO Box 722022 (APD)
Houston, TX 77272-2022
800-321-1096
713-995-6110
and:
Methodist Hospital Library
1701 Senate Blvd. (APD)
Indianapolis, IN 46202
317-929-8021
and:
N.E.E.D.S.
527 Charles Ave. 12A (APD)
Syracuse, NY 13209
800-634-1380
Fax 800-295-NEED (6333)
and:
Priorities®
70 Walnut St. (APD)
Wellesley, MA 02181
800-553-5398
and:
Vermont Country Store®, The
PO Box 3000 (APD)
Manchester Center, VT 05255-3000
802-362-2400
Fax 802-362-0285

Micro-Fresh™ System

Combination of high filtration paper bag lined with electrostatically charged fibers and filter pad to retain dander, fine dust and pollen particles

Controlling Your Environment
Dust and Pollen Control

down to 0.1 micron; fits Royal and Dirt Devil vacuum cleaners; fits some models of Eureka, Royal, Kenmore, Singer, Hoover, Concept One & Two, Decade 80, Elite/II, Legacy I & II, Innovation

Mop Cover
Cloth treated to attract and hold dust; greaseless, lint-free; odor-free; washable; fits over dry mop; 10-1/2"x15"
Available from:
Allergy Control Products, Inc.
96 Danbury Rd. (APD)
PO Box 793 (APD)
Ridgefield, CT 06877
800-422-DUST (3878)
203-438-9580
Fax 203-431-8963

One-Wipe® Dust Cloth
Static charged fabric attracts dust; wax-free, chemical-free; machine washable; safe for surfaces; also use as mop cover
Available from:
Allergy Asthma Technology
4151 N. Kedzie (APD)
PO Box 18398 (APD)
Chicago, IL 60618
800-621-5545
312-465-8020
Fax 312-465-7619
and:
Allergy Control Products, Inc.
96 Danbury Rd. (APD)
PO Box 793 (APD)
Ridgefield, CT 06877
800-422-DUST (3878)
203-438-9580
Fax 203-431-8963
and:
Allergy Relief Products
9 Renata Ct. (APD)
Dundas, ON L9H 6X1
Canada
905-628-5324 ?416
Fax 416-628-1734

HOUSEKEEPING AIDS
STORAGE
Acrylic Storage
Lidded containers store toiletries, nursery items, bath items
Available from:
Lillian Vernon Corp.
(APD)
Virginia Beach, VA 23479-0002
800-285-5555
Fax 804-430-1500
TDD/ITTY

Add-A-Closet™
Steel frame holds vinyl storage bag for garment storage in attic, basement, spare room; 3 zippers
Available from:
Solutions®
PO Box 6878 (APD)
Portland, OR 97228
800-342-9988
Fax 503-643-1973

Garment Bag
Zippered cotton canvas bags hold dresses, gowns, suits
Available from:
Hold Everything
PO Box 7807 (APD)
San Francisco, CA 94120-7807
800-421-2264
415-421-4242
Fax 415-421-5153

Portable Storage Bin
Three bin polypropylene trolley with doors holds clothing, towels, toys; casters; 28-1/2" high
Available from:
Lillian Vernon Corp.
(APD)
Virginia Beach, VA 23479-0002
800-285-5555
Fax 804-430-1500
TDD/ITTY

Controlling Your Environment

Dust and Pollen Control

Stacking Drawers

See-through polypropylene rectangular boxes of varying sizes fit on 2-drawer or 4-drawer frame; stores clothing, lingerie, shoes
Available from:
Solutions®
PO Box 6878 (APD)
Portland, OR 97228
800-342-9988
Fax 503-643-1973

Vinyl Clothing Storage

Hanging bags store suits and dresses in closets; shelf pack stores handbags, sweaters; floor bag stores blankets, out-of-season clothing; zippers
Available from:
Lillian Vernon Corp.
(APD)
Virginia Beach, VA 23479-0002
800-285-5555
Fax 804-430-1500
TDD/ITTY

Vinyl Clothing Storage

Hanging bags store suites and dresses in closets; shelf pack stores handbags, sweaters; floor bag stores blankets, out-of-season clothing; zippers, steel frame, clear vinyl front with poly/cotton and polyester fabric
Available from:
Hold Everything
PO Box 7807 (APD)
San Francisco, CA 94120-7807
800-421-2264
415-421-4242
Fax 415-421-5153

Vinyl Storage Pack

Stores infrequently used china in vinyl packs sized for 4-dish protection, 6-cup/saucer, serving bowls; stemware; zipper
Available from:
Lillian Vernon Corp.
(APD)
Virginia Beach, VA 23479-0002

800-285-5555
Fax 804-430-1500
TDD/ITTY

Zippered Storage Bag

Clear vinyl front with nylon backing bags store blankets, comforters, dresses, blankets, sweaters
Available from:
Hold Everything
PO Box 7807 (APD)
San Francisco, CA 94120-7807
800-421-2264
415-421-4242
Fax 415-421-5153

SCREENS AND FILTERS

30/30® Filter

Disposable, medium efficiency pleated air filter; use alone or as prefilter; fits most holding frames and side access housings; lofted, non-woven cotton and synthetic media, bonded to a 16-gauge galvanized steel frame with gaskets and four spring-type positive sealing fasteners to minimize air bypass; average efficiency of 25 to 30T on ASHRAE Test Standard 52 to 76; average arrestance of 90 to 92%; can be installed in banks; commercial, industrial, and residential uses; various sizes; custom sizes
Available from:
Farr Co.
PO Box 92187 (APD)
Airport Station
Los Angeles, CA 90009
800-333-7320
Fax 800-441-0003
and
Farr Co.
500 S. Main Street (APD)
Crystal Lake, IL 60014
800-777-5260
Fax 800-441-0103

Controlling Your Environment
Dust and Pollen Control

30/30® SA Filter

Disposable, medium efficiency pleated air filter with 4" extra depth; use alone or as prefilter; fits most holding frames and side access housings; lofted, non-woven cotton and synthetic media, bonded to a welded wire grid to minimize air bypass; average efficiency of 25 to 30% on ASHRAE Test Standard 52 to 76; average arrestance of 90 to 92%; can be installed in banks; commercial and industrial uses in side access housings; various sizes
Available from:
Farr Co.
PO Box 92187 (APD)
Airport Station
Los Angeles, CA 90009
800-333-7320
Fax 800-441-0003
and
Farr Co.
500 S. Main Street (APD)
Crystal Lake, IL 60014
800-777-5260
Fax 800-441-0103

3M Filtrete™ Air Conditioner Filter

Disposable electret filter for room air conditioners, replaces foam filters; captures dust, mold, pollen, smoke, and dander; 15"x24" filter can be cut to size
Available from:
3M Company
PO Box 33275 (APD)
St. Paul, MN 55133-3275
3M Center Bldg.(APD)
St. Paul, MN 55144-1000
Medical information 800-328-0255
Medical information local 612-736-4930
Customer service 800-423-5197
Outside CA 800-423-5146
In CA 818-341-1300
and:
Allergy Control Products, Inc.
96 Danbury Rd. (APD)

PO Box 793 (APD)
Ridgefield, CT 06877
800-422-DUST (3878)
203-438-9580
Fax 203-431-8963
and:
Allergy Control Products, Inc.
96 Danbury Rd. (APD)
PO Box 793 (APD)
Ridgefield, CT 06877
800-422-DUST (3878)
203-438-9580
Fax 203-431-8963
and:
E.L. Foust Co., Inc.
PO Box 105 (APD)
Elmhurst, IL 60126
800-225-9549
708-834-4952
Fax 708-834-5341

3M Filtrete™ Filter

Replaces standard furnace ir air conditioner filter; electrostatically-charged fibers attract and hold dust, pollen, mold, smoke, and dander; pleated for greater surface area; replaceable; various sizes
Available from:
3M Company
PO Box 33275 (APD)
St. Paul, MN 55133-3275
3M Center Bldg.(APD)
St. Paul, MN 55144-1000
Medical information 800-328-0255
Medical information local 612-736-4930
Customer service 800-423-5197
Outside CA 800-423-5146
In CA 818-341-1300
and:
Allergy Control Products, Inc.
96 Danbury Rd. (APD)
PO Box 793 (APD)
Ridgefield, CT 06877
800-422-DUST (3878)
203-438-9580
Fax 203-431-8963
and:
Allergy Control Products, Inc.

Controlling Your Environment

Dust and Pollen Control

96 Danbury Rd. (APD)
PO Box 793 (APD)
Ridgefield, CT 06877
800-422-DUST (3878)
203-438-9580
Fax 203-431-8963
and:
Allergy Solutions
4909 W. Park Blvd. #169 (APD)
Plano, TX 75093
800-380-SNEEZ (7633)
214-612-4188
Fax 214-985-5573
and:
Allergy-Asthma Shopper™
PO Box 239 (APD)
Fate, TX 75132
800-447-1100
Fax 903-883-4513
and:
E.L. Foust Co., Inc.
PO Box 105 (APD)
Elmhurst, IL 60126
800-225-9549
708-834-4952
Fax 708-834-5341

600 HEPA SHIELD

Removes 99.97% of all airborne particles 0.3 micron and larger; filters pollen, bacteria, fungi, dust, mold, dander, and tobacco smoke; connects to forced air furnace or air conditioning system; disposable pre-filter, activated carbon filter
Available from:
Pure Air Systems, Inc.
425 Duffey St. (APD)
PO Box 418 (APD)
Plainfield, IN 46168
800-869-8025
317-839-9135
Fax 317-839-8567

Absolute Electrostatic Air Filter

Washable, self-charging electrostatic air filter replaces standard furnace filter; traps dust, pollen, mold, dander; ozone-free
Available from:

Absolute Environmental's Allergy Store
2615 S. University Dr. (APD)
Davie, FL 33328
Nationwide 800-771-ACHOO (2246)
In FL 800-329-3773
Broward 305-472-3773
Fax 305-474-0133

Aeropleat® II Filter

Disposable, medium efficiency pleated air filter; use alone or as prefilter; fits most holding frames and side access housings; lofted, non-woven cotton and synthetic media, bonded to a welded wire grid to minimize air bypass; average efficiency of 25 to 30T on ASHRAE Test Standard 52 to 76; average arrestance of 90%; various sizes
Available from:
Farr Co.
PO Box 92187 (APD)
Airport Station
Los Angeles, CA 90009
800-333-7320
Fax 800-441-0003
and
Farr Co.
500 S. Main Street (APD)
Crystal Lake, IL 60014
800-777-5260
Fax 800-441-0103

AirMedic+

Replaces standard furnace filter; electrostatically-charged fibers attract and hold dust, pollen, mold, smoke, and dander; pleated for greater surface area; replaceable;
Available from
Hardware stores, home improvement stores, warehouse-type stores

Aller-Tech™ Vent Guard

Cut to fit air supply vents; 85% efficient at 10 micron; in warm weather used over screens and window air conditioners to trap pollen and mold spores; installs with magnetic velcro strips; installation kit

Controlling Your Environment
Dust and Pollen Control

Available from:
Allergy Asthma Technology
4151 N. Kedzie (APD)
PO Box 18398 (APD)
Chicago, IL 60618
800-621-5545
312-465-8020
Fax 312-465-7619

Allergen™

Disposble, pleated panel, alluminum frame filter made with unblended Filtrete™ filters pollen, tobacco smoke, dust, spores, dander, mildew; various sizes
Available from:
Allergen™ Air Filter Corp.
5205 Ashbrook (APD)
Houston, TX 77081
800-333-8880
In TX 713-668-2371

Allerx 84 Electrostatic Air Filter

Aluminum frame; electrostatic prefilter fits in window air conditioning unit or use as prefilter in electronic air cleaners; traps dust, pollen, mold, lint; washable; standard and custom sizes
Available from:
Allergy-Asthma Shopper™
PO Box 239 (APD)
Fate, TX 75132
800-447-1100
Fax 903-883-4513

Allerx Deluxe Filter

Washable, electrostatic air filter replaces standard heating or central air conditioning filter; traps up to 93% of dust, pollen, mold, lint; captures 21% of particles down to 0.3-6 micron; ASHRAE 52-76 standard test; standard and custom sizes
Available from:
Allergy-Asthma Shopper™
PO Box 239 (APD)
Fate, TX 75132
800-447-1100
Fax 903-883-4513

Allerx Disposable Charcoal Filter

Replaceable activated charcoal filter adsorbs odors and fumes; polyester filter adsorbs smoke and household odors; 89.3% effective with allergens; CADR=300; aluminum frame with 3 carbon pads; standard and custom sizes
Available from:
Allergy-Asthma Shopper™
PO Box 239 (APD)
Fate, TX 75132
800-447-1100
Fax 903-883-4513

Allerx Electrostatic Air Filter

Washable filter removes up to 90% of allergens; replaces standard heating filter; standard and custom sizes
Available from:
Allergy-Asthma Shopper™
PO Box 239 (APD)
Fate, TX 75132
800-447-1100
Fax 903-883-4513

Allerx Vent Filter Kit

Washable 8"x12" cover of made high efficiency polyester material; covers central air system vent to trap dust; velcro attachments; use on only one vent at a time to avoid damage to system
Available from:
Allergy-Asthma Shopper™
PO Box 239 (APD)
Fate, TX 75132
800-447-1100
Fax 903-883-4513

Basket Guard Furnace Filter

For Lennox style furnaces, cut to size and place in filter basket; replaceable; 3'x6'
Available from:
Allergy Asthma Technology
4151 N. Kedzie (APD)
PO Box 18398 (APD)
Chicago, IL 60618
800-621-5545

Controlling Your Environment

Dust and Pollen Control

312-465-8020
Fax 312-465-7619

BioKontrol

Replaces standard furnace filter; electrostatically-charged fibers attract and hold dust, pollen, mold, smoke, and dander; pleated for greater surface area; replaceable;
Available from
Hardware stores, home improvement stores, warehouse-type stores

Contractors Choice

Static-prone materials accept static charge to attract airborne pollutants; washable; average peak dust arrestance of 86% by weight on particles .001 to 80 micron; ozone-free; helps control bacteria, mold spores, and mildew on filter surface; standard and custom sizes
Available from:
Newtron Products
PO Box 27175 (APD)
3874 Virginia Ave. (APD)
Cincinnati, OH 45227-0175
800-543-9149
In OH 800-544-3753
513-561-7373
Fax 513-561-3673

Dust Eater®

Washable filter by Permatron ® removes pollen, dust, and airborne pollutants; up to 93% arrestance efficiency; filter material creates electrostatic charge; ozone-free; replaces standard heating filter; custom sizes
Available from:
Allergy Shop, Ltd.
3420 Cardston Crescent N.W. (APD)
Calgary, AB T2L 0S6
Canada
403-289-9052
and:
National Allergy Supply, Inc.
4400 Georgia Hwy. 120 (APD)
PO Box 1658 (APD)

Duluth, GA 30136
800-522-1448
In Atlanta 404-623-8077
Fax 404-623-5568
and:
Permatron Corp.
11400 Melrose St. (APD)
Franklin Park, IL 60131-1325
800-882-8012
708-451-0999
and:
Priorities®
70 Walnut St. (APD)
Wellesley, MA 02181
800-553-5398

Dust Guard Furnace Filter

Three layers trap and hold particles; soft edges fill in gaps at edge to prevent air bypass; 99% efficient; no custom fitting needed; replaceable; various sizes
Available from:
Allergy Asthma Technology
4151 N. Kedzie (APD)
PO Box 18398 (APD)
Chicago, IL 60618
800-621-5545
312-465-8020
Fax 312-465-7619

Dust Plus®

Permatron (P) filter with washable front panel is a woven, electrostatic fabric for dust and pollen; replaceable back panel is charcoal or zeolite for odors and fumes; removes odors (tobacco smoke, fuel, cleaning solvent) and non-toxic fumes; fits furnace or air conditioning system
Available from:
National Allergy Supply, Inc.
4400 Georgia Hwy. 120 (APD)
PO Box 1658 (APD)
Duluth, GA 30136
800-522-1448
In Atlanta 404-623-8077
Fax 404-623-5568
and:

Controlling Your Environment

Dust and Pollen Control

Permatron Corp.
11400 Melrose St. (APD)
Franklin Park, IL 60131-1325
800-882-8012
708-451-0999

DUST-Magnet 90

Washable electrostatic air filter; removes 90% of air-borne particles, 90 to 99% of most pollen and plant spores; replaces heater or air conditioner filter; aluminum frame; standard or custom sizes
Available from:
Allergy Clean Environments
501 Station Ave. (APD)
Haddon Heights, NJ 08035
800-882-4110
In NJ 609-546-1101
Fax 609-546-1466
URL:
http:\\WWW.infomall.com\allergy.html
and:
Allergy Supply Co.
11994 Star Court (APD)
Herndon, VA 22071
800-323-6744
Metropolitan DC 703-391-2011
Fax 703-391-2014
BBS 703-521-0638
Royal Appliance Mfg. Co.
650 Alpha Dr. (APD)
Cleveland, OH 44143-2172
800-321-1134 Ext. 533
216-449-6150
Fax 216-449-7806

Electronic Air Cleaner Filters

Layers of electrostatic fabric media trap airborne particles like dust, pollen, and dirt; arrestance efficiency of 72%; washable with either flexible vinyl or stainless steel edge; standard and custom sizes; optional, disposable odor removal filters
Model H for heating/cooling systems
Model R prefilter for electronic air cleaners
Available from:

Permatron Corp.
11400 Melrose St. (APD)
Franklin Park, IL 60131-1325
800-882-8012
708-451-0999

Electrostatic Air Filter

Removes approximately 90% to 99% of airborne particles; washable; furnace and air conditioning systems; standard and custom sizes
Available from:
Allergy Clean Environments
501 Station Ave. (APD)
Haddon Heights, NJ 08035
800-882-4110
In NJ 609-546-1101
Fax 609-546-1466
URL:
http:\\WWW.infomall.com\allergy.html

EZ-2000

Replaces disposable filter in wall grille, self-contained unit, or window unit; ozone-free; low air flow resistance; filters up to 96% of pollen, dust, allergens, smoke and other irritants
Available from:
Clean Air Services
2402 Elm St. (APD)
Allentown, PA 18104
215-435-4355
Fax 215-435-4295

Hi-Tech Filter

Washable filter replaces standard filter in furnace and air conditioner; ozone-free, polypropylene woven filaments creates own electrostatic charge; low air flow resistance; traps dust pollen, mold, air borne irritants; 99.9% efficient to 10 micron; can be used as prefilter for HEPA filter; aluminum frame; various standard sizes and custom sizes
Available from:
Aller-Guard,® Inc.
Southgate Office Park
1645 S.W. 41st St. (APD)

Controlling Your Environment

Dust and Pollen Control

Topeka, KS 66609-1250
800-234-0816
913-267-9333
Fax 913-267-0072
and:
Allergy Control Products, Inc.
96 Danbury Rd. (APD)
PO Box 793 (APD)
Ridgefield, CT 06877
800-422-DUST (3878)
203-438-9580
Fax 203-431-8963
and:
Allergy Solutions
4909 W. Park Blvd. #169 (APD)
Plano, TX 75093
800-380-SNEEZ (7633)
214-612-4188
Fax 214-985-5573
and:
Environtrol® Corporation
PO Box 31313 (APD)
St. Louis, MO 63131
800-423-1982
In St. Louis 314-966-6886
and:
Hi-Tech Filter Corp. of America
80 Myrtle St. (APD)
N. Quincy, MA 02171
800-448-3249
In MA 617-328-7756
Fax 617-773-4192
and:
Skin & Allergy Shop,™The
310 E. Broadway (APD)
Louisville, KY 40202
800-366-6483
In KY 502-585-4824
Fax 502-589-3429

Honeywell Media Air Filter

Pleated, nonwoven, reinforced cotton fabric traps pollen, dust, dander; cabinet installs in gas, oil, or electric forced air system; filters replaceable; various air flow ratings; various sizes
Locally available
Available from:
Honeywell, Inc.

Home and Building Control
Honeywell Plaza
PO Box 524 (APD)
Minneapolis, MN 55440-0524
612-951-1000
and
Honeywell, Inc.
740 Ellesmere Rd. (APD)
Scarborough, ON, M1P 2V9
Canada

King-Aire® Pro Pak

Woven polyester fiber furnace filter; reduces dust; replaces standard furnace filters; various sizes
Available from:
King-Aire®
1121 S.R. 32 E. (APD)
Noblesville, IN 46060
Mail to PO Box 398 (APD)
Noblesville, IN 46060-0398
800-999-KING (5464)
317-776-1600

Koch Multi-Pleat Air Filter

Pleated for greater area and absorption; use in heating and cooling units; replaces standard filters; various sizes
Available from:
Environtrol® Corporation
PO Box 31313 (APD)
St. Louis, MO 63131
800-423-1982
In St. Louis 314-966-6886
and:
Skin & Allergy Shop,™The
310 E. Broadway (APD)
Louisville, KY 40202
800-366-6483
In KY 502-585-4824
Fax 502-589-3429

Newtron Whistle Air

Washable, electrostatic air filter whistles when cleaning is required; standard and custom sizes
Available from:
Allergy Clean Environments
501 Station Ave. (APD)

Controlling Your Environment
Dust and Pollen Control

Haddon Heights, NJ 08035
800-882-4110
In NJ 609-546-1101
Fax 609-546-1466
URL:
http:\\WWW.infomall.com\allergy.html
and:
Newtron Products
PO Box 27175 (APD)
3874 Virginia Ave. (APD)
Cincinnati, OH 45227-0175
800-543-9149
In OH 800-544-3753
513-561-7373
Fax 513-561-3673

Newtron® Air Cleaner

Static-prone materials accept static charge to attract airborne pollutants; washable; removes up to 88.3% of particulates in the 0 to 5 micron range; ozone-free; helps control bacteria, mold spores, and mildew on filter surface; replaces furnace filter; standard and custom sizes
Available from:
Newtron Products
PO Box 27175 (APD)
3874 Virginia Ave. (APD)
Cincinnati, OH 45227-0175
800-543-9149
In OH 800-544-3753
513-561-7373
Fax 513-561-3673

Permastatic II Filter

Filters pollen, dust, other particulates; replaces existing disposable filter; washable; standard and custom filter sizes
Available from:
Allergy Relief Shop,™ Inc.
3371 Whittle Springs Rd. (APD)
Knoxville, TN 37917
Orders 800-626-2810
Questions 615-522-2795
and:
Allergy Resources
Mail: PO Box 888 (APD)
UPS: 264 Brookridge Ave. (APD)

Palmer Lake, CO 80133
Orders 800-USE-FLAX (873-3529)
Company plans to move; use 800 #
and:
AllerMed Corp.
31 Steel Rd. (APD)
Wylie, TX 75098
214-442-4898
Fax 214-442-4897
and:
Flowright Int'l Products
1495 N.W. Gilman Blvd. #4 (APD)
Issaquah, WA 98027
206-392-8357
and:
N.E.E.D.S.
527 Charles Ave. 12A (APD)
Syracuse, NY 13209
800-634-1380
Fax 800-295-NEED (6333)

Pro-Pak Furnace Filter

Replaceable, woven polyester filter replaces standard furnace filters; dust filtration; various sizes
Available from:
King-Aire®
1121 S.R. 32 E. (APD)
Noblesville, IN 46060
Mail to PO Box 398 (APD)
Noblesville, IN 46060-0398
800-999-KING (5464)
317-776-1600

Purity® Air Filter

Replaces furnace filter; removes 97% of pollen, 99% lint, 70% of dust, 20% of smoke; replaceable
Available from:
Skin & Allergy Shop,™ The
310 E. Broadway (APD)
Louisville, KY 40202
800-366-6483
In KY 502-585-4824
Fax 502-589-3429

Purolator® Puro Pleat

Replaces standard furnace filter; electrostatically-charged fibers attract and hold dust, pollen, mold, smoke,

Controlling Your Environment
Dust and Pollen Control

and dander; pleated for greater surface area; replaceable;
Available from
Hardware stores, home improvement stores, warehouse-type stores

Register Cover

Blend of small and large fibers in a 16"x60" roll; cuts with scissors to fit; optional velcro® mounting kit
Available from:
Allergy Supply Co.
11994 Star Court (APD)
Herndon, VA 22071
800-323-6744
Metropolitan DC 703-391-2011
Fax 703-391-2014
BBS 703-521-0638

REMIND-AIR

Independent filter screens accumulate dust, pollen, and mold; washable; average peak dust arrestance of 86% by weight on particles .001 to 80 micron; ozone-free; helps control bacteria, mold spores, and mildew on filter surface; standard and custom sizes
Available from:
Newtron Products
PO Box 27175 (APD)
3874 Virginia Ave. (APD)
Cincinnati, OH 45227-0175
800-543-9149
In OH 800-544-3753
513-561-7373
Fax 513-561-3673

Riga-Flo®/100PH Filters

Replaceable filter; all-metal enclosing frame, diagonal support braces, pleated stabilizers, welded wire grid, rigid construction for variable volume systems up to 500 fpm; average efficiency of 80 to 85% on ASHRAE Test Standard 52 to 76; average arrestance of 98%; media filter is a high density microfine glass fiber, forming a lofted filter blanket

laminated to a reinforced backing; commercial and industrial uses
Available from:
Farr Co.
PO Box 92187 (APD)
Airport Station
Los Angeles, CA 90009
800-333-7320
Fax 800-441-0003
and
Farr Co.
500 S. Main Street (APD)
Crystal Lake, IL 60014
800-777-5260
Fax 800-441-0103

Riga-Flo®/10PH Filters

Replaceable filter; all-metal enclosing frame, diagonal support braces, pleated stabilizers, welded wire grid, rigid construction for variable volume systems up to 500 fpm; average efficiency of 40 to 45% on ASHRAE Test Standard 52 to 76; average arrestance of 90%; media filter is a cotton/polyester with a non-woven microfiber on the air exiting side
Available from:
Farr Co.
PO Box 92187 (APD)
Airport Station
Los Angeles, CA 90009
800-333-7320
Fax 800-441-0003
and
Farr Co.
500 S. Main Street (APD)
Crystal Lake, IL 60014
800-777-5260
Fax 800-441-0103

Riga-Flo®/15PH Filters

Replaceable filter; all-metal enclosing frame, diagonal support braces, pleated stabilizers, welded wire grid, rigid construction for variable volume systems up to 500 fpm; average efficiency of 60 to 65% on ASHRAE Test Standard 52 to 76; average arrestance of 97%; media filter

Controlling Your Environment
Dust and Pollen Control

is a high density microfine glass fiber, forming a lofted filter blanket laminated to a reinforced backing; commercial and industrial uses
Available from:
Farr Co.
PO Box 92187 (APD)
Airport Station
Los Angeles, CA 90009
800-333-7320
Fax 800-441-0003
and
Farr Co.
500 S. Main Street (APD)
Crystal Lake, IL 60014
800-777-5260
Fax 800-441-0103

Riga-Flo®/200PH Filters

Replaceable filter; all-metal enclosing frame, diagonal support braces, pleated stabilizers, welded wire grid, rigid construction for variable volume systems up to 500 fpm; average efficiency of 90 to 95% on ASHRAE Test Standard 52 to 76; average arrestance of 99%; media filter is a high density microfine glass fiber, forming a lofted filter blanket laminated to a reinforced backing; commercial and industrial uses
Available from:
Farr Co.
PO Box 92187 (APD)
Airport Station
Los Angeles, CA 90009
800-333-7320
Fax 800-441-0003
and
Farr Co.
500 S. Main Street (APD)
Crystal Lake, IL 60014
800-777-5260
Fax 800-441-0103

Riga-Flo®/XLPH Filters

Replaceable filter; all-metal enclosing frame, diagonal support braces, pleated stabilizers, welded wire grid, rigid construction for variable

volume systems up to 500 fpm; average efficiency of 40 to 45% on ASHRAE Test Standard 52 to 76; average arrestance of 96%; media filter is a high density microfine glass fiber, forming a lofted filter blanket laminated to a reinforced backing; commercial and industrial uses
Available from:
Farr Co.
PO Box 92187 (APD)
Airport Station
Los Angeles, CA 90009
800-333-7320
Fax 800-441-0003
and
Farr Co.
500 S. Main Street (APD)
Crystal Lake, IL 60014
800-777-5260
Fax 800-441-0103

Safeguard Window Ventilator or Window Guard

Filtering screen for dirt, dust, pollen fits on double-hung windows; aluminum frame; washable; various sizes, adjustable
Available from:
Allergy Asthma Technology
4151 N. Kedzie (APD)
PO Box 18398 (APD)
Chicago, IL 60618
800-621-5545
312-465-8020
Fax 312-465-7619
and:
Allergy Clean Environments
501 Station Ave. (APD)
Haddon Heights, NJ 08035
800-882-4110
In NJ 609-546-1101
Fax 609-546-1466
URL:
http:\\WWW.infomall.com\allergy.html
and:
Brookstone Co.
5 Vose Farm Road (APD)
Peterborough, NH 03458
800-926-7000

Controlling Your Environment

Dust and Pollen Control

Fax 603-924-0093

Self-charging Electrostatic Air Filter

One-inch thick filters with rigid frame for existing system; 1/4 inch thick filters with non-rigid frame for window air conditioners, wall or floor vents; washable; standard and custom sizes; no wiring; ozone-free
Available from:
Allergy Control Products, Inc.
96 Danbury Rd. (APD)
PO Box 793 (APD)
Ridgefield, CT 06877
800-422-DUST (3878)
203-438-9580
Fax 203-431-8963
and:
Allergy Relief Products
9 Renata Ct. (APD)
Dundas, ON L9H 6X1
Canada
905-628-5324 ?416
Fax 416-628-1734

SERV-Aire

Disposable air filter rated 30 to 35% efficiency and 93% average arrestance; pleated; standard, custom sizes
Available from:
Allergy Supply Co.
11994 Star Court (APD)
Herndon, VA 22071
800-323-6744
Metropolitan DC 703-391-2011
Fax 703-391-2014
BBS 703-521-0638

Space-Gard® 2200

Installs in forced air heating/cooling system; traps dust, tobacco smoke, pollen, spores, pet dander, hair and dust larger than 1 micron; average efficiency of 65% at 1,200 CFM; particles from 0.01 to 30 micron; ozone-free; replaceable filter media; filtering area 78.6 sq. ft.;

capacity 600 to 2,000 CFM; under 28 lbs.
Available from:
Research Products Corp.
1015 E. Washington Ave. (APD)
PO Box 1467 (APD)
Madison, WI 53701-1467
800-545-2219
608-257-8801
Fax 608-257-4357

Space-Gard® 2250

Replaces the return air grille of the central heating/cooling system; wall or ceiling; residential capacity 600 to 2,000 CFM; filtering area 78.6 sq. ft.; under 32 lbs.
Available from:
Research Products Corp.
1015 E. Washington Ave. (APD)
PO Box 1467 (APD)
Madison, WI 53701-1467
800-545-2219
608-257-8801
Fax 608-257-4357

VACU-FILT™

Vacuum exhaust filter with imbedded electrostatic charges placed in vacuum canister over the exhaust grille; 8"x10" sheets cut to size with scissors; used for canister style or hard encased uprights
Available from:
Allergy Control Products, Inc.
96 Danbury Rd. (APD)
PO Box 793 (APD)
Ridgefield, CT 06877
800-422-DUST (3878)
203-438-9580
Fax 203-431-8963
and:
Allergy Relief Products
9 Renata Ct. (APD)
Dundas, ON L9H 6X1
Canada
905-628-5324 ?416
Fax 416-628-1734
and:
N.E.E.D.S.

Controlling Your Environment
Dust and Pollen Control

527 Charles Ave. 12A (APD)
Syracuse, NY 13209
800-634-1380
Fax 800-295-NEED (6333)

Vent and Grille Filter

Non-rigid, 1/4" thick Hi-Tech filter fits behind air supply vent and outlet grille in walls and floors and window air conditioner units
Available from:
Environtrol® Corporation
PO Box 31313 (APD)
St. Louis, MO 63131
800-423-1982
In St. Louis 314-966-6886
and:
Hi-Tech Filter Corp. of America
80 Myrtle St. (APD)
N. Quincy, MA 02171
800-448-3249
In MA 617-328-7756
Fax 617-773-4192

Vent Filtration Kit

High efficiency polyester filters trap dust from ductwork; filters fit over or under central air system air-supply vent; velcro attachment; cut to size from roll of material; use on only one vent at a time to avoid damage to system
Available from:
American Allergy Supply
PO Box 722022 (APD)
Houston, TX 77272-2022
800-321-1096
713-995-6110
and:
National Allergy Supply, Inc.
4400 Georgia Hwy. 120 (APD)
PO Box 1658 (APD)
Duluth, GA 30136
800-522-1448
In Atlanta 404-623-8077
Fax 404-623-5568

Vent-Pro™

Disposable heating vent filter; electrostatically enhanced media filters with low air flow resistance; cut to size and place behind vent cover; 20"x24" sheet
Available from:
Allergy Control Products, Inc.
96 Danbury Rd. (APD)
PO Box 793 (APD)
Ridgefield, CT 06877
800-422-DUST (3878)
203-438-9580
Fax 203-431-8963

Web, The

Electret filter traps up to 99% of pollen and up to 94% of dust and dander; ozone-free; adjustable to various filter sizes; washable; optional carbon pad for smoke and odor
Available from:
A-Plus Allergy Equipment & Supply
8325 Regis Way (APD)
Los Angeles, CA 90045-2646
Orders 800-86-ALLER (862-5537)
310-337-7468
Fax 310-337-1971

TOYS

Cotton Teddy Bear

Washable, non-fuzzy bear, 10-inches tall; cotton stuffing
Available from:
A-Plus Allergy Equipment & Supply
8325 Regis Way (APD)
Los Angeles, CA 90045-2646
Orders 800-86-ALLER (862-5537)
310-337-7468
Fax 310-337-1971

Foundlings®

Cotton-stuffed animals with embroidered eyes; no pull-out parts
Available from:
Allergy Solutions
4909 W. Park Blvd. #169 (APD)
Plano, TX 75093
800-380-SNEEZ (7633)
214-612-4188
Fax 214-985-5573

Controlling Your Environment
Dust and Pollen Control

Gund® Washable Stuffed Animals

Machine washable for dust control; range from 6" to 17" high
Available from:
Allergy Control Products, Inc.
96 Danbury Rd. (APD)

PO Box 793 (APD)
Ridgefield, CT 06877
800-422-DUST (3878)
203-438-9580
Fax 203-431-8963

HELP US TO HELP YOU

When writing to the companies and organizations listed here, be sure to use the initials (APD) as part of the address and tell them you saw them listed in *Allergy Products Directory*.

If you call, be sure to tell them you found them in *Allergy Products Directory*.

This is important to you because:

1. Lets the company know that its listings have helped you.

2. Encourages the company to keep *Allergy Products Directory* informed of its new products so that we can keep you informed.

3. Enables us to keep our listings accurate and up-to-date for you on the latest products, services, and innovations.

4. Enables us to keep the Directory price low for you.

Thank you for your help.

Controlling Your Environment
Fighting Mold and Mildew

FIGHTING MOLD AND MILDEW

CLEANERS AND REMOVERS

AFM Safety Clean

Odor-free, effective in the general control of bacteria, mold and mildew; tubs, tile, sauna
Available from:
AFM Enterprises, Inc.
1960 Chicago E7 (APD)
Riverside, CA 92507
909-781-6860
909-781-6861
Fax 909-781-6892
and:
Allergy Relief Shop™, Inc.
3371 Whittle Springs Rd. (APD)
Knoxville, TN 37917
Orders 800-626-2810
Questions 615-522-2795
and:
Allergy Resources
Mail: PO Box 888 (APD)
UPS: 264 Brookridge Ave. (APD)
Palmer Lake, CO 80133
Orders 800-USE-FLAX (873-3529)
Company plans to move; use 800 #
and:
Allergy-Asthma Shopper™
PO Box 239 (APD)
Fate, TX 75132
800-447-1100
Fax 903-883-4513
and:
Flowright Int'l Products
1495 N.W. Gilman Blvd. #4 (APD)
Issaquah, WA 98027
206-392-8357
and:
N.E.E.D.S.
527 Charles Ave. 12A (APD)
Syracuse, NY 13209
800-634-1380
Fax 800-295-NEED (6333)
and:
Priorities®
70 Walnut St. (APD)

Wellesley, MA 02181
800-553-5398

AFM X-158 Mildew Control

Liquid cleaner for mildew resistance in shower stalls, tub enclosures, and bathroom walls; does not remove existing mildew
Available from:
AFM Enterprises, Inc.
1960 Chicago E7 (APD)
Riverside, CA 92507
909-781-6860
909-781-6861
Fax 909-781-6892
and:
Allergy Relief Shop™, Inc.
3371 Whittle Springs Rd. (APD)
Knoxville, TN 37917
Orders 800-626-2810
Questions 615-522-2795
and:
Allergy Resources
Mail: PO Box 888 (APD)
UPS: 264 Brookridge Ave. (APD)
Palmer Lake, CO 80133
Orders 800-USE-FLAX (873-3529)
Company plans to move; use 800 #
and:
Allergy-Asthma Shopper™
PO Box 239 (APD)
Fate, TX 75132
800-447-1100
Fax 903-883-4513
and:
Flowright Int'l Products
1495 N.W. Gilman Blvd. #4 (APD)
Issaquah, WA 98027
206-392-8357
and:
N.E.E.D.S.
527 Charles Ave. 12A (APD)
Syracuse, NY 13209
800-634-1380
Fax 800-295-NEED (6333)
and:
Priorities®

Controlling Your Environment

Fighting Mold and Mildew

70 Walnut St. (APD)
Wellesley, MA 02181
800-553-5398

Aller-Tech™ REP10 Mold Remover

Kills mold and mildew in bathrooms, window sills, basement walls, humdidifiers, and air conditioners
Available from:
Allergy Asthma Technology
4151 N. Kedzie (APD)
PO Box 18398 (APD)
Chicago, IL 60618
800-621-5545
312-465-8020
Fax 312-465-7619

Damp Rid®

Tray with moisture absorber pulls humidity from the air
Available from:
Allergy-Asthma Shopper™
PO Box 239 (APD)
Fate, TX 75132
800-447-1100
Fax 903-883-4513

Damp Rid® Mildew and Mold Control

Spray prevents mildew growth for up to 28 days on fabrics and non-porous surfaces; use in shower stalls and on shower curtains
Available from:
Allergy Control Products, Inc.
96 Danbury Rd. (APD)
PO Box 793 (APD)
Ridgefield, CT 06877
800-422-DUST (3878)
203-438-9580
Fax 203-431-8963

Goodwrench® A/C System Disinfectant

Eliminates mold and bacteria in car air conditioners; treatment leaves no residual chemicals in the car's system; need for repeat treatment depends on: humidity levels, dust and dirt levels in the air, and weather; professional application available from Cadillac, Oldsmobile, Chevrolet, Pontiac and Buick dealers, part #25533404

Impregon Bacteriostat

Concentrated liquid that inhibits mold growth in humidifiers, air conditioners, shower stalls, basement walls, other damp places; does not kill existing mold; "non-allergenic"
Available from:
Absolute Environmental's Allergy Store
2615 S. University Dr. (APD)
Davie, FL 33328
Nationwide 800-771-ACHOO (2246)
In FL 800-329-3773
Broward 305-472-3773
Fax 305-474-0133
and:
Allergy Alternative
440 Godfrey Dr. (APD)
Windsor, CA 95492
800-838-1514
and:
Allergy Asthma Technology
4151 N. Kedzie (APD)
PO Box 18398 (APD)
Chicago, IL 60618
800-621-5545
312-465-8020
Fax 312-465-7619
and:
Allergy Clean Environments
501 Station Ave. (APD)
Haddon Heights, NJ 08035
800-882-4110
In NJ 609-546-1101
Fax 609-546-1466
URL:
http:\\WWW.infomall.com\allergy.html
and:
Allergy Resources
Mail: PO Box 888 (APD)
UPS: 264 Brookridge Ave. (APD)
Palmer Lake, CO 80133
Orders 800-USE-FLAX (873-3529)
Company plans to move; use 800 #

Controlling Your Environment

Fighting Mold and Mildew

and:
Allergy Supply Co.
11994 Star Court (APD)
Herndon, VA 22071
800-323-6744
Metropolitan DC 703-391-2011
Fax 703-391-2014
BBS 703-521-0638
and:
Allergy-Asthma Shopper™
PO Box 239 (APD)
Fate, TX 75132
800-447-1100
Fax 903-883-4513
and:
Skin & Allergy Shop,™The
310 E. Broadway (APD)
Louisville, KY 40202
800-366-6483
In KY 502-585-4824
Fax 502-589-3429

M-1 Sure Cote

Wipe, brush, or spray on hard or soft surfaces in showers, basements, closets, fabrics, concrete, glass to protect against mildew and mold
Available from:
Aller-Guard,® Inc.
Southgate Office Park
1645 S.W. 41st St. (APD)
Topeka, KS 66609-1250
800-234-0816
913-267-9333
Fax 913-267-0072

Mildew Away™

Sprays on canvas, vinyl, tile, ceramic, fiberglass, boat tops, life jackets; rinse off; effective up to 9 months
Available from:
Home Trends
1450 Lyell Ave. (APD)
Rochester, NY 14606-2184
716-254-6520
Fax 716-458-9245
and:
Solutions®
PO Box 6878 (APD)

Portland, OR 97228
800-342-9988
Fax 503-643-1973

Mildew Remover X-14

Protection on curtains, slip covers, and shower curtains and non-porous surfaces in homes, trailers, boat and car interiors; can be used on walls, glass, tile, and wallpaper
Available from:
Allergy Clean Environments
501 Station Ave. (APD)
Haddon Heights, NJ 08035
800-882-4110
In NJ 609-546-1101
Fax 609-546-1466
URL:
http:\\WWW.infomall.com\allergy.html
and:
Allergy Control Products, Inc.
96 Danbury Rd. (APD)
PO Box 793 (APD)
Ridgefield, CT 06877
800-422-DUST (3878)
203-438-9580
Fax 203-431-8963

Mold Zapper

Passes mold spores by convection through a heating chamber to kill them; serves 1000 cu. ft.; silent operation
Available from:
Allergy Control Products, Inc.
96 Danbury Rd. (APD)
PO Box 793 (APD)
Ridgefield, CT 06877
800-422-DUST (3878)
203-438-9580
Fax 203-431-8963

Motorcraft® A/C System Disinfectant

Eliminates mold and bacteria in car air conditioners; treatment leaves no residual chemicals in the car's system; need for repeat treatment depends on: humidity levels, dust and dirt levels in the air, and weather;

Controlling Your Environment

Fighting Mold and Mildew

professional application available from Ford and Lincoln-Mercury dealers, part #YN-8

No More Mildew™

Odorless liquid spray prevents mold re-growth up to two years, depending on surface and conditions; use for bathroom tile, curtains, ceilings, walls, basement walls, joists, ceilings, outdoor furniture and cushions, boat decks, seats, canvas, and interiors, RV's, wooden decks, tile, brick
Available from:
National Allergy Supply, Inc.
4400 Georgia Hwy. 120 (APD)
PO Box 1658 (APD)
Duluth, GA 30136
800-522-1448
In Atlanta 404-623-8077
Fax 404-623-5568
and:
West Coast Shoe Co.
52828 N.W. Shoe Factory Ln. (APD)
PO Box 607 (APD)
Scappoose, OR 97056-0607
800-326-2711
503-543-7114
Fax 503-543-7110

RenNew-A/C® Car Air Conditioning

Eliminates mold and bacteria in car air conditioners; treatment leaves no residual chemicals in the car's system; need for repeat treatment depends on: humidity levels, dust and dirt levels in the air, and weather; professional application available from auto mechanics with product availability from Murray Corp. and NAPA distributors, part #209948
Available from:
Alcide Corp.
1 Willard Rd. (APD)
Norwalk, CT 06851
800-543-2133
203-847-2555

REP-70 Mold Preventer

Prevents mold growth for up to six months; non-toxic spray for air conditioners, heat pumps; refrigerator coils
Available from:
Allergy Asthma Technology
4151 N. Kedzie (APD)
PO Box 18398 (APD)
Chicago, IL 60618
800-621-5545
312-465-8020
Fax 312-465-7619
and:
Allergy Solutions
4909 W. Park Blvd. #169 (APD)
Plano, TX 75093
800-380-SNEEZ (7633)
214-612-4188
Fax 214-985-5573

REP60 Mold Preventer

Spray for bathroom tile, refridgerator coils, air conditioning ducts, and basement walls; inquire for automobile air conditioner use
Available from:
Allergy Asthma Technology
4151 N. Kedzie (APD)
PO Box 18398 (APD)
Chicago, IL 60618
800-621-5545
312-465-8020
Fax 312-465-7619

Sporicidan

"Hypoallergenic," disinfectant aerosol, with odor, protects against odor-causing organsisms, viruses, fungi, and bacteria
Available from:
IDE Interstate Dental Supply Catalog
1500 New Horizons Blvd. (APD)
Amityville, NY 11701-1130
800-666-8100
Fax 516-957-1678

Sterling A/C System Disinfectant

Eliminates mold and bacteria in car air conditioners; treatment leaves

Controlling Your Environment
Fighting Mold and Mildew

no residual chemicals in the car's system; need for repeat treatment depends on: humidity levels, dust and dirt levels in the air, and weather; professional application available from Sterling dealers, part #985 985300 10

PRODUCTS FOR HOUSEHOLD USE

Aeroallergen Assessments

Detects presence of D. pteronyssinus, D. farinae, cat, cockroach, and a mold spore count from your dust sample
Available from:
Allergy Clean Environments
501 Station Ave. (APD)
Haddon Heights, NJ 08035
800-882-4110
In NJ 609-546-1101
Fax 609-546-1466
URL:
http:\\WWW.infomall.com\allergy.html

Airlet™ 500

Humidity controlled fresh air inlet; grille has a humidity sensitive strip which opens the damper to increase airflow when room humidity rises and contracts to decrease airflow when room humidity falls
Available from:
American ALDES Ventilation Corp.
Northgate Center Business Park
4537 Northgate Ct. (APD)
Sarasota, FL 34234-2124
800-255-7749
In FL 813-351-3441
Fax 813-351-3442

Aldes VMP-K Multi-Point

Outside air is vented into the bedroom, dining room, and living room while inside air is vented from the bathroom and kitchen; kitchen extract rates are 35 CFM to 120 CFM; no ventilation fans needed in bathrooms; .2 hour timer (to increase kitchen

exhaust), 1,800 rpm speeed fan; for super-insulated home, not appropriate where pollen allergy or outside pollution is a problem; only for mold and mildew control
Available from:
American ALDES Ventilation Corp.
Northgate Center Business Park
4537 Northgate Ct. (APD)
Sarasota, FL 34234-2124
800-255-7749
In FL 813-351-3441
Fax 813-351-3442

Boot and Shoe Dryer

Electric units delivers warm air that circulates through boots and shoes, drying them; appropriate for leather, plastic, rubber, vinyl, cloth, Gore-Tex®, and canvas; optional 6-inch extenders for knee boots; optional 12-inch extenders for ship and chest waders
Available from:
Gempler's
211 Blue Mounds Rd. (APD)
PO Box 270 (APD)
Mt. Horeb, WI 53572
800-382-8473
Fax 800-551-1128

Breathable Shower Curtain

Tyvek® DuPont fabric allows moisture to escape for more rapid drying; sewn hang holes
Available from:
Brookstone Co.
5 Vose Farm Road (APD)
Peterborough, NH 03458
800-926-7000
Fax 603-924-0093

Electric Shoe/Boot Dryer

Double columns hold pair of shoes or boots; slow heat radiates to the inside of footwear with less damage to material; suitable for leather or sport shoes, boots, or gloves; 2-1/2 lbs.
Available from:
Sporty's® Preferred Living

Controlling Your Environment

Fighting Mold and Mildew

Clermont County Airport (APD)
Batavia, OH 45103-9747
800-543-8633
Fax 513-732-6560

Electric Towel Warmer

Steel tubing heated by enclosed electrical element; household current; floor model; brass or chrome plate
Available from
Home Decorators Collection
2025 Concourse Dr. (APD)
St. Louis, MO 63146-4178
800-245-2217

Electric Towel Warmer

Steel tubing heat heated by circulating oil; floor model uses household current; wall model required hard-wire electricl installation; brass or chrome plate
Available from:
Hammacher Schlemmer
147 E. 57th St. (APD)
New York, NY 10022
800-543-3366
212-421-9000
and:
Sporty's® Preferred Living
Clermont County Airport (APD)
Batavia, OH 45103-9747
800-543-8633
Fax 513-732-6560

Host® Sponges™

Dry carpet cleaner for spots and spills; does not promote mold; scented
Available from:
Allergy Clean Environments
501 Station Ave. (APD)
Haddon Heights, NJ 08035
800-882-4110
In NJ 609-546-1101
Fax 609-546-1466
URL:
http:\\WWW.infomall.com\allergy.html

Johns Hopkins Dust Mite Test Kit

Indictes dust mite allergen, cat allergen, cockroach allergen levels, mold spores in your home
Available from:
Allergy-Asthma Shopper™
PO Box 239 (APD)
Fate, TX 75132
800-447-1100
Fax 903-883-4513

Mildew-Resistant Shower Curtain

Mildew-resistant vinyl; heavy gauge; reinforced top, rustproof grommets; bath and shower stall
Available from:
Colonial Garden Kitchens®
PO Box 66 (APD)
Hanover, PA 17333-0066
800-752-5552
Fax 800-338-1635
and:
Harriet Carter®
Dept. 11 (APD)
N. Wales, PA 19455
215-361-5151
and:
Improvements ™
4944 Commerce Pkwy. (APD)
Cleveland, OH 44128
800-642-2112
Fax 216-464-6764
and:
Solutions®
PO Box 6878 (APD)
Portland, OR 97228
800-342-9988
Fax 503-643-1973

Mold Resistant Shower Curtain

Mold and bacteria resistant shower curtain made of white vinyl; mold-proof SnapUps® in place of curtain rings; use alone or as liner; clean with damp cloth; two sizes
Available from:
Allergy Asthma Technology
4151 N. Kedzie (APD)
PO Box 18398 (APD)
Chicago, IL 60618

Controlling Your Environment
Fighting Mold and Mildew

800-621-5545
312-465-8020
Fax 312-465-7619

Molecular Adsorber™
Refillable zeolite container attracts odors into non-powered unit; wall mount or pedestal
Available from:
Allergy Asthma Technology
4151 N. Kedzie (APD)
PO Box 18398 (APD)
Chicago, IL 60618
800-621-5545
312-465-8020
Fax 312-465-7619
and:
Allergy-Asthma Shopper™
PO Box 239 (APD)
Fate, TX 75132
800-447-1100
Fax 903-883-4513

Polytuf™ Tarp
Mildew-proof salvage or utility cover of woven polyethylene lamined with poly film; reinforced hem; 12'x14' and 14'x18'
Available from:
Eddie Bauer, Inc.
5th & Union (APD)
Box 3700 (APD)
Seattle, WA 98130
800-426-8020

Portable Clothes Dryer
Base heating element sets up convection current to dry wet clothes, towels; warms towels; household current; welded steel, white enamel finish
Available from:
Sporty's® Preferred Living
Clermont County Airport (APD)
Batavia, OH 45103-9747
800-543-8633
Fax 513-732-6560

Shower Curtain
All cotton, washable; 6'x6' for tubs, 3'x6' for shower stalls; special sizes or colors available from some suppliers
Available from:
Allergy Relief Shop™, Inc.
3371 Whittle Springs Rd. (APD)
Knoxville, TN 37917
Orders 800-626-2810
Questions 615-522-2795
and:
Allergy Resources
Mail: PO Box 888 (APD)
UPS: 264 Brookridge Ave. (APD)
Palmer Lake, CO 80133
Orders 800-USE-FLAX (873-3529)
Company plans to move; use 800 #
and:
Cotton Place, The
2986 Talisman Dr. (APD)
PO Box 59721 (APD)
Dallas, TX 75229
800-451-8866
214-243-14941
and:
Janice Corp.
198 US Hwy. 46 (APD)
Budd Lake, NJ 07828-3001
800-JANICES (526-4237)
Fax 201-691-5459

Shower Curtain
Cotton canvas shower curtain; 10 oz. cotton duck; brass-coated, non-rusting grommets; dries quickly to prevent mildew; undyed; use with liner; machine wash and dry
Available from:
L.L. Bean, Inc.
Freeport, ME 04033
800-221-4221

Shower Splash Guard
Plastic triangle fits at corner of tub and shower head wall; prevents water splash that can cause mold
Available from:
Lillian Vernon Corp.
(APD)

Controlling Your Environment
Fighting Mold and Mildew

Virginia Beach, VA 23479-0002
800-285-5555
Fax 804-430-1500
TDD/ITTY

Water Eater®

Thin, 3-ft. long, nontoxic, highly absorbent strip for placement at a leaky tub, toilet, or window; absorbs water to prevent damage and mold until problem is corrected; reusable for water-based spill; let dry
Available from:
Solutions®
PO Box 6878 (APD)
Portland, OR 97228
800-342-9988
Fax 503-643-1973

VENTILATORS
ALDES DHV

Ventilating dehumidifier filters 95% of particles 1 micron and larger. Supplies and filters up to 100 CFM fresh air, filters indoor air, dehumidifiers to control indoor humidity levels. Operates continuously for ventilation or by timer or in response to humidity level. Portable unit with casters or connect to forced air system
Available from:
American ALDES Ventilation Corp.
Northgate Center Business Park
4537 Northgate Ct. (APD)
Sarasota, FL 34234-2124
800-255-7749
In FL 813-351-3441
Fax 813-351-3442

ALDES VMP-H

Ventilation system with heat recovery; exhausts indoor air and excess humidity from kitchen, laundry, and up to 4 bathrooms and supplies outdoor air heated by the air being exhausted to the living, dining, family, and bedrooms; 2-speed motor, fan operates at 970 rpm or 1,700 rpm; heat exchange surface is 160 sq. ft.; core encased in painted, galvanized sheet metal case with drain system; eliminates ventilating fans in bathrooms
Available from:
American ALDES Ventilation Corp.
Northgate Center Business Park
4537 Northgate Ct. (APD)
Sarasota, FL 34234-2124
800-255-7749
In FL 813-351-3441
Fax 813-351-3442

Berner AQ Plus+™

Filters gases, dust, and pollen; pollen/dust efficiency 90% to 5 micron, 60% to 1.5 micron; balances humidity; installs with 6" diameter air duct, household current; CFM up to 165; 27-1/2"x11"x17"; 55 lbs.; Berner Air Products, Inc. no longer manufactures AQ Plus+; however replacement filters are still available
Available from:
Allergy Relief Shop™, Inc.
3371 Whittle Springs Rd. (APD)
Knoxville, TN 37917
Orders 800-626-2810
Questions 615-522-2795

E-Z-AIRE® Light Commercial Models Series 70

Counterflow air-to-air plate type heat exchanger; deals with radon, formaldehyde, gas, particulate pollutants, ozone, cigarette smoke, and humidity; self-contained; air flow ranges 600-4000 CFM; 70% effectiveness; weight ranges 390 to 1,900 lbs.
Available from:
Des Champs Laboratories, Inc.
66 Okner Pkwy. (APD)
Livingston, NJ 07039
201-535-8300
Fax 201-535-0537

Controlling Your Environment
Fighting Mold and Mildew

E-Z-AIRE® Light Commercial Models Series 85

Counterflow air-to-air plate type heat exchanger; deals with radon, formaldehyde, gas, particulate pollutants, ozone, cigarette smoke, and humidity; self-contained; air flow ranges 600-4000 CFM; 85% effectiveness; weight ranges 510 to 2,200 lbs.
Available from:
Des Champs Laboratories, Inc.
66 Okner Pkwy. (APD)
Livingston, NJ 07039
201-535-8300
Fax 201-535-0537

E-Z-Vent® EZV-II

Rated air flow 240; ventilation system for radon pollutants, odors, and humidity; condensate rain; dual, variable-speed motor controls; under 80 lbs.
Available from:
Des Champs Laboratories, Inc.
66 Okner Pkwy. (APD)
Livingston, NJ 07039
201-535-8300
Fax 201-535-0537

E-Z-Vent® Series 300

Air-to-air plate type heat exchanger (heat recovery ventilator) for pollutants, odors, and high humidity; 2-speed blowers; two washable filters; insulated heat exchanger; optional remote switch, humidistat, time control. EZV-310: rated air flow 110-145; 115 lbs. EZV-320: rated air flow 165-220; 115 lbs. EZV-340: rated air flow 310-415; 150 lbs.
Available from:
Des Champs Laboratories, Inc.
66 Okner Pkwy. (APD)
Livingston, NJ 07039
201-535-8300
Fax 201-535-0537

ERV 3615

Moisture transferred in vapor phase, eliminating wet surfaces, condensate drain, bacterial growth; winter humidification requirements reduced; downflow or horizontal flow; rooftop or pad mount; 500 to 1,500 CFM for commercial, industrial, institutional applications
Available from:
Airxchange, Inc.
401 V.F.W. Dr. (APD)
Rockland, MA 02370
617-871-4816
Fax 617-871-3029

ERV 400/500

Moisture transferred in vapor phase, eliminating wet surfaces, condensate drain, bacterial growth; winter humidification requirements reduced; wall or ceiling mount; 150 to 500 CFM; small commercial use; provides 15 CFM/person for 33 occupants
Available from:
Airxchange, Inc.
401 V.F.W. Dr. (APD)
Rockland, MA 02370
617-871-4816
Fax 617-871-3029

ERV 5230 Series

Moisture transferred in vapor phase, eliminating wet surfaces, condensate drain, bacterial growth; winter humidification requirements reduced; downflow or horizontal flow; rooftop or pad mount; 1,500 to 3,000 CFM for commercial, industrial, institutional applications
Available from:
Airxchange, Inc.
401 V.F.W. Dr. (APD)
Rockland, MA 02370
617-871-4816
Fax 617-871-3029

Controlling Your Environment

Fighting Mold and Mildew

EZV-AIRE®

Various models with rated air flows of 600-4000; weights vary 390-2200 lbs.
Available from:
Des Champs Laboratories, Inc.
66 Okner Pkwy. (APD)
Livingston, NJ 07039
201-535-8300
Fax 201-535-0537

Filter-Vent™

Fresh air ventilator pulls air through standard media, extended surface filter 90 to 95% efficient (ASHRAE 52-76 Dust spot test); carbon filter with non-woven polyester base; optional media filter of pleated glass fiber paper; seven-day timer with 2-hour intervals; floor or hanging joist installation; standard outlet
Available from:
Therma-Stor Products
Div. of DEC Int'l., Inc.
1919 S. Stoughton Rd. (APD)
PO Box 8050 (APD)
Madison, WI 53708
800-533-7533
608-222-5301
Fax 608-222-1447

Honeywell Energy Recovery Ventilator ER100 Series

Mount in basement utility room, closet or suspend from outside wall or ceiling; dehumidistat, variable speed ventilation rate, 2 fan speeds; line voltage fresh air control; ER100-A1001 capacity of 70 to 185 cu. ft./min., handles .3 air changes per hour in 4,500 sq. ft., 80% efficiency; ER100-A1019 (available in Canada only) capacity of 70 to 130 cu. ft./min., handles .3 air changes per hour in 3,000 sq. ft., 80% efficiency, frost control; ER100-A1027 capacity of 70 to 185 cu. ft./min., handles .3 air changes per hour in 4,500 sq. ft., 80% efficiency, frost control; ER100-A1035 (available in U.S. only) capacity of 70 to 185 cu. ft./min., handles .3 air changes per hour in 4,500 sq. ft., 80% efficiency, frost control
Available locally in various department and home center stores and
Available from:
Honeywell, Inc.
Home and Building Control
Honeywell Plaza
PO Box 524 (APD)
Minneapolis, MN 55440-0524
612-951-1000
and
Honeywell, Inc.
740 Ellesmere Rd. (APD)
Scarborough, ON, M1P 2V9
Canada

Honeywell Energy Recovery Ventilator ER200 Series

Mount in basement utility room, closet or suspend from outside wall or ceiling; dehumidistat, variable speed ventilation rate, 2 fan speeds; line voltage fresh air control; ER200-A1000 capacity of 80 to 250 cu. ft./min., handles .3 air changes per hour in 6,200 sq. ft., 85% efficiency, no frost control; ER200-A1018 capacity of 80 to 250 cu. ft./min., handles .3 air changes per hour in 6,200 sq. ft., 85% efficiency, frost control
Available locally in various department and home center stores and
Available from:
Honeywell, Inc.
Home and Building Control
Honeywell Plaza
PO Box 524 (APD)
Minneapolis, MN 55440-0524
612-951-1000
and
Honeywell, Inc.
740 Ellesmere Rd. (APD)
Scarborough, ON, M1P 2V9
Canada

Controlling Your Environment

Fighting Mold and Mildew

Honeywell Energy Recovery Ventilator ER90 Series

Mount in basement utility room, closet or suspend from outside wall or ceiling; optional dehumidistat, variable speed ventilation rate, 2 fan speeds; line voltage fresh air control; ER90-A1004 and A1012 (available in Canada only) capacity of 70 to 185 cu. ft./min., handles .3 air changes per hour in 4,500 sq. ft., 77% efficiency; A1020 has frost control
Available locally in various department and home center stores and
Available from:
Honeywell, Inc.
Home and Building Control
Honeywell Plaza
PO Box 524 (APD)
Minneapolis, MN 55440-0524
612-951-1000
and
Honeywell, Inc.
740 Ellesmere Rd. (APD)
Scarborough, ON, M1P 2V9
Canada

LIFEBREATH™ 100 DEF

Heat exchange core of thermally efficient aluminum has cleanable air filter in exhaust and fresh air streams; optional remote dehumidistat; 2 fans, 2 motors; 5 position speed control; 82% maximum temperature recovery; damper defrost; Model 100ND as above without defrost
Available from:
Therma-Stor Products
Div. of DEC Int'l., Inc.
1919 S. Stoughton Rd. (APD)
PO Box 8050 (APD)
Madison, WI 53708
800-533-7533
608-222-5301
Fax 608-222-1447

LIFEBREATH™ 150 MAX

Heat exchange core of thermally efficient aluminum has cleanable air filter in exhaust and fresh air streams;

optional remote dehumidistat; built-in humidistat; 5 position speed control; 80% maximum temperature recovery; damper defrost
Available from:
Therma-Stor Products
Div. of DEC Int'l., Inc.
1919 S. Stoughton Rd. (APD)
PO Box 8050 (APD)
Madison, WI 53708
800-533-7533
608-222-5301
Fax 608-222-1447

LIFEBREATH™ 150 SP

Heat exchange core of thermally efficient aluminum has cleanable air filter in exhaust and fresh air streams; optional remote dehumidistat; 3 position speed control; 80% maximum temperature recovery; electric defrost
Available from:
Therma-Stor Products
Div. of DEC Int'l., Inc.
1919 S. Stoughton Rd. (APD)
PO Box 8050 (APD)
Madison, WI 53708
800-533-7533
608-222-5301
Fax 608-222-1447

LIFEBREATH™ 195 DCS

Heat exchange core of thermally efficient aluminum has cleanable air filter in exhaust and fresh air streams; optional remote dehumidistat; built-in humidistat; 5 position speed control; 94% maximum temperature recovery; damper defrost
Available from:
Therma-Stor Products
Div. of DEC Int'l., Inc.
1919 S. Stoughton Rd. (APD)
PO Box 8050 (APD)
Madison, WI 53708
800-533-7533
608-222-5301
Fax 608-222-1447

Controlling Your Environment

Fighting Mold and Mildew

LIFEBREATH™ 200 MAX

Heat exchange core of thermally efficient aluminum has cleanable air filter in exhaust and fresh air streams; optional remote dehumidistat; built-in humidistat; 5 position speed control; 80% maximum temperature recovery; damper defrost
Available from:
Therma-Stor Products
Div. of DEC Int'l., Inc.
1919 S. Stoughton Rd. (APD)
PO Box 8050 (APD)
Madison, WI 53708
800-533-7533
608-222-5301
Fax 608-222-1447

LIFEBREATH™ 200 STD

Heat exchange core of thermally efficient aluminum has cleanable air filter in exhaust and fresh air streams; optional remote dehumidistat; built-in humidistat; 3 position speed control; 80% maximum temperature recovery; electric preheat defrost
Available from:
Therma-Stor Products
Div. of DEC Int'l., Inc.
1919 S. Stoughton Rd. (APD)
PO Box 8050 (APD)
Madison, WI 53708
800-533-7533
608-222-5301
Fax 608-222-1447

LIFEBREATH™ 300 DCS

Heat exchange dual core of thermally efficient aluminum has cleanable air filter in exhaust and fresh air streams; optional remote dehumidistat; built-in humidistat; 5 position speed control; 94% maximum temperature recovery; damper defrost
Available from:
Therma-Stor Products
Div. of DEC Int'l., Inc.
1919 S. Stoughton Rd. (APD)
PO Box 8050 (APD)
Madison, WI 53708

800-533-7533
608-222-5301
Fax 608-222-1447

LIFEBREATH™ Commercial Models

Models 700, 1200, 1000; heat exchange core of thermally efficient aluminum has cleanable air filter in exhaust and fresh air streams
Available from:
Therma-Stor Products
Div. of DEC Int'l., Inc.
1919 S. Stoughton Rd. (APD)
PO Box 8050 (APD)
Madison, WI 53708
800-533-7533
608-222-5301
Fax 608-222-1447

QDT SAE 150

Modular thermal recovery unit; built-in condensation; positive seal between exhaust and fresh air flows; automatic defrost cycle; 2-speed fans; casing is 24-gauge galvenized steel; heat recovery module is aluminum and alloys; air-flow partition is galvenized steel; exterior coating is industrial enamal; internally insulated; 94 lbs.
Available from:
QDT, Ltd.
1000 Singleton Blvd.
Dallas, TX 75212-5214
214-741-1993
Fax 214-747-3614

Quiet-Vent®

Programmable, central exhaust ventilation system; lowers humidity; 2-speed motor; remote control; cleanable filter
Available from:
Therma-Stor Products
Div. of DEC Int'l., Inc.
1919 S. Stoughton Rd. (APD)
PO Box 8050 (APD)
Madison, WI 53708
800-533-7533
608-222-5301

Controlling Your Environment
Fighting Mold and Mildew

Fax 608-222-1447

RTU 1000 Series

Moisture transferred in vapor phase, eliminating wet surfaces, condensate drain, bacterial growth; winter humidification requirements reduced; rooftop ventilator supplies 500 to 1000 CFM; 15 CFM/person for 66 occupants
Available from:
Airxchange, Inc.
401 V.F.W. Dr. (APD)
Rockland, MA 02370
617-871-4816
Fax 617-871-3029

DEHUMIDIFIERS

Dri-Out

Moisture absorbing flakes remove water from the air; reservoir holds 1/2 gal. of water; closets or small enclosed areas up to 1,000 cu. ft.
Available from:
Allergy Control Products, Inc.
96 Danbury Rd. (APD)
PO Box 793 (APD)
Ridgefield, CT 06877
800-422-DUST (3878)
203-438-9580
Fax 203-431-8963
and:
Allergy Relief Products
9 Renata Ct. (APD)
Dundas, ON L9H 6X1
Canada
905-628-5324 ?416
Fax 416-628-1734
and:
Improvements (TM0
4944 Commerce Pkwy. (APD)
Cleveland, OH 44128
800-642-2112
Fax 216-464-6764
and:
Lillian Vernon Corp.
(APD)
Virginia Beach, VA 23479-0002

800-285-5555
Fax 804-430-1500
TDD/ITTY

Electric Dehumidifier

Plugs into household current, warms air from floor level; warm air rises and cooler air is forced down to be warmed; steel with baked enamel finish; no moving parts, continuous operation; small size for boats, small closets, engine compartments, storage closets; larger size for areas up to 1,000 cu. ft.
Available from:
Herrington
3 Symmes Dr. (APD)
Londonderry, NH 03053
800-622-5221
In NH 603-437-4939
603-437-4638
and:
Home Trends
1450 Lyell Ave. (APD)
Rochester, NY 14606-2184
716-254-6520
Fax 716-458-9245
and:
Solutions®
PO Box 6878 (APD)
Portland, OR 97228
800-342-9988
Fax 503-643-1973
and:
Sporty's® Preferred Living
Clermont County Airport (APD)
Batavia, OH 45103-9747
800-543-8633
Fax 513-732-6560

Electric Mildew Fighter

Plugs into household current; warms air from floor level; warm air rises and cooler air is forced down to be warmed; no moving parts, continuous operation; steel, baked enamel finish; Model 500 for boats, small closets, engine compartments, storage closets; Model 1000 for areas up to 1,000 cu. ft. (Model 1000 only

Controlling Your Environment

Fighting Mold and Mildew

available from Allergy Asthma
Technology)
Available from:
Allergy Asthma Technology
4151 N. Kedzie (APD)
PO Box 18398 (APD)
Chicago, IL 60618
800-621-5545
312-465-8020
Fax 312-465-7619
and:
Herrington
3 Symmes Dr. (APD)
Londonderry, NH 03053
800-622-5221
In NH 603-437-4939
603-437-4638
and:
Home Trends
1450 Lyell Ave. (APD)
Rochester, NY 14606-2184
716-254-6520
Fax 716-458-9245
and:
Sporty's® Preferred Living
Clermont County Airport (APD)
Batavia, OH 45103-9747
800-543-8633
Fax 513-732-6560

HI-E Dry 100

Removes 7 pints of water per
kilowatt hour; at 90 o F. and 90%
humidity, removes 178 pints per day;
commercial capacity
Available from:
Therma-Stor Products
Div. of DEC Int'l., Inc.
1919 S. Stoughton Rd. (APD)
PO Box 8050 (APD)
Madison, WI 53708
800-533-7533
608-222-5301
Fax 608-222-1447

HI-E Dry 200

Removes over 200 lbs. of water per
day; standard outlet; at 90 o F. and
90% humidity, removes 297 pints per
day; commercial capacity

Available from:
Therma-Stor Products
Div. of DEC Int'l., Inc.
1919 S. Stoughton Rd. (APD)
PO Box 8050 (APD)
Madison, WI 53708
800-533-7533
608-222-5301
Fax 608-222-1447

Hydrosorbent

Container of silica gel
hydrosorbent to absorb excess
moisture in camera cases, display
cases, silver drawrs, tool boxes;
reusable, color change indicator for
reactivation
Available from:
Improvements (TM0
4944 Commerce Pkwy. (APD)
Cleveland, OH 44128
800-642-2112
Fax 216-464-6764

Quiet Dry™

Constant drain hook-up or
automatic turn-off when full;
adjustable humidistat; for bedroom or
basement; 57 lbs.
Available from:
Allergy Control Products, Inc.
96 Danbury Rd. (APD)
PO Box 793 (APD)
Ridgefield, CT 06877
800-422-DUST (3878)
203-438-9580
Fax 203-431-8963

Sahara Ultra Efficient

Uses refrigerant to cool incoming
air to remove moixture; dehumidifer
setting from 20 to 80%; blower switch;
removes 85 to 104 lbs. or 100 pints of
water per 24 hours; standard outlet; 6-
foot drain hose; 110 lbs., portable
Attaches to existing forced air
system with filter for mold, mildew,
and mite control
Available from:
Therma-Stor Products

Div. of DEC Int'l., Inc.
1919 S. Stoughton Rd. (APD)
PO Box 8050 (APD)
Madison, WI 53708
800-533-7533
608-222-5301
Fax 608-222-1447

WATERPROOFING PAINTS

Penetrating Water Seal

Odor-free; reduces water absorption; helps control efflorescence; for porous bricks, some pavers, concrete, raw wood
Available from:
AFM Enterprises, Inc.
1960 Chicago E7 (APD)
Riverside, CA 92507
909-781-6860
909-781-6861
Fax 909-781-6892
and:
Allergy Relief Shop™, Inc.
3371 Whittle Springs Rd. (APD)
Knoxville, TN 37917
Orders 800-626-2810
Questions 615-522-2795
and:
Allergy Resources
Mail: PO Box 888 (APD)
UPS: 264 Brookridge Ave. (APD)
Palmer Lake, CO 80133
Orders 800-USE-FLAX (873-3529)
Company plans to move; use 800 #
and:
Flowright Int'l Products
1495 N.W. Gilman Blvd. #4 (APD)
Issaquah, WA 98027
206-392-8357
and:
N.E.E.D.S.
527 Charles Ave. 12A (APD)
Syracuse, NY 13209
800-634-1380
Fax 800-295-NEED (6333)

Paver Seal .003

Seals porous tile, conrete, and grout; helps control efflorescence
Available from:
AFM Enterprises, Inc.
1960 Chicago E7 (APD)
Riverside, CA 92507
909-781-6860
909-781-6861
Fax 909-781-6892
and:
Allergy Relief Shop™, Inc.
3371 Whittle Springs Rd. (APD)
Knoxville, TN 37917
Orders 800-626-2810
Questions 615-522-2795
and:
N.E.E.D.S.
527 Charles Ave. 12A (APD)
Syracuse, NY 13209
800-634-1380
Fax 800-295-NEED (6333)

Water Base Mexe Seal

Protects pavers from stain; applies to saltillo pavers, adobe, adoquin, grout, granite, concrete quarry tile, fired and unfired porcelain
Available from:
AFM Enterprises, Inc.
1960 Chicago E7 (APD)
Riverside, CA 92507
909-781-6860
909-781-6861
Fax 909-781-6892
and:
Allergy Relief Shop™, Inc.
3371 Whittle Springs Rd. (APD)
Knoxville, TN 37917
Orders 800-626-2810
Questions 615-522-2795
and:
N.E.E.D.S.
527 Charles Ave. 12A (APD)
Syracuse, NY 13209
800-634-1380
Fax 800-295-NEED (6333)

Controlling Your Environment
Fighting Mold and Mildew

Water Seal

Seals grout, tile, and concrete; coats porous surfaces, bare wood, painted surfaces, drywall, paneling, cabinets
Available from:
AFM Enterprises, Inc.
1960 Chicago E7 (APD)
Riverside, CA 92507
909-781-6860
909-781-6861
Fax 909-781-6892
and:
Allergy Relief Shop™, Inc.
3371 Whittle Springs Rd. (APD)
Knoxville, TN 37917
Orders 800-626-2810
Questions 615-522-2795
and:
Flowright Int'l Products
1495 N.W. Gilman Blvd. #4 (APD)
Issaquah, WA 98027
206-392-8357
and:
N.E.E.D.S.
527 Charles Ave. 12A (APD)
Syracuse, NY 13209
800-634-1380
Fax 800-295-NEED (6333)

Dyno Seal

A liquid copolymer for use as a sealer and waterproof membrane; can be used below grade, under shower stalls and tubs, to repair or coat roofs; adheres to concrete, block, metal, wood, or asphalt shingles
Available from:
AFM Enterprises, Inc.
1960 Chicago E7 (APD)
Riverside, CA 92507
909-781-6860
909-781-6861
Fax 909-781-6892
and:
Allergy Relief Shop ™, Inc.
3371 Whittle Springs Rd. (APD)
Knoxville, TN 37917
Orders 800-626-2810
Questions 615-522-2795
and:
Flowright Int'l Products
1495 N.W. Gilman Blvd. #4 (APD)
Issaquah, WA 98027
206-392-8357
and:
N.E.E.D.S.
527 Charles Ave. 12A (APD)
Syracuse, NY 13209
800-634-1380
Fax 800-295-NEED (6333)

ENVIRONMENTAL IRRITANTS

No matter how a product is formulated, there is the potential that someone can react to it. All a manufacturer can do is try to remove as many known irritants as possible.

Remember, even products marked unscented probably have scents known as masking scents.

The importance of any single source of pollution depends on how much pollutant it emits and how hazardous that emission is. It is important to maintain and adjust equipment properly to control emissions and use it in a well-ventilated area.

HOUSEHOLD IRRITANTS

Some sources like building materials, furnishings, and household products like air fresheners release pollutants just about all the time.

Other sources related pollutants intermittently: smoking, poorly vented or malfunctioning stoves, furnaces, or space heaters; using solvents while cleaning or hobby activities, paint strippers when redecorating; use of cleaning products. Sometimes pollutant concentrations can remain in the home for long periods after these activities.

Homes need to "leak" or allow an exchange of stale, indoor air with fresh outdor air.

Homes need to "leak" or allow an exchange of stale, indoor air with fresh, outdoor air. The more airtight homes are (and newer ones are very airtight) the more you need to depend on ventilation systems to keep pollutant levels down.

Many substances in the environment can cause problems for sensitive individuals. Most of these are proteins, which can sensitize such as house dust mite, cockroach, and mold. Chemicals, like cleaning agents and bug killers, are usually irritants, but they can also be allergens.

Controlling Your Environment

Environmental Irritants

APARTMENTS AND OFFICE BUILDINGS

Apartments and office buildings have indoor air problems similar to homes because of furnishings, equipment, building materials, and cleaning products.

They have other problems caused by emissions from copiers and laser printers and ventilation controls designed to cut down on expenses. Newer buildings are very airtight and most do not allow for window opening. Facilities are cleaned nightly with strong products are used. During the day, multiple pollutant sources are at work.

Solutions here require eliminating or controlling sources of pollution, increasing ventilation, installing air cleaning devices.

THREE BASICS FOR CONTROLLING IRRITANTS AND ALLERGENS

Medication is not always helpful because as exposure continues, your sensitivity may increase and you may require more and more medication or your medication may stop working. So, the question becomes, what *can* you do?

1. CONTROL THE SOURCE

If you can eliminate a source of pollution or reduce its emissions, you've made an effective change in pollution level. Controlling the source of the pollution is the most effective solution.

Sources that contain asbestos can be sealed or enclosed; gas stoves can be adjusted; appliances can be vented outside. Generally, good maintenance can solve many problems.

Activities like painting, kerosene heating, cooking, welding, and soldering temporarily cause a higher pollution level. You should prepare for these by increasing ventilation in the area or by working outdoors if possible.

2. IMPROVE VENTILATION

Most home heating and air conditioning systems do not bring fresh air into the house. Newer homes are very airtight, only allowing low levels of fresh air exchange. Air-to-air heat exchangers are energy-efficient heat recovery ventilators that bring outdoor air into the home after warming it with outgoing, warm house air.

If you can, open a window or door or use a window or attic fan. Air conditioners can help as well. When using lavatory or kitchen facilities, use the fan.

3. USE AIR CLEANERS

Air cleaners, discussed in-depth in, *Controlling Your Environment: Improving Air Quality in Your Home*, are generally not effective in removing gaseous pollutants. They can be very effective particle removers, but how long they remain effective depends on how well you maintain them. Follow manufacturers instructions for maintenance and replacement.

WHAT ARE THE SOURCES OF IRRITANTS?

The following sources discuss various pollutants found in homes that can effect your health. Information indicating at what levels of pollution health effects will occur is limited. Most of us live in our homes without apparent problems. However, for those with sensitivities or other health problems, pollutant tolerance levels are lower.

SMOKING

Environmental tobacco smoke is considered a major indoor contaminant. The problem lies in the smoke rising from the burning end of a cigarette, pipe, or cigar and from exhaled smoke. More than 40 of the compounds in exhaled smoke are known to cause cancer and other compounds are strong irritants.

This environmental tobacco smoke is also called secondhand smoke and exposure to it is called passive smoking.

WHAT CAN YOU DO?

Do not allow smoking in your home. Avoid whenever possible being in enclosed environments with smokers. Be sure that your children are not exposed to environmental smoke in day care, baby sitting, play, or extra-curricular activities. See the chapter on *Smoking* for a more comprehensive discussion of this problem.

Controlling Your Environment

Environmental Irritants

ALLERGIC AND BIOLOGICAL CONTAMINANTS

These contaminants are the molds, mildew, animal dander, and saliva proteins, house dust mites, pollen, and cockroaches that swirl through your home environment.

Sources are plants, people, animals, soil, plant debris, pets, mice, central air handling systems, and humidifiers.

Some biological contaminants cause allergic reactions such as hypersensitivity pneumonitis, allergic rhinitis, and some types of asthma. Symptoms of these contaminants are sneezing, watery eyes, coughing, shortness of breath, dizziness, lethargy, and fever.

WHAT CAN YOU DO?

If you can control the relative humidity level in your home, you can somewhat control the growth of some of these contaminants.

Air cleaners, air conditioners, and air filters are of help. The chapter on *Controlling Your Environment: Your Home Environment* gives specific steps you can take to lower the contaminant levels of your home.

Exhaust fans vented outdoors in your kitchen and bathroom eliminate the moisture that supports mold, mildew, and bacteria.

Try for a 30 to 50 percent relative humidity level. If you use a humidifier, keep it scrupulously clean to prevent bacteria and mold growth. Also, clean evaporation trays in air conditioners, dehumidifiers and refrigerators frequently.

Install and use exhaust fans vented outdoors in your kitchen and bathroom, and vent clothes dryers outdoors. There are two benefits to this. First, these fans and vents eliminate the moisture that supports mold, mildew, and bacterial growth. Second, these fans can reduce the levels of organic pollutants that vaporize from hot water.

Hotel non-smoking rooms may still allow pets.

Normal hotel cleaning does not clear a room of pet dander.

Ventilate attic and crawl spaces. If there is a leak or spill on a carpet, clean and dry (with fans, if necessary) the carpeting and underlying pad as quickly as possible to prevent mold growth.

Eliminating animals from your home further decreases contaminant levels

Controlling Your Environment
Environmental Irritants

Hotel chains have varying policies on pets in their rooms. You may have a non-smoking room and yet be in a room that allows pets. Check with the hotel before making a reservation. Dander is a difficult substance to clear from a room, and normal hotel cleaning, no matter how thorough, cannot clear a room of pet dander.

IRRITANTS THAT INCITE OR AGGRAVATE ASTHMA

If you have asthma, your lungs are very reactive. Some inhalants may irritate you and cause bronchoconstriction and ongoing airway inflammation. Fumes, from perfumes, cosmetics, (or flowers) may cause problems.

These inhalant particles are extremely small and are less likely to be cleared from a room using a mechanical air purifier. Irritants like perfume, spray deodorant hair spray, air fresheners, cosmetics can cause allergic reactions, non-allergic reactions, or irritation.

WHAT CAN YOU DO?

Electrostatic precipitators and HEPA filters (ozone-free) can generally handle these particles that are smaller than pollen and are unlikely to be cleared from a room using a mechanical air purifier.

Try to eliminate the source of the irritant. Do not use perfumes and personal care items that cause you to react.

A SAMPLING OF PROBLEMS IN THE WORK PLACE

PAPAIN

an enzyme used in brewing beer and in formulating meat tenderizers, can cause immediate asthmatic symptoms

ANIMAL DANDERS

are a problem for veterinarians and lab workers, farmers, jockeys, and others who work around animals. Animal saliva and urine are also problems.

PROTEIN SECRETIONS

from birds have caused asthma and other problems for bird breeders.

FOOD

contaminants like insects or mold and even an allergy to wheat flour can cause asthma. People working as food

Controlling Your Environment

Environmental Irritants

processors have developed sensitivity to green coffee beans, tea, garlic, and soybeans.

CASTOR BEANS

in fertilizer can cause asthma in workers and also in those living in the area.

SAWDUSTS

can cause asthma in workers.

TEXTILES

like cotton, hemp, and flax can cause asthma.

ANTIBIOTICS

can cause asthma in industry workers.

PLATINUM AND NICKEL

can sensitize workers and welders.

FORMALDEHYDE

is an irritant that can cause various problems both in those working in manufacturing and in those using the finished products.

POLYVINYL CHLORIDE

is the film that wraps meat and some individuals react when the film is heated for wrapping.

MOLDY HAY

can cause farmer's lung.

MALT WORKER'S DISEASE

from fungus spores.

WOOD-PULP WORKER'S DISEASE

from moldy logs.

According to Dr. Leslie Grammer, management consists of controlling exposure: changing jobs or retraining, moving from the area, ventilating efficiently, extracting dust and vapor efficiently.

Even if exposure levels are below legal limits, immunologic reactions may still occur.

Even if exposure levels are below legal limits, immunologic reactions may still occur. The goal should be prevention by improving ventilation and appropriate equipment, being aware of threshold limits, and education.

Controlling Your Environment
Environmental Irritants

STOVES, FIREPLACES, HEATERS

Combustion products are produced indoors by unvented gas space heaters, gas ranges, ovens, furnaces, gas water heaters, gas clothes dryers, charcoal grills, wood, gas, or coal-burning stoves, and fireplaces, improperly installed or maintained chimneys and flues, and from cracks in heat exchangers.

How much pollutant is released depends on the type of appliance, the fuel it uses, its installation, maintenance, and ventilation. Are vents and chimneys inspected?

Combustion releases water vapor that can cause high humidity, encouraging house dust mites, molds, and bacteria.

The combustion pollutants are particles or gases that result from burning fuels like gas, kerosene, wood, or coal in various appliances. These products of combustion are carbon monoxide, nitrogen dioxide, particles, sulfur dioxide, unburned hydrocarbons, and aldehydes.

These gases can cause discomfort or illness even if you are healthy. Effects can range from headache and breathing difficulties to death from the carbon monoxide of faulty heaters. Effects may be immediate or become apparent after long exposure. Effects depend on age and health.

If you have asthma or respiratory disease, this type of exposure is particularly damaging. Further, combustion also releases water vapor that can cause high humidity, encouraging house dust mites, molds, and bacteria.

WHAT CAN YOU DO?

VENT OUTDOORS

Appliances should be vented outdoors to prevent the noxious by-products of combustion from flowing throughout your living and working areas. Be sure all pilot lights burn blue, a sign of cleaner, complete combustion; a yellow flame indicates a need for adjustment.

BUY SAFE HEATERS AND APPLIANCES

Oil heaters should have a UL label. Gas appliances should have an AGA or UL label.

IMPROVE INDOOR VENTILATION

If you must use unvented kerosene or gas space heaters, follow instructions very carefully. Be sure all pilot lights burn blue. Keep a safety screen around any appliances

Controlling Your Environment

Environmental Irritants

with an open flame. Keep the door opened and open a window.

USE FUEL APPROPRIATELY

Use only the correct fuel for each appliance. Never try to increase a fire with kerosene or gasoline. When you must refill an oil or kerosene unit, don't overfill it. The oil expands as it warms and can flood the burner. Do not fill the heater while it is burning. Store fuels outside of the house in the correct containers.

INSTALL HOODS

Install stove hoods with fans vented outdoors. If you can't install a hood in your kitchen, use an exhaust fan. Do not use a gas stove for heat. If you are purchasing a new gas stove, consider one with a pilotless ignition, called an electronic ignition.

USE WOODSTOVES SAFELY

Your woodstove should be air tight and meet EPA emission standards. Use aged wood and follow manufacturer's instructions. Look for asbestos-free replacement gaskets made of fiberglass. Inspect chimneys and keep them clean.

KEEP CENTRAL AIR SYSTEM IN REPAIR

Have a professional inspect your central air handling systems and repair any damage. Check to see that your gas heater has a safety shut-off.

For more information, call your local American Lung Association in the white pages of the phone book.

HOUSEHOLD PRODUCTS

Remember that we use many chemicals on a daily basis: cleaning, disinfecting, cosmetic, and hobby products. For safety reasons, store these items in well ventilated areas out of the reach of children and, preferably, in locked cabinets.

WHAT CAN YOU DO?

Work in well-ventilated areas, or open a door and windows, or work outdoors. Safely dispose of old containers, unneeded containers, or containers that are almost empty. Buy only quantities that you need for the project at hand. Read and follow all health hazard information and precautions. Dress in work clothes that

Controlling Your Environment
Environmental Irritants

can be removed when the job is done. Wear an appropriate mask.

Professional dry cleaners use perchloroethylene which can be inhaled from clothing that has been dry cleaned. Do not accept clothing with a strong smell. It should have been properly dried by the cleaner. Request that this be done.

FORMALDEHYDE

Formaldehyde is used in building materials and household products. It is also a by-product of combustion from unvented gas stoves or kerosene space heaters.

Formaldehyde is used in permanent press clothing and drapes, in glues and adhesives and in some paints. If your home has furniture or cabinets made from pressed wood that use urea-formaldehyde adhesives, those products will

---

Formaldehyde is used in building materials and household products.

It is also a by-product of combustion from unvented gas stoves or kerosene space heaters.

---

emit formaldehyde. These products are: particleboard (subflooring and shelving), hardwood plywood paneling, fiberboard (drawer fronts, cabinets, furniture tops). Other sources of formaldehyde are: carpeting, paper goods, household cleaners, and water repellents.

In the 1970's, urea-formaldehyde foam insulation was installed in many homes as added insulation, resulting in high indoor concentrations of formaldehyde. This problem was reported on and followed by American Allergy Association since many symptom complaints had been received.

In March, 1980, the National Academy of Sciences concluded that formaldehyde did pose a serious health problem "even at extremely low airborne concentrations"

Formaldehyde vaporizes at low temperatures. Off-gassing releases vapors that can cause a variety of symptoms. In March, 1980, the National Academy of Sciences concluded that formaldehyde did pose a serious health problem: "even at extremely low airborne concnentrations" it will irritate the eyes, nose, and throat of some individuals. The quantity of formaldehyde emission decreases with age of product, lower temperatures, and humidity.

Controlling Your Environment

Environmental Irritants

Since 1985, the Department of Housing and Urban Development (HUD) has restricted plywood and particle board for mobile homes only to those materials that conform to specific formaldehyde emission limits.

WHAT CAN YOU DO?

Ask about formaldehyde content of pressed wood products, building materials, and furniture before buying. There is a possibility that coating pressed wood products with polyurethane may reduce emissions for some length of time, but every surface area, including edges must be covered. You may also want to investigate the possibility of covering the cabinets with Formica®. Try to keep heat and humidity levels down.

INDOOR PLANTS

Not all sources of pollution are chemical or high-tech. Indoor plants in home or office are a source of mold. Large plants with large leaves can become dust collectors. Their leaves need regular cleaning. If you have enough plants, misting them will raise humidity levels somewhat and watering them will cause carpet damage and mold from water spills.

WHAT CAN YOU DO?

Don't over-water houseplants because you will encourage mold and microorganism growth on the soil. If you are sensitive to mold, don't have house plants, especially in your bedroom. Mold can even grow on the sides of the pots.

The notion that houseplants can help improve air quality because of their oxygen output is subject to disussion. We've heard said that it would take a greenhouse worth of plants to supply sufficient oxygen – but then we'd have a greenhouse worth of mold and very high humidity levels to pamper house dust mites.

PESTICIDES

We use pesticides at home to kill insects, termites, and as disinfectants. We also use them on the lawn and garden. These products are sold as sprays, powders, crystals, liquids, balls, and foggers. It is easy to track these around

Controlling Your Environment
Environmental Irritants

the house and children are major victims of pesticide poisonings.

Symptoms are irritation to your eyes, nose and throat. Higher exposures to certain insecticides have caused various symptoms: headache and nausea.

> EPA has concern that exposure to cyclodienes might cause long-term liver damage and central nervous system damage. For these reasons, cyclodienes are not permitted to be sold any longer; neither are chlordane, aldrin, dieldrin, and heptachlor. If you have any products so labeled, dispose of them immediately and safely.

WHAT CAN YOU DO?

When you garden, try wearing clothes and shoes that you use only for gardening. When you finish, take your shoes off and put them away somewhere outside the main house. Take your clothes and socks off immediately to be washed so that pesticide residues are not brought indoors.

Follow manufacturer's instructions. If you must dilute a product, do it outdoors. Apply it according to directions and don't over use. If you must use products like these indoors, open doors and windows. If you must spray house plants or pets, do so outdoors.

Do not buy more than you need.

It is better to use and then dispose of these products safely, according to their directions.

Do not store these products in your home. Do not store them within reach of children. Keep these products in locked, ventilated cabinets. Do not buy more than you need. It is better to use and then dispose of these products safely, according to their directions.

National Pesticides Telecommunications Network, 800-858-PEST (7378), in Texas, 806-743-3091, 8:00 am to 6 pm central time, provides information about pesticides and pesticide exposure to the public and to physicians.

ASBESTOS

Asbestos becomes a problem when it begins to deteriorate or is damaged in some way. It is found in insulation, acoustic materials, floor tiles, and the door gaskets of wood-burning stoves. Older homes are more

Controlling Your Environment

Environmental Irritants

likely to have asbestos in furnace insulation, shingles, millboard, textured paints, and floor tiles.

Fibers in the air are inhaled and can cause cancers or scarring of the lungs years after exposure. Fibers from exposures outside the home can cling to clothing and be brought home.

WHAT CAN YOU DO?

If asbestos is not damaged or crumbling, EPA recommends that it is best to leave it alone. Don't start projects requiring any abrasion of asbestos. Such projects will release fibers into the air. Only qualified contractors should be used to remove asbestos or to handle it in any way.

EPA has an assistance line: 202-554-1404. Call it to find out if your state has a training and certification program for asbestos removal contractors.

LEAD

Lead-based paint is a common pollutant source in older home. Exposure can result in serious problelms: lethargy, kidney, nervous system, and blood cell problems, coma, and convulsions. Children effected by lead can show mental and physical developmental delays, lower IQ levels, decreased attention spans, and behavioral problems. A developing fetus can be seriously harmed.

WHAT CAN YOU DO?

Keep play areas as clean as you can. Pay special attention to window sills and ledges, cribs, banisters, any painted surface. Wash them with a solution of high phosphate, powdered, automatic dishwasher detergent and warm water. (Be sure to protect your hands.) Keep toys and stuffed animals washed. Wash children's hands before they eat, before they go to bed, and as soon as they come inside after playing outdoors.

Do not burn painted wood since the paint may be leaded.

Do not sand or scrape lead paint because you can inhale particles.

Do not burn painted wood since the paint may be leaded. Do not sand or scrape lead paint because you can inhale the particles. If any work needs to be done involving the removal or sanding of lead paint, keep away from the premises until the work is finished and the area is clean.

Controlling Your Environment
Environmental Irritants

For help in finding an agency that can test for lead, try your state's department of health or housing department. You'll need someone trained to remove lead-based paints.

Another method requiring a professional is encapsulation in which a film is sprays over the lead-

---

If you work in construction, demolition, in a radiator repair shop, or use lead in your hobby, you may be bringing it home on your hands and on your clothing.

---

painted walls. The film is cured and a finish coat put over it. This finish coat can then be painted.

If you work in construction, in demolition, in a radiator repair shop, or use lead in your hobby, you may be bringing it home on your hands and on your clothing. The best defense is to change your clothes before you go home. Wash these clothes separately.

OTHER CHEMICALS

Many chemicals can irritate the lungs and cause wheezing. Chemicals that are generally considered irritants are ammonia, chlorine, formaldehyde, hydrogen chloride, nitrous oxide, ozone, phosgene, sulphur dioxide, and toluene in dyes can also cause irritation. Strong odors like aerosol sprays, perfumes, cleansers, and room fresheners can also be problems.

At home, avoidance is the main control; containment of the odor, if possible or a high-efficiency filtration system.

ODORS

Your negative response to an odor depends on how your trigeminal nerve perceives the odor as an irritant. Most people react negatively to irritating smells like ammonia but allergic individuals may wheeze or have drippy noses or hives as a response to odors that don't bother other people. (See "The role of odors and vapors in allergic disease" by A. J. Horesh in the *Journal of Asthma Research* 4:125, 1966 for a comprehensive listing of indoor odors.)

Allergic individuals may wheeze or have drippy noses or hives as a response to odors that don't bother other people.

At home, irritants can be strong odors like perfumes, room fresheners, cleansers, deodorant sprays, and aerosol sprays. Some mattress and pillow encasings used for house

Controlling Your Environment

Environmental Irritants

dust mite control have a very strong odor. Mothballs and flakes, kerosene fumes, insecticide sprays, floor wax, newly printed newspapers, cleaners with chlorine and ammonia, brass polishers, tobacco smoke are all examples of fumes that can make allergic rhinitis or asthma worse.

While driving, be aware that fumes in heavy traffic, particularly in states or coutries without smog control devices on cars can be highly irritating. Driving in tunnels and in cities or being stuck in traffic can provoke symptoms.

At home, irritants can be strong odors like room fresheners, deodorant sprays, and aerosol sprays.

The odors of certain foods being fried can cause problems for sensitive individuals, while burning wood and kerosene used for heating produce particulates and fumes.

Do it yourselfers run into difficulties with paints, paint cleaners, paint thinners, paint removers, varnishes.

Odors are hard enough to avoid when you know about the source. When they come upon you unaware, they are more difficult to cope with. For some time now, magazines have been produced with scent strips in advertisements. Department store bills can also arrive with scent-saturated adds.

Department store bills can arrive with scent-saturated strips.

The strips either have a scratch strip or are sealed in a packet. Both the scratch strip and the packet are supposed to keep the odor controlled until either the strip is scratched or the packet is opened to release the smell.

Unfortunately, the scents are so powerful that the odor is strongly obvious as soon as the magazine or envelope arrives. Reactions to these strong odors range from stinging eyes to tearing or headache.

WHAT CAN YOU DO?

The prime source of relief is to avoid odors. Do not use perfumes and air fresheners. Avoid products with smells that irritate you and look for alternatives.

Avoidance is not always within your power. You cannot control the perfume worn by the stranger who sits beside you on a bus, but you can move. You need not prepare certain foods. You can sit in non-smoking sections. You can tell your friends not to smoke when they are with you

Controlling Your Environment

Environmental Irritants

or at your home. Smoke odor is very difficult to eradicate from drapes, carpets, and upholstered furniture.

If you can't avoid frying foods that cause problems, turn on the vents and open windows and doors. If you are not doing the frying, leave.

Products with strong smells should be safely stored outside and away from the house. If you find that your new mattress encasing has an objectionable odor, air it outside until the odor is no longer a problem.

Air out carpeting in your garage or some sheltered area before installation.

Air out carpeting in your garage or some sheltered area before installation. New furniture and any new building materials may need airing. When bringing these new items inside, be sure doors and windows are opened.

Avoid traveling during rush hour if possible. If that is unavoidable, keep your car windows closed. Use a car air conditioner that recirculates inner air. Keep your windows closed during pollen season. Try covering the car's air vents with cheese cloth when operating the air conditioner to trap some of the mold growth in the system.

Try not to exercise when air pollution levels are high. Don't exercise near heavily used roads, especially if traffic is stalled.

Problems with the strong smells that permeate a magazine or bill because of enclosed advertising scent strips are more difficult to handle because the problem comes to you. You have to pay the bill or you want to read the magazine.

Some magazines companies are able to identify a subscriber and eliminate the scent strip because their computer system is sophisticated.

(Writer's Note: The fragrance was still strong through the plastic wrap of a magazine that arrived at our home over eight months ago and left un opened as a test.)

Write to the publisher and request elimination of the strips from your magazines. Write to the department store and request that strips be eliminated from your bills or that a warning be printed on the envelope of the bill so someone else can open and respond to it. Request that packaging be used that does not allow odor to escape until opened.

Controlling Your Environment

Environmental Irritants

Some magazines companies are responsive to complaints from individual consumers because they are able to identify a particular subscriber and eliminate the scent strip from that particular magazine because of the sophistication of the computer systems they use. Others find the cost of such action extremely costly.

If there is no result in relief, state that you are canceling your subscription after many years of readership. Then say exactly why you are doing so. Write the advertiser to say that you will not buy the product and clearly state why.

If the problem is with department store bills and your request has not gotten results, you can cancel your account and clearly state why.

We urge everyone who has to contend with scent-strips to speak up. As more of us speak up, we will be heard.

CARS

Some makes of cars pull outside air in through their air conditioning systems. Although an advantage in clean air situations, these car air conditioners can be a problem when driving in heavy traffic or behind cars with particularly dirty exhausts because the air conditioning system can draw the fumes into your car.   Exhaust fumes from your car can enter your home from an attached garage.

WHAT CAN YOU DO?

If possible, try not to drive during rush hours when traffic is heavy. If unavoidable, keep the car windows closed. Select a car that recirculates car air through the conditioning system or discuss a car filter with your doctor. Also ask about mold control services through Ford and General Motors dealers.

A garage that is attached to your home should treated as part of your home. Never run the car's engine with the garage door closed or with the connecting door to your home opened.

In fact, be safe. Don't run the car inside the garage at all. If you must make repairs, pull the car outside. Fumes from the car's exhaust can enter your home even with the connecting door closed.

Controlling Your Environment
Environmental Irritants

For some of the information in this article we are indebted to

American Lung Assn.
US Consumer Product Safety Commission
US Environmental Protection Agency

HOUSE HOLD CLEANING TIPS:

Although we've collected these cleaning tips over the years from a variety of sources, we cannot vouch for them because individuals have differing needs and requirements. Remember, some of these approaches will be more effective than others and most of them require a great deal of elbow grease.

We're always looking for more tips, so write and tell us what you've discovered.

1. Clean brass with a mixture of equal parts of salt and flour and a few drops of vinegar. Or squeeze lemon juice on a soft cloth and apply; rinse off with warm water and dry. Or apply a cut lemon directly.

2. Clean copper with a squeeze of lemon juice on a soft cloth and apply; rinse off with warm water and dry.

3. Clean silver with baking soda and water and rub. Or 1 tsp salt and 1 tbsp baking soda to one quart of water; boil for 3 minutes in an aluminum pan or pot lined with aluminum foil; use with a soft cloth

4. Clean plastic laminate cabinets with club soda

5. Garbage Can Mold, Bacteria: pour some borax inside the can

6. Air Fresheners: baking soda is a good odor absorbent

7. Tile and Glass Cleaners: clean with baking soda on a dampened cloth and rinse

8. Lubricants: use castor oil instead of oil lubricants. Check with the manufacturer first, since you don't want to damage the motor.

9. Ammonia-based Cleaner: substitute vinegar, salt, water

10. Furniture Polish: lemon juice with twice as much vegetable oil or 3 parts olive oil and 1 part white vinegar.

11. Drain Cleaner: boiling water with 1/4 cup baking soda and 1/4 cup vinegar plus a plunger.

HOUSEHOLD MAINTENANCE

This chapter presents a selection of cleaning and repair products that may be less likely to irritate lungs and skin. As always, what works for someone else may not work for you and what does not irritate you may not do quite the job you envision.

CLEANING AIDS

AFM SafeChoice Carpet Shampoo

Dye-free, odorless; do not use on wool carpeting
Available from:
Allergy Resources
Mail: PO Box 888 (APD)
UPS: 264 Brookridge Ave. (APD)
Palmer Lake, CO 80133
Orders 800-USE-FLAX (873-3529)
Company plans a move; use 800 #
and:
Allergy-Asthma Shopper™
PO Box 239 (APD)
Fate, TX 75132
800-447-1100
Fax 903-883-4513

AFM Super Clean

Odor-free, dye-free all-purpose cleaner for grease, dirt, oil, film; use on floors, woodwork, walls, countertops, tubs, tile, furniture, rugs, fabrics, laundry
Available from:
AFM Enterprises, Inc.
1960 Chicago E7 (APD)
Riverside, CA 92507
909-781-6860
909-781-6861
Fax 909-781-6892
and:
Allergy Relief Shop,™Inc.
3371 Whittle Springs Rd. (APD)
Knoxville, TN 37917
Orders 800-626-2810
Questions 615-522-2795
and:
Allergy Resources
Mail: PO Box 888 (APD)
UPS: 264 Brookridge Ave. (APD)

Palmer Lake, CO 80133
Orders 800-USE-FLAX (873-3529)
Company plans a move; use 800 #
and:
Allergy-Asthma Shopper™
PO Box 239 (APD)
Fate, TX 75132
800-447-1100
Fax 903-883-4513
and:
Flowright Int'l Products
1495 N.W. Gilman Blvd. #4 (APD)
Issaquah, WA 98027
206-392-8357
and:
N.E.E.D.S.
527 Charles Ave. 12A (APD)
Syracuse, NY 13209
800-634-1380
Fax 800-295-NEED (6333)

All Purpose Polish and Wax

Liquid or paste to clean and polish furniture, most floors and vinyl, and metal finishes on automobiles and applliances
Available from:
Allergy Relief Shop,™Inc.
3371 Whittle Springs Rd. (APD)
Knoxville, TN 37917
Orders 800-626-2810
Questions 615-522-2795
and:
Flowright Int'l Products
1495 N.W. Gilman Blvd. #4 (APD)
Issaquah, WA 98027
206-392-8357
and:
N.E.E.D.S.
527 Charles Ave. 12A (APD)
Syracuse, NY 13209
800-634-1380

Controlling Your Environment
Household Maintenance

Fax 800-295-NEED (6333)

Allersearch X-Mite™ All-in-One

Controls dust mites, mite allergen, and animal dander; can be used on carpets and some fabrics; moist powder based on tannic acid; covers 115 sq. ft. of carpet
Available from:
American Allergy Supply
PO Box 722022 (APD)
Houston, TX 77272-2022
800-321-1096
713-995-6110
and:
National Allergy Supply, Inc.
4400 Georgia Hwy. 120 (APD)
PO Box 1658 (APD)
Duluth, GA 30136
800-522-1448
In Atlanta 404-623-8077
Fax 404-623-5568

Ar-Ex® Safe Suds

"Hypo-allergenic;" lanolin-free; unscented; soap-free
Available from:
Ar-Ex Ltd.
156 N. Jefferson St. #205 (APD)
Chicago, IL 60661
312-879-0017
Fax 312-879-0019

Arm & Hammer® Detergent

Detergent, perfume, and dye free
Available from
Supermarkets

Automatic Dish Washing Machine Detergent

Biodegradeable agent for removing oil, grease, and food products; spot-free
Available from:
Allergy Relief Shop,™Inc.
3371 Whittle Springs Rd. (APD)
Knoxville, TN 37917
Orders 800-626-2810
Questions 615-522-2795

Bissell® Carpet Care Allergen Control

Eliminates allergens in carpets and upholstery; suitable for non-cartridge carpet cleaners
Available from:
Priorities®
70 Walnut St. (APD)
Wellesley, MA 02181
800-553-5398

Capture® Carpet Care

Dry carpet cleaner; moisture-free use does not support mold growth; includes spot cleaner and brush
Available from:
Allergy Asthma Technology
4151 N. Kedzie (APD)
PO Box 18398 (APD)
Chicago, IL 60618
800-621-5545
312-465-8020
Fax 312-465-7619
and:
Allergy Control Products, Inc.
96 Danbury Rd. (APD)
PO Box 793 (APD)
Ridgefield, CT 06877
800-422-DUST (3878)
203-438-9580
Fax 203-431-8963

Carpet Shampoo

Use as cleaner; removes grease, dirt, oil films; any carpet cleaning equipment
Available from:
AFM Enterprises, Inc.
1960 Chicago E7 (APD)
Riverside, CA 92507
909-781-6860
909-781-6861
Fax 909-781-6892
and:
Allergy Relief Shop,™Inc.
3371 Whittle Springs Rd. (APD)
Knoxville, TN 37917
Orders 800-626-2810
Questions 615-522-2795
and:

Controlling Your Environment

Household Maintenance

Flowright Int'l Products
1495 N.W. Gilman Blvd. #4 (APD)
Issaquah, WA 98027
206-392-8357

Deodorizing Pouch

Fragrance-free zeolite in a 9"x9" mesh pouch adsorbs odors; for enclosed spaces, closets, basements, and cars; reusable, reactivates with sun exposure; company notes that there is minimal residual dust only upon opening seal
Available from:
Absolute Environmental's Allergy Store
2615 S. University Dr. (APD)
Davie, FL 33328
Nationwide 800-771-ACHOO (2246)
In FL 800-329-3773
Broward 305-472-3773
Fax 305-474-0133
and:
Allergy Resources
Mail: PO Box 888 (APD)
UPS: 264 Brookridge Ave. (APD)
Palmer Lake, CO 80133
Orders 800-USE-FLAX (873-3529)
Company plans a move; use 800 #
and:
Signatures
19465 Brennan Ave. (APD)
Perris, CA 92599
800-777-0327
909-943-2021

Dip-N-Glow

Jewelry cleaner
Available from:
Flowright Int'l Products
1495 N.W. Gilman Blvd. #4 (APD)
Issaquah, WA 98027
206-392-8357

Dishwashing Liquid

Color-free, fragrance-free, alcohol-free
Available from:
Janice Corp.
198 US Hwy. 46 (APD)
Budd Lake, NJ 07828-3001

800-JANICES (526-4237)
Fax 201-691-5459

DRI-APP™

Applicator for cleaning powders
Available from:
Allergy Control Products, Inc.
96 Danbury Rd. (APD)
PO Box 793 (APD)
Ridgefield, CT 06877
800-422-DUST (3878)
203-438-9580
Fax 203-431-8963

Dust Grabber™

Fabric with permanent electrostatic surface charge; washable; odor-free, chemical-free; does not feel tacky; leaves no film; 14x14 cloth stretchable, can be clipped to mop head
Available from:
National Allergy Supply, Inc.
4400 Georgia Hwy. 120 (APD)
PO Box 1658 (APD)
Duluth, GA 30136
800-522-1448
In Atlanta 404-623-8077
Fax 404-623-5568

E-Z-On Shoe Polish

Self-polishing, little or no buffing; no petroleum distillates; white, black, brown
Available from:
Flowright Int'l Products
1495 N.W. Gilman Blvd. #4 (APD)
Issaquah, WA 98027
206-392-8357

E.Z. Maid

Dish washing and all-purpose liquid; unscented; non-abrasive
Available from:
Allergy Resources
Mail: PO Box 888 (APD)
UPS: 264 Brookridge Ave. (APD)
Palmer Lake, CO 80133
Orders 800-USE-FLAX (873-3529)
Company plans a move; use 800 #

Controlling Your Environment
Household Maintenance

and:
Flowright Int'l Products
1495 N.W. Gilman Blvd. #4 (APD)
Issaquah, WA 98027
206-392-8357

Ivory Snow®

Clinically proven to be mild to skin
Available from
Supermarkets

Laundry Detergent

Color-free, fragrance-free, alcohol-free
Available from:
Janice Corp.
198 US Hwy. 46 (APD)
Budd Lake, NJ 07828-3001
800-JANICES (526-4237)
Fax 201-691-5459

Libwipes

Edge sealed limited linting cotton for scratch-free wiping; does not attract air-borne particles with electrostatic charges; high absorbency
Available from:
Liberty Industries, Inc.
133 Commerce St. (APD)
E. Berlin, CT 06023
800-828-5656
In CT 828-6361
Fax 203-828-8879

Like Nu Rust Remover

Removes rust from metal and concrete surfaces; can remove water spots from tile
Available from:
Allergy Relief Shop,™Inc.
3371 Whittle Springs Rd. (APD)
Knoxville, TN 37917
Orders 800-626-2810
Questions 615-522-2795
and:
Flowright Int'l Products
1495 N.W. Gilman Blvd. #4 (APD)
Issaquah, WA 98027
206-392-8357
and:

N.E.E.D.S.
527 Charles Ave. 12A (APD)
Syracuse, NY 13209
800-634-1380
Fax 800-295-NEED (6333)

Nature Clean All Purpose Cleaning Lotion

Free of fragrance; "hypo-allergenic"
Available from:
Allergy Shop, Ltd.
3420 Cardston Crescent N.W. (APD)
Calgary, AB T2L 0S6
Canada
403-289-9052

Nature Clean Window/Glass Cleaner

Free of ammonia, dyes, perfumes, chlorine bleach, enzymes
Available from:
Allergy Shop, Ltd.
3420 Cardston Crescent N.W. (APD)
Calgary, AB T2L 0S6
Canada
403-289-9052

Power Plus

Laundry concentrate; no fragrances
Available from:
Allergy Alternative
440 Godfrey Dr. (APD)
Windsor, CA 95492
800-838-1514
and:
Allergy Resources
Mail: PO Box 888 (APD)
UPS: 264 Brookridge Ave. (APD)
Palmer Lake, CO 80133
Orders 800-USE-FLAX (873-3529)
Company plans a move; use 800 #
and:
Flowright Int'l Products
1495 N.W. Gilman Blvd. #4 (APD)
Issaquah, WA 98027
206-392-8357
and:
N.E.E.D.S.
527 Charles Ave. 12A (APD)

Controlling Your Environment
Household Maintenance

Syracuse, NY 13209
800-634-1380
Fax 800-295-NEED (6333)

Power Scrubber
Keeps hands out of gloves and away from soap and water; three rotating brushes (nylon, stainless steel sponge, bristle) clean pots and pans; water resistant; requires 3 C batteries
Available from:
Home Trends
1450 Lyell Ave. (APD)
Rochester, NY 14606-2184
716-254-6520
Fax 716-458-9245

Shingle Protek
Flame retardant for wood shingled roofs; water resistant
Available from:
Allergy Relief Shop,™Inc.
3371 Whittle Springs Rd. (APD)
Knoxville, TN 37917
Orders 800-626-2810
Questions 615-522-2795
and:
Flowright Int'l Products
1495 N.W. Gilman Blvd. #4 (APD)
Issaquah, WA 98027
206-392-8357
and:
N.E.E.D.S.
527 Charles Ave. 12A (APD)
Syracuse, NY 13209
800-634-1380
Fax 800-295-NEED (6333)

Soft N' Fresh Fabric Softener
Fragrance-free; citrus-free
Available from:
Allergy Resources
Mail: PO Box 888 (APD)
UPS: 264 Brookridge Ave. (APD)
Palmer Lake, CO 80133
Orders 800-USE-FLAX (873-3529)
Company plans a move; use 800 #

Soil Away
Fabric stain remover for ink, blood, crayon, mud, lipstick; no synthetic fragrance or color
Available from:
Allergy Resources
Mail: PO Box 888 (APD)
UPS: 264 Brookridge Ave. (APD)
Palmer Lake, CO 80133
Orders 800-USE-FLAX (873-3529)
Company plans a move; use 800 #
and:
Flowright Int'l Products
1495 N.W. Gilman Blvd. #4 (APD)
Issaquah, WA 98027
206-392-8357
and:
N.E.E.D.S.
527 Charles Ave. 12A (APD)
Syracuse, NY 13209
800-634-1380
Fax 800-295-NEED (6333)

Spray Cleaner
Color-free, fragrance-free, alcohol-free
Available from:
Janice Corp.
198 US Hwy. 46 (APD)
Budd Lake, NJ 07828-3001
800-JANICES (526-4237)
Fax 201-691-5459

Super Clean
All-purpose cleaner without fumes; non-irritating to skin
Available from:
Allergy Resources
Mail: PO Box 888 (APD)
UPS: 264 Brookridge Ave. (APD)
Palmer Lake, CO 80133
Orders 800-USE-FLAX (873-3529)
Company plans a move; use 800 #
and:
N.E.E.D.S.
527 Charles Ave. 12A (APD)
Syracuse, NY 13209
800-634-1380
Fax 800-295-NEED (6333)
and:

Priorities®
70 Walnut St. (APD)
Wellesley, MA 02181
800-553-5398

Twice as Gentle

Liquid detergent free of perfume, coloring, brighteners, emulsifiers, no strong alkalis, enzymes, phosphates, fillers
Available from
Boots Chemists, England

Ultra Safe

Air cleaner with vacuum attachment for computers, reading boxes; 350 CFM; filters 650 sq. ft.; filtered motor, intake has washable prefilter and exhaust chamber has prefilter, carbon filter; HEPA filter; blower; commercial use, stainles steel case, casters; 27"x25"x12"
Available from:
Allergy Relief Shop,™Inc.
3371 Whittle Springs Rd. (APD)
Knoxville, TN 37917
Orders 800-626-2810
Questions 615-522-2795
and:
AllerMed Corp.
31 Steel Rd. (APD)
Wylie, TX 75098
214-442-4898
Fax 214-442-4897

Woolworths Home Brand Laundry Soap

"Less irritating" laundry soap; available in local groceries and markets in Australia and New Zealand

Zeolite® Odor Neutralizer

Non-toxic, non allergenic powder attracts odors; fragrance-free; for carpets and upholstery
Available from:
Absolute Environmental's Allergy Store
2615 S. University Dr. (APD)
Davie, FL 33328
Nationwide 800-771-ACHOO (2246)

In FL 800-329-3773
Broward 305-472-3773
Fax 305-474-0133

REPAIRS AND MAINTENANCE AIDS

3 in 1 Adhesive

Odor-free, bonds ceramic, vinyl, and parquet tiles; use test application
Available from:
AFM Enterprises, Inc.
1960 Chicago E7 (APD)
Riverside, CA 92507
909-781-6860
909-781-6861
Fax 909-781-6892
and:
Allergy Relief Shop,™Inc.
3371 Whittle Springs Rd. (APD)
Knoxville, TN 37917
Orders 800-626-2810
Questions 615-522-2795
and:
Allergy Resources
Mail: PO Box 888 (APD)
UPS: 264 Brookridge Ave. (APD)
Palmer Lake, CO 80133
Orders 800-USE-FLAX (873-3529)
Company plans a move; use 800 #
and:
Flowright Int'l Products
1495 N.W. Gilman Blvd. #4 (APD)
Issaquah, WA 98027
206-392-8357
and:
N.E.E.D.S.
527 Charles Ave. 12A (APD)
Syracuse, NY 13209
800-634-1380
Fax 800-295-NEED (6333)

Acrylacq
Replaces lacquer; clear, high gloss for gym floors, stair railings, hardwood floors
Available from:
AFM Enterprises, Inc.
1960 Chicago E7 (APD)

Controlling Your Environment

Household Maintenance

Riverside, CA 92507
909-781-6860
909-781-6861
Fax 909-781-6892
and:
Allergy Relief Shop,™ Inc.
3371 Whittle Springs Rd. (APD)
Knoxville, TN 37917
Orders 800-626-2810
Questions 615-522-2795
and:
Flowright Int'l Products
1495 N.W. Gilman Blvd. #4 (APD)
Issaquah, WA 98027
206-392-8357
and:
N.E.E.D.S.
527 Charles Ave. 12A (APD)
Syracuse, NY 13209
800-634-1380
Fax 800-295-NEED (6333)

AFM Caulking Compound
Use as putty for windows, cracks, and repairs
Available from:
Flowright Int'l Products
1495 N.W. Gilman Blvd. #4 (APD)
Issaquah, WA 98027
206-392-8357
and:
N.E.E.D.S.
527 Charles Ave. 12A (APD)
Syracuse, NY 13209
800-634-1380
Fax 800-295-NEED (6333)

Almighty Adhesive
Bonds wood, plastic, marble, ceramic, some pavers, slate, metal, carpet, parquet, furniture, and cork
Available from:
AFM Enterprises, Inc.
1960 Chicago E7 (APD)
Riverside, CA 92507
909-781-6860
909-781-6861
Fax 909-781-6892
and:
Allergy Relief Shop,™ Inc.

3371 Whittle Springs Rd. (APD)
Knoxville, TN 37917
Orders 800-626-2810
Questions 615-522-2795

Carpet Adhesive
For installing textiles and various carpet floor coverings
Available from:
Allergy Relief Shop,™ Inc.
3371 Whittle Springs Rd. (APD)
Knoxville, TN 37917
Orders 800-626-2810
Questions 615-522-2795
and:
Flowright Int'l Products
1495 N.W. Gilman Blvd. #4 (APD)
Issaquah, WA 98027
206-392-8357
and:
N.E.E.D.S.
527 Charles Ave. 12A (APD)
Syracuse, NY 13209
800-634-1380
Fax 800-295-NEED (6333)

Cem Bond Paint
Odor-free; coats and seals concrete and masonry surfaces and exterior or interior wood trim
Available from:
AFM Enterprises, Inc.
1960 Chicago E7 (APD)
Riverside, CA 92507
909-781-6860
909-781-6861
Fax 909-781-6892
and:
Allergy Relief Shop,™ Inc.
3371 Whittle Springs Rd. (APD)
Knoxville, TN 37917
Orders 800-626-2810
Questions 615-522-2795
and:
Allergy Resources
Mail: PO Box 888 (APD)
UPS: 264 Brookridge Ave. (APD)
Palmer Lake, CO 80133
Orders 800-USE-FLAX (873-3529)
Company plans a move; use 800 #

Controlling Your Environment

Household Maintenance

and:
Flowright Int'l Products
1495 N.W. Gilman Blvd. #4 (APD)
Issaquah, WA 98027
206-392-8357

Drain Gun

Compressed air pump clears clogged drains without chemicals; sinks, toilets, bathtubs
Available from:
Brookstone Co.
5 Vose Farm Road (APD)
Peterborough, NH 03458
800-926-7000
Fax 603-924-0093

Dura Stain

Interior and exterior protective coating; shades of oak, maple, mahogany, walnut, birch, redwood, cedar, and clear
Available from:
AFM Enterprises, Inc.
1960 Chicago E7 (APD)
Riverside, CA 92507
909-781-6860
909-781-6861
Fax 909-781-6892
and:
Allergy Relief Shop,™ Inc.
3371 Whittle Springs Rd. (APD)
Knoxville, TN 37917
Orders 800-626-2810
Questions 615-522-2795
and:
Flowright Int'l Products
1495 N.W. Gilman Blvd. #4 (APD)
Issaquah, WA 98027
206-392-8357
and:
N.E.E.D.S.
527 Charles Ave. 12A (APD)
Syracuse, NY 13209
800-634-1380
Fax 800-295-NEED (6333)

Dyno Flex Caulking Compound

Use as putty for windows, cracks, and repairs; can be applied over

asphalt shingles, roll roofing; repair seams and leaks on metal roofs and heating and air ducts
Available from:
AFM Enterprises, Inc.
1960 Chicago E7 (APD)
Riverside, CA 92507
909-781-6860
909-781-6861
Fax 909-781-6892
and:
Allergy Relief Shop,™ Inc.
3371 Whittle Springs Rd. (APD)
Knoxville, TN 37917
Orders 800-626-2810
Questions 615-522-2795
and:
Flowright Int'l Products
1495 N.W. Gilman Blvd. #4 (APD)
Issaquah, WA 98027
206-392-8357

Dyno Flex

Water emulsion synthetic polymer system for use as a sealant and mastic compound; seals and repairs seams and leaks on metal roofs; natural, gray, and white
Available from:
AFM Enterprises, Inc.
1960 Chicago E7 (APD)
Riverside, CA 92507
909-781-6860
909-781-6861
Fax 909-781-6892
and:
Allergy Relief Shop,™ Inc.
3371 Whittle Springs Rd. (APD)
Knoxville, TN 37917
Orders 800-626-2810
Questions 615-522-2795
and:
N.E.E.D.S.
527 Charles Ave. 12A (APD)
Syracuse, NY 13209
800-634-1380
Fax 800-295-NEED (6333)

Controlling Your Environment

Household Maintenance

Dyno Seal

A liquid copolymer for use as a sealer and waterproof membrane; can be used below grade, under shower stalls and tubs, to repair or coat roofs; adheres to concrete, block, metal, wood, or asphalt shingles
Available from:
AFM Enterprises, Inc.
1960 Chicago E7 (APD)
Riverside, CA 92507
909-781-6860
909-781-6861
Fax 909-781-6892
and:
Allergy Relief Shop,™ Inc.
3371 Whittle Springs Rd. (APD)
Knoxville, TN 37917
Orders 800-626-2810
Questions 615-522-2795
and:
Flowright Int'l Products
1495 N.W. Gilman Blvd. #4 (APD)
Issaquah, WA 98027
206-392-8357
and:
N.E.E.D.S.
527 Charles Ave. 12A (APD)
Syracuse, NY 13209
800-634-1380
Fax 800-295-NEED (6333)

GT1000 Flat Latex Wall Paint

Formulated without slow releasing compounds or airborne fungicide; when dry, the preservative does not become airborne or leach out of the paint; low odor; "hypo-allergenic"; 9 stock colors, light tint bases
Available from:
Murco Wall Products, Inc.
300 N.E. 21st St. (APD)
Ft. Worth, TX 76106-8528
817-626-1987

Hard Seal

Odor-free, medium gloss sealer applies over previously painted surfaces to seal fumes and as finish coat on floors and cabinets

Available from:
AFM Enterprises, Inc.
1960 Chicago E7 (APD)
Riverside, CA 92507
909-781-6860
909-781-6861
Fax 909-781-6892
and:
Allergy Relief Shop,™ Inc.
3371 Whittle Springs Rd. (APD)
Knoxville, TN 37917
Orders 800-626-2810
Questions 615-522-2795
and:
Allergy Resources
Mail: PO Box 888 (APD)
UPS: 264 Brookridge Ave. (APD)
Palmer Lake, CO 80133
Orders 800-USE-FLAX (873-3529)
Company plans a move; use 800 #
and:
Flowright Int'l Products
1495 N.W. Gilman Blvd. #4 (APD)
Issaquah, WA 98027
206-392-8357
and:
N.E.E.D.S.
527 Charles Ave. 12A (APD)
Syracuse, NY 13209
800-634-1380
Fax 800-295-NEED (6333)

Interior Flat Latex 6450

Low odor; low biocide, produced without adding additional biocides during manufacture; free of fungicide and solvent; use on drywall, concrete, cement block, or primed wood; 8% gloss
Available from:
Miller Paint Co.
317 S.E. Grand Ave. (APD)
Portland, OR 97214
503-233-4021
Fax 503-238-6289

Interior Satin Latex 1450

Low odor; low biocide, produced without adding additional biocides during manufacture; free of fungicide

Controlling Your Environment

Household Maintenance

and solvent; walls and ceilings; 15% gloss
Available from:
Miller Paint Co.
317 S.E. Grand Ave. (APD)
Portland, OR 97214
503-233-4021
Fax 503-238-6289

Interior Semi-Gloss Latex 2850

Low odor; low biocide, produced without adding additional biocides during manufacture; free of fungicide and solvent; walls and trim; kitchens, bathrooms; 50% gloss
Available from:
Miller Paint Co.
317 S.E. Grand Ave. (APD)
Portland, OR 97214
503-233-4021
Fax 503-238-6289

Joint Compound

Low odor joint and patching compound, low shrinkage; asbestos-free, fiber-free
Available from:
AFM Enterprises, Inc.
1960 Chicago E7 (APD)
Riverside, CA 92507
909-781-6860
909-781-6861
Fax 909-781-6892
and:
Allergy Relief Shop,™ Inc.
3371 Whittle Springs Rd. (APD)
Knoxville, TN 37917
Orders 800-626-2810
Questions 615-522-2795
and:
Flowright Int'l Products
1495 N.W. Gilman Blvd. #4 (APD)
Issaquah, WA 98027
206-392-8357
and:
N.E.E.D.S.
527 Charles Ave. 12A (APD)
Syracuse, NY 13209
800-634-1380
Fax 800-295-NEED (6333)

Klear Seal

Interior/exterior metal, masonry, and concrete sealer; glossy finish
Available from:
Flowright Int'l Products
1495 N.W. Gilman Blvd. #4 (APD)
Issaquah, WA 98027
206-392-8357
and:
N.E.E.D.S.
527 Charles Ave. 12A (APD)
Syracuse, NY 13209
800-634-1380
Fax 800-295-NEED (6333)

LE1000 High Gloss Latex Enamel

For kitchen, bathroom, woodwork; free of fungicide; low odor; "hypo-allergenic"; 9 stock colors, light tint bases
Available from:
Murco Wall Products, Inc.
300 N.E. 21st St. (APD)
Ft. Worth, TX 76106-8528
817-626-1987

Lift Off

Paint stripper; can be neutralized with water; removes paint, polymers, wax, asphalt, PVC plastics, fiber glass, adhesives, resins
Available from:
AFM Enterprises, Inc.
1960 Chicago E7 (APD)
Riverside, CA 92507
909-781-6860
909-781-6861
Fax 909-781-6892
and:
Allergy Relief Shop,™ Inc.
3371 Whittle Springs Rd. (APD)
Knoxville, TN 37917
Orders 800-626-2810
Questions 615-522-2795
and:
N.E.E.D.S.
527 Charles Ave. 12A (APD)
Syracuse, NY 13209
800-634-1380
Fax 800-295-NEED (6333)

Controlling Your Environment

Household Maintenance

M-100 Hypo Joint Compound

Powdered, joint cement and texture compound; inert fillers, natural binders; free of preservatives, slow releasing compounds, asbestos; low odor; "hypo-allergenic"
Available from:
Murco Wall Products, Inc.
300 N.E. 21st St. (APD)
Ft. Worth, TX 76106-8528
817-626-1987

One Step Seal & Shine

Industrial/domestic sealer-polish; dries clear
Available from:
Flowright Int'l Products
1495 N.W. Gilman Blvd. #4 (APD)
Issaquah, WA 98027
206-392-8357
and:
N.E.E.D.S.
527 Charles Ave. 12A (APD)
Syracuse, NY 13209
800-634-1380
Fax 800-295-NEED (6333)

Paver Seal .003

Seals porous tile, conrete, and grout; helps control efflorescence
Available from:
AFM Enterprises, Inc.
1960 Chicago E7 (APD)
Riverside, CA 92507
909-781-6860
909-781-6861
Fax 909-781-6892
and:
Allergy Relief Shop,™ Inc.
3371 Whittle Springs Rd. (APD)
Knoxville, TN 37917
Orders 800-626-2810
Questions 615-522-2795
and:
N.E.E.D.S.
527 Charles Ave. 12A (APD)
Syracuse, NY 13209
800-634-1380
Fax 800-295-NEED (6333)

Penetrating Water Seal

Odor-free; reduces water absorption; helps control efflorescence; for porous bricks, some pavers, concrete, raw wood
Available from:
AFM Enterprises, Inc.
1960 Chicago E7 (APD)
Riverside, CA 92507
909-781-6860
909-781-6861
Fax 909-781-6892
and:
Allergy Relief Shop,™ Inc.
3371 Whittle Springs Rd. (APD)
Knoxville, TN 37917
Orders 800-626-2810
Questions 615-522-2795
and:
Allergy Resources
Mail: PO Box 888 (APD)
UPS: 264 Brookridge Ave. (APD)
Palmer Lake, CO 80133
Orders 800-USE-FLAX (873-3529)
Company plans a move; use 800 #
and:
Flowright Int'l Products
1495 N.W. Gilman Blvd. #4 (APD)
Issaquah, WA 98027
206-392-8357
and:
N.E.E.D.S.
527 Charles Ave. 12A (APD)
Syracuse, NY 13209
800-634-1380
Fax 800-295-NEED (6333)

Polyuraseal

Odor-free, clear gloss coating for floors, cabinets, and woodwork, metal, vinyl coated fabrics, plastic surfaces; substitute for polyurathane
Available from:
AFM Enterprises, Inc.
1960 Chicago E7 (APD)
Riverside, CA 92507
909-781-6860
909-781-6861
Fax 909-781-6892
and:
Allergy Relief Shop,™ Inc.

Controlling Your Environment

Household Maintenance

3371 Whittle Springs Rd. (APD)
Knoxville, TN 37917
Orders 800-626-2810
Questions 615-522-2795
and:
Allergy Resources
Mail: PO Box 888 (APD)
UPS: 264 Brookridge Ave. (APD)
Palmer Lake, CO 80133
Orders 800-USE-FLAX (873-3529)
Company plans a move; use 800 #
and:
Flowright Int'l Products
1495 N.W. Gilman Blvd. #4 (APD)
Issaquah, WA 98027
206-392-8357
and:
N.E.E.D.S.
527 Charles Ave. 12A (APD)
Syracuse, NY 13209
800-634-1380
Fax 800-295-NEED (6333)

Safecoat™ All Purpose Enamel

Water-base gloss enamel for interior and exterior walls, trim, woodwork, metal; water resisitant; white, bone
Available from:
AFM Enterprises, Inc.
1960 Chicago E7 (APD)
Riverside, CA 92507
909-781-6860
909-781-6861
Fax 909-781-6892
and:
Allergy Relief Shop,™ Inc.
3371 Whittle Springs Rd. (APD)
Knoxville, TN 37917
Orders 800-626-2810
Questions 615-522-2795
and:
Flowright Int'l Products
1495 N.W. Gilman Blvd. #4 (APD)
Issaquah, WA 98027
206-392-8357
and:
N.E.E.D.S.
527 Charles Ave. 12A (APD)
Syracuse, NY 13209

800-634-1380
Fax 800-295-NEED (6333)

Safecoat™ Enamel

Odor-free, water-base semi-gloss enamel; bathroom, kitchen; white or bone, can be tinted
Available from:
AFM Enterprises, Inc.
1960 Chicago E7 (APD)
Riverside, CA 92507
909-781-6860
909-781-6861
Fax 909-781-6892
and:
Allergy Relief Shop,™ Inc.
3371 Whittle Springs Rd. (APD)
Knoxville, TN 37917
Orders 800-626-2810
Questions 615-522-2795
and:
Allergy Resources
Mail: PO Box 888 (APD)
UPS: 264 Brookridge Ave. (APD)
Palmer Lake, CO 80133
Orders 800-USE-FLAX (873-3529)
Company plans a move; use 800 #
and:
Flowright Int'l Products
1495 N.W. Gilman Blvd. #4 (APD)
Issaquah, WA 98027
206-392-8357
and:
N.E.E.D.S.
527 Charles Ave. 12A (APD)
Syracuse, NY 13209
800-634-1380
Fax 800-295-NEED (6333)

Safecoat™ Paint

Low odor, non-reactive sealant and flat finish coat for walls and woodwork. Water base copolymer emulsion, odor-free; white, bone, and eight pastel colors; white can be tinted locally with Universal Tinting System.
Available from:
AFM Enterprises, Inc.
1960 Chicago E7 (APD)
Riverside, CA 92507

Controlling Your Environment

Household Maintenance

909-781-6860
909-781-6861
Fax 909-781-6892
and:
Allergy Relief Shop,™ Inc.
3371 Whittle Springs Rd. (APD)
Knoxville, TN 37917
Orders 800-626-2810
Questions 615-522-2795
and:
Flowright Int'l Products
1495 N.W. Gilman Blvd. #4 (APD)
Issaquah, WA 98027
206-392-8357
and:
N.E.E.D.S.
527 Charles Ave. 12A (APD)
Syracuse, NY 13209
800-634-1380
Fax 800-295-NEED (6333)

Safecoat™ Primer
Odor-free, water-base primer for walls, woodwork
Available from:
Allergy Resources
Mail: PO Box 888 (APD)
UPS: 264 Brookridge Ave. (APD)
Palmer Lake, CO 80133
Orders 800-USE-FLAX (873-3529)
Company plans a move; use 800 #
and:
AFM Enterprises, Inc.
1960 Chicago E7 (APD)
Riverside, CA 92507
909-781-6860
909-781-6861
Fax 909-781-6892
and:
Allergy Relief Shop,™ Inc.
3371 Whittle Springs Rd. (APD)
Knoxville, TN 37917
Orders 800-626-2810
Questions 615-522-2795
and:
Allergy Resources
Mail: PO Box 888 (APD)
UPS: 264 Brookridge Ave. (APD)
Palmer Lake, CO 80133
Orders 800-USE-FLAX (873-3529)

Company plans a move; use 800 #
and:
Flowright Int'l Products
1495 N.W. Gilman Blvd. #4 (APD)
Issaquah, WA 98027
206-392-8357
and:
N.E.E.D.S.
527 Charles Ave. 12A (APD)
Syracuse, NY 13209
800-634-1380
Fax 800-295-NEED (6333)

Sanding Sealer
Helps prevent bleed through of oils, turpentines, and resins and raising grain on wood when water-base products are applied
Available from:
AFM Enterprises, Inc.
1960 Chicago E7 (APD)
Riverside, CA 92507
909-781-6860
909-781-6861
Fax 909-781-6892
and:
Allergy Relief Shop,™ Inc.
3371 Whittle Springs Rd. (APD)
Knoxville, TN 37917
Orders 800-626-2810
Questions 615-522-2795
and:
N.E.E.D.S.
527 Charles Ave. 12A (APD)
Syracuse, NY 13209
800-634-1380
Fax 800-295-NEED (6333)

Tile Grout
Substitute for cement-type compounds; narrow joints on counter tops and bath areas
Available from:
Flowright Int'l Products
1495 N.W. Gilman Blvd. #4 (APD)
Issaquah, WA 98027
206-392-8357

Controlling Your Environment
Household Maintenance

Vinyl Block

Controls out-gassing from vinyl coverings in automobiles; liquid applies to any surface
Available from:
Flowright Int'l Products
1495 N.W. Gilman Blvd. #4 (APD)
Issaquah, WA 98027
206-392-8357

Wallpaper Adhesive

Use with wallpaper and vinyl wall covers
Available from:
Flowright Int'l Products
1495 N.W. Gilman Blvd. #4 (APD)
Issaquah, WA 98027
206-392-8357

Water Base Mexe Seal

Protects pavers from stain; applies to saltillo pavers, adobe, adoquin, grout, granite, concrete quarry tile, fired and unfired porcelain
Available from:
AFM Enterprises, Inc.
1960 Chicago E7 (APD)
Riverside, CA 92507
909-781-6860
909-781-6861
Fax 909-781-6892
and:
Allergy Relief Shop,™ Inc.
3371 Whittle Springs Rd. (APD)
Knoxville, TN 37917
Orders 800-626-2810
Questions 615-522-2795

and:
N.E.E.D.S.
527 Charles Ave. 12A (APD)
Syracuse, NY 13209
800-634-1380
Fax 800-295-NEED (6333)

Water Seal

Seals grout, tile, and concrete; coats porous surfaces, bare wood, painted surfaces, drywall, paneling, cabinets
Available from:
AFM Enterprises, Inc.
1960 Chicago E7 (APD)
Riverside, CA 92507
909-781-6860
909-781-6861
Fax 909-781-6892
and:
Allergy Relief Shop,™ Inc.
3371 Whittle Springs Rd. (APD)
Knoxville, TN 37917
Orders 800-626-2810
Questions 615-522-2795
and:
Flowright Int'l Products
1495 N.W. Gilman Blvd. #4 (APD)
Issaquah, WA 98027
206-392-8357
and:
N.E.E.D.S.
527 Charles Ave. 12A (APD)
Syracuse, NY 13209
800-634-1380
Fax 800-295-NEED (6333)

Controlling Your Environment

Air Quality

IMPROVING YOUR AIR QUALITY

Air cleaners and filters draw in pollutants and allergens like pollens and dander that are airborne. Some units may have more than one filter in order to trap particulates and chemicals of different sizes. Particulates that are settled on carpeting or can become a problem if they are stirred into the air (when you walk or sit or your children play). From the air they can settle on your mucous membranes before the purifier can pull them in or if they rise too far from your filter for it to be effective.

For these reasons, the speed and power with which your filter works become important. But, do not expect an air purifier to work miracles for you. Air cleaners alone cannot adequately remove all of the pollutants usually found in indoor air. No air purifier will help you if you do not also follow your doctor's advice in environmental control procedures.

Air filters do not work miracles.

Follow your doctor's advice.

Most air cleaners for home use are recirculating. A fan pulls air through some form of entrapment like a filter and it should be able to do this faster than air enters the room.

In general, units that sit on tables may have about a 75% efficiency for pollen. HEPA filter are efficient to 99.97% at 0.3 micron. Pleated filters trap up to 95% of particles to 0.3 micron. Air conditioner filters trap about 30% at 10 micron. The types of air conditioners and the terms used to describe them are described in detail in this chapter.

FILTER EFFICIENCY (PARTICLE CAPTURE)

The DOP (dioctylphthalate) test measures (at MILSPEC which are military specifications) the efficiency of an air cleaner at 0.3 micron because that is the size most likely to pass through your own lung filtering system into your lungs. It is also the particle size that is the most difficult for air cleaners to capture.

A filter's efficiency is expressed in percentage, indicating how many micron are captured and how many pass through. If three, 0.3 micron particles out of 10,000 pass through, that means that .03% pass through. This also means that 99.97% or 9,997 out of 10,000 are captured.

HEPA filter standards are efficiencies of 99.97% at 0.3 micron. Pleated filters trap up to 95% of particles to 0.3 micron. Air conditioner filters trap about 30% at 10 micron.

CLEAN AIR DELIVERY RATE

CADR or clean air delivery rate assesses air flow/volume and filter efficiency. The numbers are based on tests used by the Association of Home Appliance Manufacturers (AHAM), although not all products have been tested.

> CADR number is the amount of clean air (in cubic feet per minute) that the air cleaner can return to a room for a **specific particle.** The higher the CADR, the faster the performance and the faster clean air returns to the room.

The tests give numbers for dust, smoke, and pollen. CADR ratings for dust can range from 10 to 350; for tobacco smoke, 10 to 300, for pollen, 25 to 400. The numbers are based on the percentage of particles removed and the speed with which they are removed.

The CADR rating is printed on the seal of room air cleaner boxes along with suggested room size for the model. Performances of certified models are verified every year.

TOTAL AIR FLOW

How much air moves through the air cleaner is also important. This is the volume of the air moving through the cleaner. The larger the volume of air (cubic feet per minutes) your unit can deliver, the cleaner will be your air. The total air flow rate is a good measure to air cleaner efficiency.

BLOWERS

The blower is an important part of any filter. It should have sufficient power to draw air through the filters, including the extremely small holes in the HEPA filter that trap particles down to 0.3 micron as well as the large

Controlling Your Environment

Air Quality

mass of filtering material. Yet, the blower must be quiet enough for bedroom use.

HOW TO FIGURE YOUR AIR VOLUME NEEDS

The volume of air a filter fan can handle is rated in cubic feet per minute displacement (CFM). A filter should funnel the air volume of a room through its filters several times each hour. To be effective, its fan should be able to pull floating particulates into the filter from the far sides of the room.

> **Be sure you calculate the volume of air in your room and buy a filter that is large enough to handle that volume. A unit with insufficient CFM will not filter your entire room.**

HOW TO CALCULATE WHAT SIZE FILTER YOU NEED

1. Multiply the length of one wall times the length of the adjoining wall.

2. Multiply that answer by the height of the wall. The answer is the volume of air in your room.

3. Multiply the cubic feet per minute displacement (CFM) rating on the filter you are considering times 60 to determine cubic feet per hour.

4. Divide that number by the volume of air in your room.

5. Your answer is the number of air changes the proposed filter will provide each hour in your room.

PARTICULATES YOU CAN EXPECT YOUR FILTER TO HANDLE

Animal dander is light and stays air borne, so that filtering systems are able to remove it. Unfortunately, animal dander remains a problem. Because it is airborne for longer periods, you have time to breathe it before it is pulled into the purifier. Dander is inert but carries proteins from your pet's skin, saliva, and urine as well as dust, mold, and pollen protein.

Smoke particles are smaller than dust particles and so do not settle as quickly. Because smoke particles are airborne longer, air purifiers can lessen irritation. Not all

118

Controlling Your Environment

Air Quality

air filters solve the problem of odor. If smoke odor or gaseous pollutants bothers you, try a carbon filter for some relief.

Larger mold and pollen particulates can be partially filtered out with air conditioning systems. These units need to be kept clean and free of mold. Air filters will catch the smaller pollen and plant proteins.

There are different kind of filters and you will want to understand how they work before purchasing one.

HOW TO EVALUATE AN AIR CLEANER
✔ CHECK LIST

- Does the device mask odors with a scent?

- Is ozone emitted?

- What is its CADR? What is the amount of air handled?

- What is its DOP? How efficient is the unit?

- Does the unit have a high CFM?

- Does the unit draw air from more than one point?

- Do you need to worry about where it is placed in the room (raised table, centered in the room, near a wall)?

- Is the unit quiet when functioning? Listening to the unit in a store will not necessarily indicate how loud it will sound in your home.

- How often do filters need to be replaced? What is the cost? How easily replaced are they?

- Can I tell if the filter is working?

- What kind of dealer support is available for repair? Is repair local? Is there a guarantee? What is the average length of time for repair? What are the costs involved?

CHEMICAL FILTERS

The most common chemical filters are made of charcoal or activated carbon. Other chemical filters contain potassium permanganate, zeolite, or a similar chemical that can adsorb gases, fumes, vapors, and odors.

Chemical filters are not reusable. As the filter becomes clogged with contaminants, it should be replaced because it loses its effectiveness. Be sure that these particles cannot be redispersed into the air.

Controlling Your Environment

Air Quality

Catalysis is a chemical reaction that can change pollutants like ozone and formaldehyde into oxygen and water. Research continues in this area.

ELECTRONIC AIR CLEANERS — ELECTROSTATIC PRECIPITATOR AIR CLEANERS or ELECTRONIC AGGLOMERATORS

Electronic cleaners do not filter. They place a negative electronic charge on airborne particles entering the cleaner, pulled in by a fan. The particulates are then attracted to a positively charged plate(s) or grid(s) that should be washed frequently in a dishwasher or tub because they lose efficiency.

These cleaners may be installed in air conditioning or forced air heating systems by heating and air companies. They do not remove gases or odors and some may produce ozone which is a gas that can irritate the lungs of people with asthma.

With relatively low air resistance, they can handle relatively large volumes of air and their filters are washable. Efficiency is lowered when the plates become full, but improve with washing. It is therefore important to wash the plates frequently. Some manufacturers recommend monthly washing.

Whenever you notice a difference in your comfort level, wash your filter. Depending upon your home need, you may need to wash it weekly or more often.

ELECTRET FILTERS

Some filters do not need any wiring. They use a special polymer material that develops its own static electrical charge as air passes through and they do not produce ozone.

The filter is used in place of your fiberglass furnace filter. It should be cleaned every month. Electret filters are made of an electronically-charged, polyester mesh that traps particulates. They are very efficient initially, are ozone-free, but require filter replacement every six months or less and do not remove gases or odors.

Controlling Your Environment

Air Quality

HYBRID DEVICES

These are filters that utilize two or three particle removal devices. They may have any combination of or all three of the following: a mechanical filter, a carbon (or other medium) filter, and an electronic cleaner.

MECHANICAL FILTERS

A mechanical filter has one or more removable sheets, screens, or blankets that are made of glass fibers, fabric, plastic, wood, metal or other materials. The pores in these materials are small enough to grab particulates as the air is forced through them. Mechanical filters are not reusable. With use it needs replacing.

These are similar to and may include typical furnace filters.

TYPES OF MECHANICAL FILTERS

✔ **Panel filter** has a fibrous filter media; it is a basic unit and the type that most desktop models are. It is small and the replacement filters are not costly.

✔ **Extended surface filters** have folded or pleated media, allowing for more media surface in a given area for more surfaces to trap particles and for holding capacity.

✔ **HEPA filters** are made of closely spaced fibrous material that collect particulates. They have a minimum efficiency of 99.97 % at 0.3 micron (compared to the period at the end of a sentence which is 1000 micron wide).

HEPA FILTERS

The HEPA or high efficiency particulate arresting air filter is very efficient. It was developed to filter out radioactive dust during World War II. This filter can be coated with chemicals to kill molds, bacteria or viruses.

The HEPA filter itself is composed of a mixture of various sized glass fibers that are densely packed and achieve large surface area through pleating. It maintains its efficiency (99.97% for particles of 0.3 micron) over a two to five year life without cleaning. Gases or odors are not removed.

This type of filter generally becomes more efficient with use and is ozone-free. Its efficiency remains unimpaired

Controlling Your Environment

Air Quality

over the lifetime without cleaning or complicated maintenance.

HEPA-TYPE FILTERS

Hepa-type filters have many of the benefits of HEPA filters: they become more efficient with use, do not produce ozone, and have a filter life of two to five years. They appear similar to HEPA filters, but since the density of the fibers is lower, the efficiency is limited.

When a filter is tested in accordance with ASHRAE method 52-70, the method of testing is to look at 99% particles down to 0.5 micron. When a filter is tested in accordance with DOP method, the method of testing is to look at 99.97% at 0.3 micron.

ASHRAE and DOP are methods for testing to evaluate performance, not standards by which testing is performed.)

(According to ASHRAE (American Society of Heating, Refrigeration, and Air Conditioning Engineers), ASHRAE and DOP are methods for testing to evaluate performance, not standards by which testing is performed.) An ASHRAE standard is *how* to test. It does not *define* efficiency.

ASHRAE
1791 Tullie Cir, NE,
Atlanta, GA 30329-2398
404-636-8400

Center for Disease Control (CDC) recommends that sufficient fresh air be pulled into the system. ASHRAE Standard 62-89 calls for 20 cubic feet per minute (cfm) ventilation rate per person.

ULPA FILTERS

ULPA filters are not as available, but may become more accessible in the future. They are effective to 0.12 micron at 99.999% efficiency.

ULTRAVIOLET RADIATION CHAMBERS

Some air cleaners use ultraviolet radiation chambers to kill viruses, bacteria, and molds. Radiation is emitted from lamps in shielded chambers. Some ozone is emitted, but FDA prohibits the marketing of any medical device that emits more than 0.05 parts ozone per million parts of air circulating through the device.

Controlling Your Environment

Air Quality

HUMIDIFIERS

When winter comes, the heating system warms the air in the house. As the air becomes warmer, it has the capacity to hold more moisture, but because there actually is no extra moisture in your home, that warm air takes moisture from your body and your furniture. You may find that your lips are chapped and your skin is drier and itchy.

Do not humidify

if your house has a vapor barrier but no insulation.

If your house has no insulation and no vapor barrier (sheets with the plastic, foil, or treated paper facing the inside of the house), moisture escapes directly outdoors.

A humidifier could cause condensation on your walls. If your house was built before 1950, you may have insulation and no vapor barrier. If so, humidifying your home could ruin your insulation.

Units are rated as to how they work in a 70° environment at 30 percent relative humidity by the Association of Home Appliance Manufacturers.

> **Comfortable humidity range is considered to be between 30 and 50 percent, although some sources recommend 10 to 30 percent humidity during winter. A hygrometer measures humidity levels.**

Be careful with your humidifier. Too much moisture in the air encourages mold growth and mite proliferation so use a humidity gauge (hygrometer). Available data indicates that somewhere between 30 and 50 percent is a reasonable range for humidity.

Mites, which can be culprits in asthma and dust allergy thrive with humidity increases over 50 percent. Fungi and molds, which can be culprits in asthma and rhinitis, thrive as humidity increases past 75 percent. Excessively high humidity gives molds a welcoming environment beyond the bathroom and kitchen and into other parts of your home.

WHITE DUST COATING

If you live in a hard water area and use tap water in the humidifier, you may find that the walls and furniture are coated with fine white dust. This dust is the minerals from the water that have been dispersed into the air along

Controlling Your Environment

Air Quality

with the water droplets. This dust settles on the furniture and draperies and you can inhale it.

The Environmental Protection Agency noted that exposure to these white dust particles is a problem for those with asthma.

Distilled water may partially improve the problem. Also available are demineralization cartridges and filters. (These products are listed in the Directory in the chapter, *For the Air*, subchapter *Associated Products*.) You will want to ask about the improvement in particulate levels that these products can produce.

WHAT TO LOOK FOR IN A HUMIDIFIER
✔ CHECK LIST

- Volume controls
- Automatic humidistats
- Ease of filling through a reasonably wide opening
- Ease of cleaning
- 'On' indicator light
- Protective fuses
- Other features:

  indicator that the tank needs refilling

  a tip-over off switch

  a relative humidity gauge.

HUMIDIFIER MAINTENANCE

The water reservoirs in humidifiers can be an ideal environment for bacteria and molds (including fungi), which are then spewed into the air along with the moisture.

Clean and dry the unit whenever you fill it **and** at least weekly, preferably more often, and give it a thorough cleaning with a weak bleach mixture, letting it soak for 30 minutes. Rinse until the bleach smell disappears. If you see mineral deposits, try a fifty-fifty solution of vinegar and water and a brush.

If you have a model with an absorbent pad, rinse it regularly and consider replacing it at least annually.

Controlling Your Environment

Air Quality

Follow any other maintenance instructions the manufacturer might specify. If you have a mold allergy, have someone else do the cleaning.

Most important is to keep your humidifier clean.
Its water reservoir is a hospitable environment for molds, fungi, and bacteria.

FDA RECOMMENDATIONS FOR HUMIDIFIER SAFETY:

✔ CHECK LIST

- If you buy a heated humidifier, look for one with an automatic safety shut-off in case of overheating.

- Do not use a heated humidifier that has shown signs of overheating: smoking, sparking or causing shocks. Have it repaired.

- If the humidifier is used in conjunction with a volume ventilator, use an audible alarm that senses gas temperature in the line that delivers gas to the patient.

- Be sure you follow the service recommendation of the manufacturer. Some of these recommendations may be long term such as replacing the thermoswitch every five years.

- Check power cords for damage inside or outside the unit. Use a strain relief device inside the chassis.

EVAPORATIVE, DRUM, OR BELT CONSOLE HUMIDIFIERS

These types of evaporative humidifiers have a reservoir of water with an absorbent pad that is either on a revolving drum or on a rolling belt.

A wicking humidifier has a fan that blows air through a moisturized filter rather than a pad.

Evaporative humidifiers do not produce spray, but they must be scrupulously maintained.

Air is pulled into the humidifier from the room by a fan and pushed through the wet pad, gaining moisture, and then pushed through vents back into the room. Some units push air through a wet filter; these are wicking humidifiers.

Evaporative humidifiers do not produce spray, but their pads or filters can still breed bacteria and must be

Controlling Your Environment

Air Quality

scrupulously maintained. Their pads must also be changed periodically.

Look for humidistats, ease of cleaning, ease of filling, ease of emptying, protective, small grille openings, 'on' lights.

IMPELLERS

These cool-mist vaporizers fracture water into droplets and spray cool mist into the air. They are actually meant for use in sickrooms. They are noisy and must sit on a plastic tray to protect floors or tables.

These humidifiers spew a white dust and should be used with distilled or soft water or demineralization cartridges.

As with many humidifiers, bacteria and molds grow in their water tanks. The main problem with impellers is that they can spew these bacteria and molds into the air along with their cool mist. This can cause allergic reactions or respiratory problems.

The American Lung Association suggests that you clean the unit daily or when you refill it. Use a diluted bleach mixture.

ULTRASONIC HUMIDIFIERS

Compared to conventional humidifiers and vaporizers, they are very quiet. An electronic transducer produces a cool mist. The transducer is like a token or disk that vibrates at an extremely high rate, vaporizing the water that hits it into a very fine mist.

Ultrasonic humidifiers are very quiet, very effective at humidifying, and can efficiently raise the moisture level of your room.

A fan flings the droplets into the air and you can control the humidification rate. There are few bacteria and no molds in the mist, although there is some question about whether the bits of dead bacteria that are present can cause allergic reactions. There is also the problem of white dust which you can avoid by using distilled or soft water or demineralization cartridges.

An ultrasonic humidifier can handle about 3000 to 5000 cubic feet, depending upon how well insulated your home is. A well-insulated home will lose less of the

126

moisture produced by cooking, bathing, breathing, etc. and will require less added moisture.

You will want to protect your floor or table from moisture with a plastic tray and keep the reservoir clean.

STEAM VAPORIZERS

Steam vaporizers heat water with electrodes to create steam from boiling water. The steam kills the molds and bacteria that can flourish in the holding tanks so no health problem is posed. You can use tap water.

Vaporizers do not provide mist to the lungs. They only help moisten the nasal membranes. Very little white dust is produced because the minerals are generally left in the tank. Since the water minerals are left in the tank, the heating element needs careful cleaning.

Be cautious because of the danger posed by vaporizer steam.

These vaporizers are quiet, but you should be exceedingly cautious because of the danger posed by the steam. Keep away from the steam and be sure your vaporizer cannot be tipped over accidentally. Use extra caution when children are present. Look for child-resistant reservoir covers. Keep out of reach.

WARM MIST HUMIDIFIERS

These units boil water like the steam vaporizers, but cool the steam before allowing it into the air so that the mist is warm.

IN-DUCT HUMIDIFIERS

These humidifiers are installed in the ductwork close to your furnace. They consist of a wet sponge or pad (kept wet because it is connected to your home's water supply) that either sits in water or is constantly wetted by a moving water supply.

They function when the heating system blower is on. Although they do not need to be filled, they do need to be cleaned and can spew germs throughout the entire house.

Controlling Your Environment

Air Quality

DEHUMIDIFIERS

Dehumidifiers lower humidity in an enclosed environment by taking out water from the air. Humid air encourages mold, mildew, and house dust mite growth. This growth is especially noticeable in basements, laundry rooms, bathrooms, and where there are cement floors. With less moisture in the air, you will feel physically cooler and require less air conditioning to make you comfortable.

Depending upon their capacity, dehumidifiers can remove from 10 pints to 50 pints of moisture daily from a room.

How much capacity will you need? Your closet may only require calcium chloride suspended over a large pot. Larger areas will probably need a dehumidifier.

The capacity of a dehumidifier is rated by how many pints of water the dehumidifier can remove in one day (24 hours) at 80 degrees and 60 percent relative humidity.

Depending upon their capacity, dehumidifiers can remove from 10 pints to 50 pints of moisture daily from a room. If your room is moderately humid, you might need a unit with a 10-pint capacity. If that same room were very humid, you might need a unit with a 16-pint capacity.

Look for:

- Automatic shut-offs

- Adjustable, automatic humidistats

- Automatic overflow controls

- Warning lights that tell you when to empty the water container

- Ease of emptying

- Ease of cleaning.

AIR CONDITIONERS

Air conditioners themselves use only a relatively small amount of outside air. When you use them, you can close windows and so prevent pollen from entering your home in large numbers.

Because air conditioners also reduce the humidity level to some extent, their use will also reduce the numbers of mold spores and house dust mites. Remember to keep drip trays clean because molds will grow in them. (Refrigerant systems without drip trays that hold standing water are usually not a problem.) Air conditioner filters trap about 30% at 10 micron.

CAR AIR CONDITIONER ALERT

Some allergic rhinitis and bronchial asthma patients find that their symptoms are worse after they turn on the air conditioners in their cars. This finding was confirmed by culture measurements of mold concentration taken while the air conditioner was turned on.

Putting a filter at the entry of outside air caused a major reduction in mold concentration in the seating areas of the car. Other suggestions are to run the air conditioner for several moments before getting into the car and not aiming the air vents directly on your face.

EQUIPMENT MAINTENANCE

Doing something to the air with air conditioners, heating units, humidifiers, or dehumidifiers makes us more comfortable, but it is important to follow the manufacturer's maintenance and care directions to prevent collections of molds, fungi, and bacteria that can cause or make worse asthmatic and allergic conditions.

Moisture (humidity or water vapor in the air), darkness, and warmth make an especially welcome environment for molds, mildew and fungi indoors as well

as out. You can find them in the refrigerator, in furniture, carpeting, wallpaper, damp cellars, boats, basements, laundry rooms, bathrooms, humidifiers, and air conditioner drip trays.

Humidifiers and small vaporizers use water reservoirs that are hospitable to molds and fungi. These units should be cleaned and dried frequently.

HEAT PUMPS

Heat pumps are two-way streets: they move cold from inside your home to outside in the winter and they move heat from inside your home to outside in the summer. These are an energy-efficient system of heat recovery.

In air to air heat pumps, outside air helps warm coils holding a refrigerant gas that is then pumped indoors. In summer, inside heat is pumped outside. In both seasons,

Controlling Your Environment

Air Quality

the system tries to salvage the appropriate cool or warm air and recirculate it to cut heating or cooling or cooling. Very cold weather can ice the coils and the incoming air may feel cool; air to air heat pumps may function better in milder winter climates.

Quality of installation, reliability of installer, and reliability of maintenance personnel are of utmost importance.

For information about air to air heat exchangers:

Energy Efficiency and Renewable Energy Clearinghouse
PO Box 3048
Merrifield, VA 22116
800-523-2929

In ground source heat pumps, heat is drawn through plastic pipes buried in the ground. A very large surface area of pipes is necessary since the pipes must be buried horizontally or vertically in an area equal to about the square footage of your home.

You need to know about the cooling efficiency (a minimum of 10 for air to air heat pumps), the heating efficiency (a range of 7 to 10), and the heating output compared with the use of electricity to provide that heat (a range of 1.5 to 3.5 for either kind). The higher the number, the better.

Quality of installation and reliability of installer and maintenance personnel are of utmost importance and both should be checked out very carefully.

SUPPLEMENTAL SPACE HEATERS

Forced air heating systems can have problems. It is difficult to keep the ducts free of dust and mold. When you first start the heating system in the late fall or early winter, an accumulation of several months of dust and mold is likely to whoosh through your home. Filters can help, but sometimes it is necessary to close off the vent in a bedroom and use a supplemental heat source.

If you decide to use space heaters, look for one iwht a UL label. As a general precaution, be sure to keep a clear space at least three feet around any such heater. This includes bedding and draperies. You don't want anything to catch fire. Don't put anything on top of the heater.

The wiring in your home should be adequate for the heater's power demand. Portable heaters can use 1,200 watts or more and you don't want to overload the circuit.

Controlling Your Environment

Air Quality

If you use your heater the a bedroom, install a smoke detector.

If you must use an extension cord, be sure it is a heavy, well-insulated one with a #14 or #12 AWG tag. It should not be frayed. Unplug it if it feels hot.

If you need a heater for your bathroom, buy one especially designed for bathrooms. Do not touch it while you are wet.

Be sure your heater has tip-over switch that shuts it off if it should get knocked over or a thermostat to shut it off if it should overheat. Keep children away.

CONVECTION HEATERS

Convection heaters can give you quick room warmth and maintain it at a reasonable comfort level. Fans move room air over warm electric oil and then into the room. When you touch these units, they are not as hot as radiant units. They are small enough to be conveniently portable. Look for a safety tipover switch and an automatic shut-off for over-heating protection.

Because they are filled with oil or water that must first be warmed, liquid-filled convection heaters are heavy and slow to heat.

Surfaces tend to be hot to the touch.

LIQUID-FILLED, CONVECTION HEATERS

These heaters are able to maintain heat levels comfortably. Because they are filled with oil or water that must first be warmed, they are heavy and they are slow to heat. Surfaces tend to be hot to the touch. Look for heaters with a solid base that are less likely to be knocked over. Look for a thermostat control and safety switches.

CERAMIC HEATERS

Ceramic heaters have a ceramic (porcelain) heating element that does not become hot enough to create a fire hazard. Although ceramic heaters can heat a room quickly, they are not as effective in maintaining room temperature.

Controlling Your Environment

Air Quality

RADIANT HEATERS

For heating specific areas, raidant heaters are a good choice. They warm you quickly rather than warm the air around you (unless they have a fan that can blow out heat into the room). Surfaces are hot. Since they can also

Keep children away from radiant heaters and

Keep radiant heaters away from items that can burn

warm furniture or machinery, be careful where they face, especially towards delicate equipment or com-bustible items. Protect any vinyl tile under the unit from the heat. Vacuum the reflector. Keep it clean and dust free.

QUARTZ HEATERS

Another type of spot heater is the quartz heater. It works by heating an electric coil that is inside a quartz (colorless, transparent mineral) container. Be especially careful about using these near fabrics. Because these heaters are so efficient, fires can occur quickly. Horizontal heaters are probably less likely to fall over.

CONCLUSIONS

Devices that manipulate the air we breathe are not cure-alls. There have been few studies on how allergens in the air as opposed to allergens in furniture actually affect individuals.

Other measures of controlling your home environment (discussed in *Controlling Your Home Environment*) should be tried before deciding to buy an air cleaner, humidifier, dehumidifier, or air conditioner.

INFORMATION ON STANDARDS FOR CLEANERS

Standards for in-duct air cleaners:
Air-Conditioning and Refrigeration Institute (ARI)
1501 Wilson Blvd. 6th Flr. (APD)
Arlington, VA 22209

Standards for portable air cleaners:
Send a self-addressed, stamped envelope to:
Assn. of Home Appliance Manufacturers (AHAM)
Air Cleaner Certification Program
20 North Wacker Dr. (APD)
Chicago, IL 60606

Controlling Your Environment

FOR THE AIR

HYBRID FILTERS

Air Sentry

Prefilter traps dust and hair; HEPA filter traps 95% of particles to 0.3 micron including house dust, mold, pollen, and bacteria; carbon filter for vapor and gas control; 2-speed motor; 48 lbs.
Available from:
E.L. Foust Co., Inc.
PO Box 105 (APD)
Elmhurst, IL 60126
800-225-9549
708-834-4952
Fax 708-834-5341

AllerMed Air Purifier

HEPA type filter plus filters to control pollen, mold, dust and odors; carbon tray; steel construction; 360 degree airflow; casters
Available from:
A-Plus Allergy Equipment & Supply
8325 Regis Way (APD)
Los Angeles, CA 90045-2646
Orders 800-86-ALLER (862-5537)
310-337-7468
Fax 310-337-1971

Austin Air Health Mate Plus™

Replaceable carbon/Zeolite filter for odors (other blends available); HEPA filter filters 99.97% particles down to 0.3 micron; range of 1,500 sq. ft.; over 400 CFM; 3-speed motor; casters
Available from:
Absolute Environmental's Allergy Store
2615 S. University Dr. (APD)
Davie, FL 33328
Nationwide 800-771-ACHOO (2246)
In FL 800-329-3773
Broward 305-472-3773
Fax 305-474-0133
and:
N.E.E.D.S.

527 Charles Ave. 12A (APD)
Syracuse, NY 13209
800-634-1380
Fax 800-295-NEED (6333)

Austin Air HealthMate™ Home Air Purifier

HEPA filter removes 99.97% of airborne particles of pollen, dust, smoke, dander; carbon/zeolite filter for gases, odors, vapors; steel casing; 23-1/2"x14-1/2" square; 42 lbs;
Available from:
Allergy Resources
Mail: PO Box 888 (APD)
UPS: 264 Brookridge Ave. (APD)
Palmer Lake, CO 80133
Orders 800-USE-FLAX (873-3529)
Company plans to move; use 800 #
and:
Priorities®
70 Walnut St. (APD)
Wellesley, MA 02181
800-553-5398
and:
Self Care® Catalog
5850 Shellmound St. #390 (APD)
Emeryville, CA 94608-1901
800-345-3371
Fax 800-345-4021

Bionaire® HEPA Air Purifier CH-3550

HEPA filter removes 99.97% of pollen, mold spores, animal hair, dander, dust mites, bacteria, smoke particles, and dust; pre-filter traps larger particles; carbon filter for odors; 4-speed fan; filters 20'x24' room at high speed; 20"x10.5"x27.5"; 39 lbs. Call Bionaire for retailer availability.
Available from:
Bionaire Corp.
90 Boroline Rd. (APD)
Allendale, NJ 07401
80-253-2764
201-934-0755

Controlling Your Environment

For the Air

Bionaire® HEPA Air Purifier SH-1240

HEPA filter removes 99.97% of pollen, mold spores, animal hair, dander, dust mites, bacteria, smoke particles, and dust; pre-filter traps larger particles; carbon filter for odors; 3-speed fan; wall mounts or corner placement; filters 12'x16' room at high speed; 15"x9.4"x14.5"; 11.6 lbs.
Available from:
Bionaire Corp.
90 Boroline Rd. (APD)
Allendale, NJ 07401
80-253-2764
201-934-0755

Bionaire® HEPA Air Purifier SH-1840

HEPA filter removes 99.97% of pollen, mold spores, animal hair, dander, dust mites, bacteria, smoke particles, and dust; pre-filter traps larger particles; carbon filter for odors; 3-speed fan; wall mounts or corner placement; filters 14'x20' room at high speed; 15"x10.4"x14.5"; 12.7 lbs.
Available from:
Bionaire Corp.
90 Boroline Rd. (APD)
Allendale, NJ 07401
80-253-2764
201-934-0755

BREATHEasy 2500

Activated carbon filter and non-woven polyester filter media; HEPA borosilicate glass filter media, 99.97% effective removal of particles to 0.3 micron; optional, second carbon filter; variable air flow 50 to 175 CFM; maximum air flow rate 10,500 cu. ft.; services 200 sq. ft.; portable; hexagonal; baked enamel; 16" wide, 13.5" high; 17 lbs.
Available from:
Allergy Shop, Ltd.
3420 Cardston Crescent N.W. (APD)
Calgary, AB T2L 0S6
Canada
403-289-9052

BREATHEasy 3000

Activated carbon filter and non-woven polyester filter media; HEPA borosilicate glass filter media, 99.97% effective removal of particles to 0.3 micron; optional, second carbon filter; variable air flow 50 to 225 CFM; maximum air flow rate 13,500 cu. ft.; services 400 sq. ft.; portable; hexagonal; baked enamel; 16" wide, 23" high; 25 lbs.
Available from:
Allergy Shop, Ltd.
3420 Cardston Crescent N.W. (APD)
Calgary, AB T2L 0S6
Canada
403-289-9052

BREATHEasy 4000

Activated carbon filter and non-woven polyester filter media; HEPA borosilicate glass filter media, 99.97% effective removal of particles to 0.3 micron; optional, second carbon filter; variable air flow 75 to 300 CFM; maximum air flow rate 18,000 cu. ft.; services 700 sq. ft.; portable; hexagonal; baked enamel; 16" wide, 23" high; 25 lbs.
Available from:
Allergy Shop, Ltd.
3420 Cardston Crescent N.W. (APD)
Calgary, AB T2L 0S6
Canada
403-289-9052

Ceiling-Mount CL1020 Self-Contained

Pre-filter collects large particles; 3 speeds with efficiency range from 85% to 96%, air flow range 650 CFM to 1000 CFM; four optional charcoal filters; mounts on 16"x18" centers; 30"x30"x12 1/2"; 75 lbs.
Available from:
Tectronic Products Co., Inc.
PO Box 157 (APD)
6500 Badgley Rd. (APD)

Controlling Your Environment

For the Air

E. Syracuse, NY 13057-0157
800-227-1375
315-463-0240
Fax 315-437-7290

Chairman 800

Replaceable prefilter, HEPA filter; refillable carbon tray; filters 1,500 sq. ft.; 800 CFM; variable speed; painted or stainless cabinet on carpet casters; 25"x24"x29"
Available from:
Allergy Relief Shop,™ Inc.
3371 Whittle Springs Rd. (APD)
Knoxville, TN 37917
Orders 800-626-2810
Questions 615-522-2795
and:
Allergy Resources
Mail: PO Box 888 (APD)
UPS: 264 Brookridge Ave. (APD)
Palmer Lake, CO 80133
Orders 800-USE-FLAX (873-3529)
Company plans to move; use 800 #
and:
AllerMed Corp.
31 Steel Rd. (APD)
Wylie, TX 75098
214-442-4898
Fax 214-442-4897
and:
Flowright Int'l Products
1495 N.W. Gilman Blvd. #4 (APD)
Issaquah, WA 98027
206-392-8357
and:
N.E.E.D.S.
527 Charles Ave. 12A (APD)
Syracuse, NY 13209
800-634-1380
Fax 800-295-NEED (6333)

Champion Air Purifier

Washable filter for large particles extends pre-filter life; replaceable polyester fiber pre-filter; replaceable HEPA filter removes over 99% of particles down to .5 micron; replaceable carbon filter for smoke, carbon monoxide, and common vapors;

optional UV germicidal fifth stage filter; 300 CFM blower or 18,000 CFH; 14"x14"x23; 50 lbs.; steel cabinet on casters, laboratories, commercial
Available from:
King-Aire®
1121 S.R. 32 E. (APD)
Noblesville, IN 46060
Mail to PO Box 398 (APD)
Noblesville, IN 46060-0398
800-999-KING (5464)
317-776-1600

Cloud 9 Sterile-Aire #150

Replaceable charcoal filter for gases, odors; HEPA filter for pollen, dust, mold, fungus, bacteria, virus, 99.994% effective to 0.3 micron; for rooms up to 150 sq. ft.; 2-speed fan; 23-1/2"x13"x12"; carrying handle, 22 lbs.
Available from:
Allergy Relief Distributors
Div. of E.C.Environmental Control, Inc.
177 Telegraph Rd. #365 (APD)
Bellingham, WA 98226
206-734-1646
Fax 206-734-3696
Canadian office in Vancouver, BC
and:
Cloud 9®
Div. of Mason Engineering Corp.
777 Edgewood Ave. (APD)
Wood Dale, IL 60191
708-595-5000

Cloud 9 Sterile-Aire #300

Replaceable charcoal filter for gases, odors; HEPA filter for pollen, dust, mold, fungus, bacteria, virus, 99.994% effective to 0.3 micron; for rooms up to 300 sq. ft.; 3-speed fan; wall mounting system; 25-1/2"x21"x12"; 39 lbs.
Available from:
Allergy Relief Distributors
Div. of E.C.Environmental Control, Inc.
177 Telegraph Rd. #365 (APD)
Bellingham, WA 98226
206-734-1646

Controlling Your Environment

For the Air

Fax 206-734-3696
Canadian office in Vancouver, BC
and:
Cloud 9®
Div. of Mason Engineering Corp.
777 Edgewood Ave. (APD)
Wood Dale, IL 60191
708-595-5000

CRSI 600HS™

Prefilter for large particles; replaceable carbon filter for odors and vapors; attaches to furnace or air conditioning system; HEPA filter effective to 0.3 micron at 99.97% efficiency; removes fumes, odors, gaseous contaminants, smoke, lints, pollen, mold, spores, some viruses; 18 guage sheet metal; 100 lbs.
Available from:
Environtrol® Corporation
PO Box 31313 (APD)
St. Louis, MO 63131
800-423-1982
In St. Louis 314-966-6886

Dust Guzzler 200

Washable filter for large particles extends pre-filter life; replaceable polyester fiber pre-filter; replaceable HEPA filter removes over 99% of particles down to .5 micron; optional UV germicidal fourth stage filter; 200 CFM blower or 12,000 CFH; 13"x13"x24; 35 lbs.; steel cabinet on casters, laboratories, commercial
Available from:
King-Aire®
1121 S.R. 32 E. (APD)
Noblesville, IN 46060
Mail to PO Box 398 (APD)
Noblesville, IN 46060-0398
800-999-KING (5464)
317-776-1600

Flush-Mount FM1400 Self-Contained

Pre-filter collects large particles; 4 speeds with efficiency range from 85% to 96%, air flow range 250 CFM to 1400 CFM; two optional charcoal filters; replaces 2'x4' ceiling panel; 23 5/8"x47 5/8"x13 1/2"; 95 lbs.
Available from:
Tectronic Products Co., Inc.
PO Box 157 (APD)
6500 Badgley Rd. (APD)
E. Syracuse, NY 13057-0157
800-227-1375
315-463-0240
Fax 315-437-7290

Flush-Mount FM500 Self-Contained

Pre-filter collects large particles; 4 speeds with efficiency range from 85% to 96%, air flow range 100 CFM to 500 CFM; optional charcoal filter; replaces 2'x2' ceiling panel; 23 5/8"x25 5/8"x12"; 47 lbs.
Available from:
Tectronic Products Co., Inc.
PO Box 157 (APD)
6500 Badgley Rd. (APD)
E. Syracuse, NY 13057-0157
800-227-1375
315-463-0240
Fax 315-437-7290

Freedom Air Purifier

Replaceable polyester fiber pre-filter; replaceable HEPA filter removes over 99% of particles down to .5 micron; replaceable carbon filter for smoke, carbon monoxide, and common vapors; 200 CFM blower or 12,000 CFH; 12"x12"x22"; 30 lbs.; poplar, brass cabinet
Available from:
King-Aire®
1121 S.R. 32 E. (APD)
Noblesville, IN 46060
Mail to PO Box 398 (APD)
Noblesville, IN 46060-0398
800-999-KING (5464)

Controlling Your Environment

For the Air

317-776-1600

Guardian Air Purifier

Replaceable polyester fiber pre-filter; replaceable HEPA filter removes over 99% of particles down to .5 micron, measured by ASHRAE 52-70 method; replaceable carbon filter for smoke, carbon monoxide, and common vapors; 300 CFM blower or 18,000 CFH; 16"x16"x23"; 50 lbs.; oak, brass cabinet
Available from:
King-Aire®
1121 S.R. 32 E. (APD)
Noblesville, IN 46060
Mail to PO Box 398 (APD)
Noblesville, IN 46060-0398
800-999-KING (5464)
317-776-1600

Haven

Replaceable prefilter; odor-reduction filter; replaceable HEPA filter; 360 degrees air flow; 225 CFM; cleans up to 425 sq. ft.; wheel casters, enameled steel cabinet; 24"x16"x16"; 52 lbs.
Available from:
Allergy Resources
Mail: PO Box 888 (APD)
UPS: 264 Brookridge Ave. (APD)
Palmer Lake, CO 80133
Orders 800-USE-FLAX (873-3529)
Company plans to move; use 800 #

Hepanaire® HP50 Air Cleaner

Washable prefilter; replaceable HEPA filter efficient to 98% on .5 micron and 95% on .3 micron; replaceable, optional activated carbon filter for odors; continuously variable airflower from 100 to 200 CFM; circulates the air in a room 12x20x8 ft. 6 times per hour; ozone-free; household current; on-off switch; vinyl-clad cabinet; 19-1/2"x20-5/8"x14-5/8"; 37.5 lbs.
Available from:
Summit Hill Laboratories

Ship to 429 Highway 36 (APD)
Mail to PO Box 535 (APD)
Navesink, NJ 07752
800-922-0722
201-291-3600

Honeywell Enviracaire® 13500 Series (EV-35)

Replaceable charcoal filter; replaceable HEPA filter effective down to 0.3 micron at 99.97% efficiency; 360 degrees air intake, output; filters tobacco smoke, pollen, mold spores, bacteria, viruses, animal hair, dander, dust mite allergens; 3-speed fan to 350 CFM; ozone-free; 14" high by 16" diameter; 15.5 lbs.
Available from:
AAir Purification Systems
7340 Trade St. #C (APD)
San Diego, CA 92121-2457
800-776-6746
619-578-2825
Fax 619-578-3762
and:
Allergy Control Products, Inc.
96 Danbury Rd. (APD)
PO Box 793 (APD)
Ridgefield, CT 06877
800-422-DUST (3878)
203-438-9580
Fax 203-431-8963

Honeywell F59A Electronic Air Cleaner

Washable electronic filter traps pollen, dust, tobacco smoke, pollen; washable pre-filter screen traps larger particles; replaceable carbon filter adsorbs odors; 3-speed fan; up to 330 CFM on high speed; CADR=290 for dust, CADRE=250 for tobacco smoke, CADRE=240 for pollen; dark oak wood grain, light oak wood grain
Available from:
Honeywell, Inc.
Home and Building Control
Honeywell Plaza
PO Box 524 (APD)
Minneapolis, MN 55440-0524

Controlling Your Environment

For the Air

612-951-1000
and
Honeywell, Inc.
740 Ellesmere Rd. (APD)
Scarborough, ON, M1P 2V9
Canada

Honeywell/Enviracaire® 10500 Series EV-10

Traps pollen, mold, animal hair, dander, dust mite allergens, bactria, some viruses, tobacco smoke, odors, soot, and non-toxic fumes; HEPA filter 99.97% efficiency to 0.3 micron; replaceable polyester-based activated carbon mixture; 360 degrees airflow at 55 and 85 CFM; filters 5,100 cu. ft. per hr. or four changes per hour in a 10'x16' room; 9.5"tall by 14.5" diameter; 10 lbs.
Available locally in various department and home center stores and
Available from:
AAir Purification Systems
7340 Trade St. #C (APD)
San Diego, CA 92121-2457
800-776-6746
619-578-2825
Fax 619-578-3762
and:
Allergy Asthma Technology
4151 N. Kedzie (APD)
PO Box 18398 (APD)
Chicago, IL 60618
800-621-5545
312-465-8020
Fax 312-465-7619
and:
Allergy Control Products, Inc.
96 Danbury Rd. (APD)
PO Box 793 (APD)
Ridgefield, CT 06877
800-422-DUST (3878)
203-438-9580
Fax 203-431-8963
and:
Appliance Sales & Service Co.
655 Mission St. (APD)
San Francisco, CA 94105
800-424-6783

In 415 area call 415-362-7195

Honeywell/Enviracaire® 11500 Series EV-15

Replaceable polyester-based activated carbon mixture prefilter; HEPA filter effective down to 0.3 micron at 99.97% efficiency; 150 CFM; filter rate is 9,000 cu. ft./hr.; 360 degrees air intake, output; filters tobacco smoke, pollen, mold spores, bacteria, viruses, animal hair, dander, dust mite allergens; ozone-free; 11" high x16" diameter; 11 lbs.
Available from:
AAir Purification Systems
7340 Trade St. #C (APD)
San Diego, CA 92121-2457
800-776-6746
619-578-2825
Fax 619-578-3762
and:
Allergy Control Products, Inc.
96 Danbury Rd. (APD)
PO Box 793 (APD)
Ridgefield, CT 06877
800-422-DUST (3878)
203-438-9580
Fax 203-431-8963

Honeywell/Enviracaire® 12500 Series 12520 (EV-25)

Replaceable polyester-based activated carbon mixture prefilter; replaceable HEPA filter effective down to 0.3 micron at 99.97% efficiency; variable speed, 120 to 250 CFM; filter rate 15,000 cu. ft./hr; 360 degrees air intake, output; filters tobacco smoke, pollen, mold spores, bacteria, viruses, animal hair, dander, dust mite allergens; ozone-free; 12" high x 16" diameter; 12 lbs.
Available from:
AAir Purification Systems
7340 Trade St. #C (APD)
San Diego, CA 92121-2457
800-776-6746
619-578-2825
Fax 619-578-3762

Controlling Your Environment

For the Air

and:
Allergy Asthma Technology
4151 N. Kedzie (APD)
PO Box 18398 (APD)
Chicago, IL 60618
800-621-5545
312-465-8020
Fax 312-465-7619
and:
Allergy Control Products, Inc.
96 Danbury Rd. (APD)
PO Box 793 (APD)
Ridgefield, CT 06877
800-422-DUST (3878)
203-438-9580
Fax 203-431-8963
and:
Allergy Supply Co.
11994 Star Court (APD)
Herndon, VA 22071
800-323-6744
Metropolitan DC 703-391-2011
Fax 703-391-2014
BBS 703-521-0638
and:
Appliance Sales & Service Co.
655 Mission St. (APD)
San Francisco, CA 94105
800-424-6783
In 415 area call 415-362-7195
and:
Brookstone Co.
5 Vose Farm Road (APD)
Peterborough, NH 03458
800-926-7000
Fax 603-924-0093
and:
Honeywell/Enviracaire®
Honeywell Environmental Air Control
100 Jamison Ct. (APD)
Hagerstown, MD 21740-5185
800-332-1110
and:
National Allergy Supply, Inc.
4400 Georgia Hwy. 120 (APD)
PO Box 1658 (APD)
Duluth, GA 30136
800-522-1448
In Atlanta 404-623-8077
Fax 404-623-5568

and:
Skin & Allergy Shop,™ The
310 E. Broadway (APD)
Louisville, KY 40202
800-366-6483
In KY 502-585-4824
Fax 502-589-3429

Honeywell/Enviracaire® 13500 Series 13520 (EV-35)

Replaceable polyester-based activated carbon mixture prefilter; HEPA filter effective down to 0.3 micron at 99.97% efficiency; variable speed, 150, 250, 350 CFM; filter rate is 21,000 cu. ft./hr.; 360 degrees air intake, output; filters tobacco smoke, pollen, mold spores, bacteria, viruses, animal hair, dander, dust mite allergens; ozone-free; 14" high x 17" diameter; 14 lbs.
Available from:
Allergy Asthma Technology
4151 N. Kedzie (APD)
PO Box 18398 (APD)
Chicago, IL 60618
800-621-5545
312-465-8020
Fax 312-465-7619
and:
Allergy Control Products, Inc.
96 Danbury Rd. (APD)
PO Box 793 (APD)
Ridgefield, CT 06877
800-422-DUST (3878)
203-438-9580
Fax 203-431-8963
and:
Allergy Supply Co.
11994 Star Court (APD)
Herndon, VA 22071
800-323-6744
Metropolitan DC 703-391-2011
Fax 703-391-2014
BBS 703-521-0638
and:
American Allergy Supply
PO Box 722022 (APD)
Houston, TX 77272-2022
800-321-1096

Controlling Your Environment

For the Air

713-995-6110
and:
Appliance Sales & Service Co.
655 Mission St. (APD)
San Francisco, CA 94105
800-424-6783
In 415 area call 415-362-7195
and:
Honeywell/Enviracaire®
Honeywell Environmental Air Control
100 Jamison Ct. (APD)
Hagerstown, MD 21740-5185
800-332-1110
and:
National Allergy Supply, Inc.
4400 Georgia Hwy. 120 (APD)
PO Box 1658 (APD)
Duluth, GA 30136
800-522-1448
In Atlanta 404-623-8077
Fax 404-623-5568
and:
Skin & Allergy Shop,™ The
310 E. Broadway (APD)
Louisville, KY 40202
800-366-6483
In KY 502-585-4824
Fax 502-589-3429

Honeywell/Enviracaire® 61500

Portable room air cleaner; replaceable HEPA filter; replaceable charcoal prefilter; 2-speed fan up to 150 CFM; 10" tall by 16" diameter; 11.5 lbs.
Available from:
AAir Purification Systems
7340 Trade St. #C (APD)
San Diego, CA 92121-2457
800-776-6746
619-578-2825
Fax 619-578-3762
and:
Allergy Clean Environments
501 Station Ave. (APD)
Haddon Heights, NJ 08035
800-882-4110
In NJ 609-546-1101
Fax 609-546-1466
URL:

http:\\WWW.infomall.com\allergy.html
and:
Honeywell/Enviracaire®
Honeywell Environmental Air Control
100 Jamison Ct. (APD)
Hagerstown, MD 21740-5185
800-332-1110
and:
National Allergy Supply, Inc.
4400 Georgia Hwy. 120 (APD)
PO Box 1658 (APD)
Duluth, GA 30136
800-522-1448
In Atlanta 404-623-8077
Fax 404-623-5568

Honeywell/Enviracaire® 62500

Portable room air cleaner; replaceable HEPA filter; replaceable charcoal prefilter; 3-speed fan up to 250 CFM; 12" tall by 16" diameter; 13.5 lbs.
Available from:
AAir Purification Systems
7340 Trade St. #C (APD)
San Diego, CA 92121-2457
800-776-6746
619-578-2825
Fax 619-578-3762
and:
Allergy Clean Environments
501 Station Ave. (APD)
Haddon Heights, NJ 08035
800-882-4110
In NJ 609-546-1101
Fax 609-546-1466
URL:
http:\\WWW.infomall.com\allergy.html
and:
Honeywell/Enviracaire®
Honeywell Environmental Air Control
100 Jamison Ct. (APD)
Hagerstown, MD 21740-5185
800-332-1110
and:
National Allergy Supply, Inc.
4400 Georgia Hwy. 120 (APD)
PO Box 1658 (APD)
Duluth, GA 30136
800-522-1448

Controlling Your Environment

For the Air

In Atlanta 404-623-8077
Fax 404-623-5568

Honeywell/Enviracaire® 63200

Charcoal prefilter; HEPA filter, CPZ™(carbon, alumina potassium permangate, zeolite) filled canister; synthetic fiber final filter for airborne pollen and mold spores, bacteria and viruses, animal hair and dander, dust, fibers, dust mite allergens, smoke; removes over 85% of gases and odors from wood smoke, formaldehyde, hair sprays and nail polishes, hydrocarbons, ammonia, smog, tobacco smoke and cooking odors, printing inks, paint, and thinners, glues and adhesives; 3-speed fan to 300 CFM; 15" tall by 16" diameter; 21 lbs.
Available from:
AAir Purification Systems
7340 Trade St. #C (APD)
San Diego, CA 92121-2457
800-776-6746
619-578-2825
Fax 619-578-3762
and:
Allergy Clean Environments
501 Station Ave. (APD)
Haddon Heights, NJ 08035
800-882-4110
In NJ 609-546-1101
Fax 609-546-1466
URL:
http:\\WWW.infomall.com\allergy.html
and:
Allergy Control Products, Inc.
96 Danbury Rd. (APD)
PO Box 793 (APD)
Ridgefield, CT 06877
800-422-DUST (3878)
203-438-9580
Fax 203-431-8963
and:
Honeywell/Enviracaire®
Honeywell Environmental Air Control
100 Jamison Ct. (APD)
Hagerstown, MD 21740-5185
800-332-1110

Honeywell/Enviracaire® 63500

Portable room air cleaner; replaceable HEPA filter; replaceable charcoal prefilter; 3-speed fan up to 350 CFM; 14" tall by 16" diameter; 15.5 lbs.
Available from:
AAir Purification Systems
7340 Trade St. #C (APD)
San Diego, CA 92121-2457
800-776-6746
619-578-2825
Fax 619-578-3762
and:
Allergy Clean Environments
501 Station Ave. (APD)
Haddon Heights, NJ 08035
800-882-4110
In NJ 609-546-1101
Fax 609-546-1466
URL:
http:\\WWW.infomall.com\allergy.html
and:
Honeywell/Enviracaire®
Honeywell Environmental Air Control
100 Jamison Ct. (APD)
Hagerstown, MD 21740-5185
800-332-1110
and:
National Allergy Supply, Inc.
4400 Georgia Hwy. 120 (APD)
PO Box 1658 (APD)
Duluth, GA 30136
800-522-1448
In Atlanta 404-623-8077
Fax 404-623-5568

Honeywell/Enviracaire® 64500

Portable room air cleaner; replaceable HEPA filter; replaceable charcoal prefilter; 3-speed fan up to 400 CFM; 16"tall by 16" diameter; 17-1/2 lbs.
Available from:
AAir Purification Systems
7340 Trade St. #C (APD)
San Diego, CA 92121-2457
800-776-6746
619-578-2825
Fax 619-578-3762

Controlling Your Environment

For the Air

and:
Allergy Asthma Technology
4151 N. Kedzie (APD)
PO Box 18398 (APD)
Chicago, IL 60618
800-621-5545
312-465-8020
Fax 312-465-7619
and:
Allergy Clean Environments
501 Station Ave. (APD)
Haddon Heights, NJ 08035
800-882-4110
In NJ 609-546-1101
Fax 609-546-1466
URL:
http:\\WWW.infomall.com\allergy.html
and:
Honeywell/Enviracaire®
Honeywell Environmental Air Control
100 Jamison Ct. (APD)
Hagerstown, MD 21740-5185
800-332-1110
and:
National Allergy Supply, Inc.
4400 Georgia Hwy. 120 (APD)
PO Box 1658 (APD)
Duluth, GA 30136
800-522-1448
In Atlanta 404-623-8077
Fax 404-623-5568

Hunter Air Purifier

Replaceable micro filtrete™
material removes up to 99.999%
airborne allergen particles; carbon
filter for odors; 3-speed fan; automatic
shut-off
Available from:
Allergy Control Products, Inc.
96 Danbury Rd. (APD)
PO Box 793 (APD)
Ridgefield, CT 06877
800-422-DUST (3878)
203-438-9580
Fax 203-431-8963

Pollenex Health Aire® PA500R

HEPA filter, 99.97% efficient at 0.3
micron; replaceable, activated carbon

pre-filter; 360 degree filter output;
cleans over 12,000 cu. ft. of air every
hour; 6 cleanings per hour for a
16'x20' room; programmable timer with
LED clock; variable speeds to 235
CFM; rollers
Available from:
Absolute Environmental's Allergy Store
2615 S. University Dr. (APD)
Davie, FL 33328
Nationwide 800-771-ACHOO (2246)
In FL 800-329-3773
Broward 305-472-3773
Fax 305-474-0133
and:
Allergy-Asthma Shopper™
PO Box 239 (APD)
Fate, TX 75132
800-447-1100
Fax 903-883-4513

Portable PT150 Table-Top

Washable pre-filter collects large
particles; replaceable charcoal filter;
removes up to 96% of dust, pollen,
smoke; variable speed with efficiency
range from 85% to 96%, air flow range
10 CFM to 150 CFM; 6"x14"x12";
standard household outlet; woodgrain
design; 18 lbs.
Available from:
Tectronic Products Co., Inc.
PO Box 157 (APD)
6500 Badgley Rd. (APD)
E. Syracuse, NY 13057-0157
800-227-1375
315-463-0240
Fax 315-437-7290

Portable PT410 Console

Washable pre-filter collects large
particles; replaceable charcoal filter;
removes up to 96% of dust, pollen,
smoke; variable speed with efficiency
range from 85% to 96%, air flow range
10 CFM to 400 CFM; portable or wall
mounted; 23"x21"x12"; standard
household outlet; woodgrain design;
45 lbs.
Available from:

Controlling Your Environment

For the Air

Tectronic Products Co., Inc.
PO Box 157 (APD)
6500 Badgley Rd. (APD)
E. Syracuse, NY 13057-0157
800-227-1375
315-463-0240
Fax 315-437-7290

Portable PT800 Console

Washable pre-filter collects large particles; replaceable charcoal filter; removes up to 96% of dust, pollen, smoke; variable speed with efficiency range from 85% to 96%, air flow range 50 CFM to 800 CFM; portable or wall mounted; 27"x24"x13"; standard household outlet; woodgrain design; 80 lbs.
Available from:
Tectronic Products Co., Inc.
PO Box 157 (APD)
6500 Badgley Rd. (APD)
E. Syracuse, NY 13057-0157
800-227-1375
315-463-0240
Fax 315-437-7290

Recessed/Wall-Mount CL1220 Self-Contained

Pre-filter collects large particles; variable speed control with efficiency range from 85% to 96%, air flow range 50 CFM to 800 CFM; two optional charcoal filters; can be recessed, on ceiling, surface, or wall-mounted, replaces 2'x2' ceiling panel; 23-5/8"x23-5/8"x12"; 48 lbs.
Available from:
Tectronic Products Co., Inc.
PO Box 157 (APD)
6500 Badgley Rd. (APD)
E. Syracuse, NY 13057-0157
800-227-1375
315-463-0240
Fax 315-437-7290

Series 400 System

Pleated prefilters, HEPA filter, and pollutant filter for pollen, tobacco smoke, mold, bacteria, formaldehyde,

ozone, smoke, and fumes; top loaded components avoids air leakage; 2-speed motor
Available from:
E.L. Foust Co., Inc.
PO Box 105 (APD)
Elmhurst, IL 60126
800-225-9549
708-834-4952
Fax 708-834-5341

Space Saver 400

Replaceable prefilter, HEPA filter; refillable carbon tray; filters 750 sq. ft.; 400 CFM; variable speed; painted or stainless cabinet on carpet casters; 12"x25"x27"
Available from:
Allergy Relief Shop,™ Inc.
3371 Whittle Springs Rd. (APD)
Knoxville, TN 37917
Orders 800-626-2810
Questions 615-522-2795
and:
Allergy Resources
Mail: PO Box 888 (APD)
UPS: 264 Brookridge Ave. (APD)
Palmer Lake, CO 80133
Orders 800-USE-FLAX (873-3529)
Company plans to move; use 800 #
and:
AllerMed Corp.
31 Steel Rd. (APD)
Wylie, TX 75098
214-442-4898
Fax 214-442-4897
and:
Flowright Int'l Products
1495 N.W. Gilman Blvd. #4 (APD)
Issaquah, WA 98027
206-392-8357

Tectronic Furnace-Mount Air Cleaner TFM 1625E, E1

Cleanable pre-filter for lint, hair, dust, and large particles; washable electronic collector; replaceable charcoal filter for gas adsorption; duct size 16"x25"; up to 1400 CFM; 35 lbs.
Available from:

Controlling Your Environment

For the Air

Tectronic Products Co., Inc.
PO Box 157 (APD)
6500 Badgley Rd. (APD)
E. Syracuse, NY 13057-0157
800-227-1375
315-463-0240
Fax 315-437-7290

Tectronic Furnace-Mount Air Cleaner TFM 2020E, E1

Cleanable pre-filter for lint, hair, dust, and large particles; washable electronic collector; replaceable charcoal filter for gas adsorption; duct size 20"x20"; up to 2000 CFM; 37 lbs.
Available from:
Tectronic Products Co., Inc.
PO Box 157 (APD)
6500 Badgley Rd. (APD)
E. Syracuse, NY 13057-0157
800-227-1375
315-463-0240
Fax 315-437-7290

Tectronic Furnace-Mount Air Cleaner TFM 2025E, E1

Cleanable pre-filter for lint, hair, dust, and large particles; washable electronic collector; replaceable charcoal filter for gas adsorption; duct size 20"x25"; up to 2000 CFM; 41 lbs.
Available from:
Tectronic Products Co., Inc.
PO Box 157 (APD)
6500 Badgley Rd. (APD)
E. Syracuse, NY 13057-0157
800-227-1375
315-463-0240
Fax 315-437-7290

Thurmond Whole House Heating/Cooling/Filtration System

High efficiency heating and cooling system with HEPA filter, 95-99.997% at 0.3 micron); charcoal and other adsorbent filters available and steam humidification and dehumidification
Available from:
Allergy-Asthma Shopper™
PO Box 239 (APD)

Fate, TX 75132
800-447-1100
Fax 903-883-4513

Ultra Aire 1000

Pre filter, post filter, carbon filter, HEPA filter; filters 1,200 sq. ft. with variable speed to 1,000 CFM
Available from:
Flowright Int'l Products
1495 N.W. Gilman Blvd. #4 (APD)
Issaquah, WA 98027
206-392-8357

Ultra Aire Central System 2000

Central home system with prefilter, carbon filter, HEPA filter
Available from:
Flowright Int'l Products
1495 N.W. Gilman Blvd. #4 (APD)
Issaquah, WA 98027
206-392-8357

Ultra Safe

Air cleaner with vacuum attachment for computers, reading boxes; 350 CFM; filters 650 sq. ft.; filtered motor, intake has washable prefilter and exhaust chamber has prefilter, carbon filter; HEPA filter; blower; commercial use, stainless steel case, casters; 27"x25"x12"
Available from:
Allergy Relief Shop,™ Inc.
3371 Whittle Springs Rd. (APD)
Knoxville, TN 37917
Orders 800-626-2810
Questions 615-522-2795
and:
AllerMed Corp.
31 Steel Rd. (APD)
Wylie, TX 75098
214-442-4898
Fax 214-442-4897
and:
Flowright Int'l Products
1495 N.W. Gilman Blvd. #4 (APD)
Issaquah, WA 98027
206-392-8357

Controlling Your Environment

For the Air

VH-300

Chemical carbon filters before and after motor; HEPA filter, prefilter; filters 250 sq. ft.; airflow 135 CFM; variable speed; stainless cabinet; 12"x12"x24"
Available from:
Allergy Relief Shop,™ Inc.
3371 Whittle Springs Rd. (APD)
Knoxville, TN 37917
Orders 800-626-2810
Questions 615-522-2795
and:
Allergy Resources
Mail: PO Box 888 (APD)
UPS: 264 Brookridge Ave. (APD)
Palmer Lake, CO 80133
Orders 800-USE-FLAX (873-3529)
Company plans to move; use 800 #
and:
AllerMed Corp.
31 Steel Rd. (APD)
Wylie, TX 75098
214-442-4898
Fax 214-442-4897
and:
Flowright Int'l Products
1495 N.W. Gilman Blvd. #4 (APD)
Issaquah, WA 98027
206-392-8357

HEPA FILTERS

600 HEPA SHIELD

Removes 99.97 % of all airborne particles 0.3 micron and larger; filters pollen, bacteria, fungi, dust, mold, dander, and tobacco smoke; connects to forced air furnace or air conditioning system; disposable pre-filter, activated carbon filter
Available from:
Pure Air Systems, Inc.
425 Duffey St. (APD)
PO Box 418 (APD)
Plainfield, IN 46168
800-869-8025
317-839-9135
Fax 317-839-8567

CompanionAire®

Travel filter; 3 stage filters with HEPA and chemical/odor filtration; filters 170 sq. ft; airflow 90 CFM; carrying handle; 3-speed motor; 12"x8"x7-1/2"' 9 lbs.
Available from:
Allergy Relief Shop,™ Inc.
3371 Whittle Springs Rd. (APD)
Knoxville, TN 37917
Orders 800-626-2810
Questions 615-522-2795
and:
Flowright Int'l Products
1495 N.W. Gilman Blvd. #4 (APD)
Issaquah, WA 98027
206-392-8357
and:
N.E.E.D.S.
527 Charles Ave. 12A (APD)
Syracuse, NY 13209
800-634-1380
Fax 800-295-NEED (6333)

Integrated Blower Filter

HEPA filter with efficiency of 99.99% on particles to 0.3 micron; prefilter; variable motor speed from 45 to 130 fpm at 65 db; blower; ceiling hang on supports or duct collar available; aluminum; 2'x4'; 48 lbs.
Available from:
Clean Room Products, Inc.
1800 Ocean Ave. (APD)
Ronkonkoma, NY 11779
516-588-7000
Fax 516-588-7863

Vitaire® Model H-200

Traps dust, pollen, mold spores, dog and cat hair, tobacco smoke, air pollution particles, many household odors; removes 99+% of all pollen and up to 99+% of other particulates; variable speed motor with automatic reset air air flow range 50 CFM to 200 CFM; cleans room up to 500 sq. ft.; wood composition with wood grain overlay; 20"x15"x14"; 31 lbs.
Available from:

Controlling Your Environment

For the Air

Aller-Guard,® Inc.
Southgate Office Park
1645 S.W. 41st St. (APD)
Topeka, KS 66609-1250
800-234-0816
913-267-9333
Fax 913-267-0072
and:
Environtrol® Corporation
PO Box 31313 (APD)
St. Louis, MO 63131
800-423-1982
In St. Louis 314-966-6886
and:
Vitaire Corp.
PO Box 88 (APD)
Elmhurst Annex, NY 11380
800-447-4344
201-473-2244

ELECTROSTATIC PRECIPITATORS

DUST-Magnet 90

Washable electrostatic air filter removes 90% of air-borne particles, 90 to 99% of most pollen and plant spores; replaces heater or air conditioner filter; aluminum frame; standard or custom sizes
Available from:
Allergy Supply Co.
11994 Star Court (APD)
Herndon, VA 22071
800-323-6744
Metropolitan DC 703-391-2011
Fax 703-391-2014
BBS 703-521-0638

Honeywell F50E Series Electronic Air Cleaner

Four sizes with capacity varying from 1,000 CFM to 2,000 CFM; up to 95% efficient; 1 or 2 electronic cells and 1 or 2 prefilters; washable cells; optional performance indicator; mounts in return air duct of a forced air heating, cooling, or ventilating system; galvanized cabinet, access door, solid state power supply
Available locally in various department and home center stores and
Available from:
Honeywell, Inc.
Home and Building Control
Honeywell Plaza
PO Box 524 (APD)
Minneapolis, MN 55440-0524
612-951-1000
and
Honeywell, Inc.
740 Ellesmere Rd. (APD)
Scarborough, ON, M1P 2V9
Canada

Smokemaster® C-12

For smoke and airborne particulates; removeable prefilters and grille; washable filters; optional wall mount kit and remote three-speed switch plate assembly; up to 1,250 CFM; effective down to .01 micron with 97% efficiency
Available from:
Air Quality Engineering, Inc.
3340 Winpark Dr. (APD)
Minneapolis, MN 55427-2083
800-328-0787
612-544-4426
Fax 612-544-4013

Smokemaster® F61

In-duct model for industrial airborne contaminates and airborne particulates in commercial uses; up to 12,000 CFM; automatic in-place wash system; weights vary depending upon number of filters
Available from:
Air Quality Engineering, Inc.
3340 Winpark Dr. (APD)
Minneapolis, MN 55427-2083
800-328-0787
612-544-4426
Fax 612-544-4013

Controlling Your Environment

For the Air

Smokemaster® F62A

Filters particulates and smoke and recirculates air; three-speed switch; up to 2,500 CFM; 2 washable filters; prefilter; vents from the bottom; commercial use; 225 lbs.
Available from:
Air Quality Engineering, Inc.
3340 Winpark Dr. (APD)
Minneapolis, MN 55427-2083
800-328-0787
612-544-4426
Fax 612-544-4013

Smokemaster® F62B

Filters particulates and smoke and recirculates air; three-speed switch; up to 2,500 CFM; 2 washable filters; prefilter; vents from the top; commercial use; 225 lbs.
Available from:
Air Quality Engineering, Inc.
3340 Winpark Dr. (APD)
Minneapolis, MN 55427-2083
800-328-0787
612-544-4426
Fax 612-544-4013

Smokemaster® F66V

Wheel-mounted for particulates and fumes; up to 1,300 CFM; washable filters; prefilter; industrial use; 396 lbs. or 528 lbs. for second work station use
Available from:
Air Quality Engineering, Inc.
3340 Winpark Dr. (APD)
Minneapolis, MN 55427-2083
800-328-0787
612-544-4426
Fax 612-544-4013

Smokemaster® X-11Q

Washable collector; three-speed motor; airborne particulates, including smoke; mounts flush in 2x4 drop ceiling panel; cleans up to 1,100 cu. ft. per minute
Available from:
Air Quality Engineering, Inc.
3340 Winpark Dr. (APD)
Minneapolis, MN 55427-2083
800-328-0787
612-544-4426
Fax 612-544-4013

Smokemaster® X-400

Washable collector; airborne particulates, including smoke; mounts flush in 2x2 drop ceiling pannel; cleans up to 400 cu. ft. per minute
Available from:
Air Quality Engineering, Inc.
3340 Winpark Dr. (APD)
Minneapolis, MN 55427-2083
800-328-0787
612-544-4426
Fax 612-544-4013

ADSORBING FILTERS

AIREOX® Air Purifier 45

Portable for gases and particles; up to 2,000 cu. ft. every 15 minutes; two-speed motor; blower; carbon; one micron particle filter, optional 0.5 micron particle filter; 125 CFM; floor or table; replaceable cartridges
Available from:
A-Plus Allergy Equipment & Supply
8325 Regis Way (APD)
Los Angeles, CA 90045-2646
Orders 800-86-ALLER (862-5537)
310-337-7468
Fax 310-337-1971
and:
Aireox Research Corp.
11015 Whitford Ave. (APD)
Riverside, CA 92505
909-689-2781
and:

Controlling Your Environment

For the Air

N.E.E.D.S.
527 Charles Ave. 12A (APD)
Syracuse, NY 13209
800-634-1380
Fax 800-295-NEED (6333)

Auto Air Purifier 160A

3 lbs. of media (customer choice) cleans 500 cu. ft. car interior; plugs into cigarette lighter; 5 amps.; 9 lbs.
Available from:
E.L. Foust Co., Inc.
PO Box 105 (APD)
Elmhurst, IL 60126
800-225-9549
708-834-4952
Fax 708-834-5341

Desktop Air Purifier 160DT

3 lbs. of media (customer choice) cleans up to 150 sq. ft.; 10 lbs.
Available from:
E.L. Foust Co., Inc.
PO Box 105 (APD)
Elmhurst, IL 60126
800-225-9549
708-834-4952
Fax 708-834-5341

Foust Room Air Purifier 160R2

7 lbs. of media (various types) cleans up to 400 sq. ft.; 75% efficient to 1 micron; 18 lbs.
Available from:
E.L. Foust Co., Inc.
PO Box 105 (APD)
Elmhurst, IL 60126
800-225-9549
708-834-4952
Fax 708-834-5341

Riga-Sorb™ 25D

Replaceable, activated, replaceable carbon filter adsorbs exhaust, bacterial, bleaching, camphor, chemicals, fish, floral, food, fumes, mold, oils, ozone, perfumes, and gas odors; 25% odor removal efficiency; side access applications for multiple filter housing

Available from:
Farr Co.
PO Box 92187 (APD)
Airport Station
Los Angeles, CA 90009
800-333-7320
Fax 800-441-0003
and
Farr Co.
500 S. Main Street (APD)
Crystal Lake, IL 60014
800-777-5260
Fax 800-441-0103

Riga-Sorb™ 25R

Rechargeable cell can be serviced in house or at factory; activated carbon filter adsorbs exhaust, bacterial, bleaching, camphor, chemicals, fish, floral, food, fumes, mold, oils, ozone, perfumes, and gas odors; 25% odor removal efficiency; side access applications for multiple filter housing
Available from:
Farr Co.
PO Box 92187 (APD)
Airport Station
Los Angeles, CA 90009
800-333-7320
Fax 800-441-0003
and
Farr Co.
500 S. Main Street (APD)
Crystal Lake, IL 60014
800-777-5260
Fax 800-441-0103

Riga-Sorb™ 80D

Replaceable, activated carbon filter adsorbs exhaust, bacterial, bleaching, camphor, chemicals, fish, floral, food, fumes, mold, oils, ozone, perfumes, and gas odors; 80% odor removal efficiency; side access applications for multiple filter housing
Available from:
Farr Co.
PO Box 92187 (APD)

Controlling Your Environment

For the Air

Airport Station
Los Angeles, CA 90009
800-333-7320
Fax 800-441-0003
and
Farr Co.
500 S. Main Street (APD)
Crystal Lake, IL 60014
800-777-5260
Fax 800-441-0103

Riga-Sorb™ 80R

Rechargeable cell can be serviced in house or at factory; activated carbon filter adsorbs exhaust, bacterial, bleaching, camphor, chemicals, fish, floral, food, fumes, mold, oils, ozone, perfumes, and gas odors; 25% odor removal efficiency; side access applications for multiple filter housing
Available from:
Farr Co.
PO Box 92187 (APD)
Airport Station
Los Angeles, CA 90009
800-333-7320
Fax 800-441-0003
and
Farr Co.
500 S. Main Street (APD)
Crystal Lake, IL 60014
800-777-5260
Fax 800-441-0103

REPLACEABLE FILTERS

30/30® Filter

Disposable, medium efficiency pleated air filter; use alone or as prefilter; fits most holding frames and side access housings; lofted, non-woven cotton and synthetic media, bonded to a 16-gauge galvanized steel frame with gaskets and four spring-type positive sealing fasteners to minimize air bypass; average efficiency of 25 to 30T on ASHRAE Test Standard 52 to 76; average arrestance of 90 to 92%; can be installed in banks;

commercial, industrial, and residential uses; various sizes; custom sizes
Available from:
Farr Co.
PO Box 92187 (APD)
Airport Station
Los Angeles, CA 90009
800-333-7320
Fax 800-441-0003
and
Farr Co.
500 S. Main Street (APD)
Crystal Lake, IL 60014
800-777-5260
Fax 800-441-0103

30/30® SA Filter

Disposable, medium efficiency pleated air filter with 4" extra depth; use alone or as prefilter; fits most holding frames and side access housings; lofted, non-woven cotton and synthetic media, bonded to a welded wire grid to minimize air bypass; average efficiency of 25 to 30% on ASHRAE Test Standard 52 to 76; average arrestance of 90 to 92%; can be installed in banks; commercial and industrial uses in side access housings; various sizes
Available from:
Farr Co.
PO Box 92187 (APD)
Airport Station
Los Angeles, CA 90009
800-333-7320
Fax 800-441-0003
and
Farr Co.
500 S. Main Street (APD)
Crystal Lake, IL 60014
800-777-5260
Fax 800-441-0103

3M Filtrete™ Air Conditioner Filter

Replaces foam filters in room-size air conditioners; electrostatically charged fibers trap dust, pollen, mold,

Controlling Your Environment

For the Air

smoke, dander; 15"x24" filter may be cut to size
Available from
3M by direct mail
Hardware stores, home centers
Available from:
3M Company
PO Box 33275 (APD)
St. Paul, MN 55133-3275
3M Center Bldg.(APD)
St. Paul, MN 55144-1000
Medical information 800-328-0255
Medical information local 612-736-4930
Customer service 800-423-5197
Outside CA 800-423-5146
In CA 818-341-1300
and:
Allergy Control Products, Inc.
96 Danbury Rd. (APD)
PO Box 793 (APD)
Ridgefield, CT 06877
800-422-DUST (3878)
203-438-9580
Fax 203-431-8963
and:
E.L. Foust Co., Inc.
PO Box 105 (APD)
Elmhurst, IL 60126
800-225-9549
708-834-4952
Fax 708-834-5341

3M Filtrete™ Furnace Filter

Replaces standard furnace filter; electrostatically charged fibers trap dust, pollen, mold, smoke, dander; pleated for greater surface area; various sizes
Available from
3M by direct mail
Hardware stores, home centers
Available from:
3M Company
PO Box 33275 (APD)
St. Paul, MN 55133-3275
3M Center Bldg.(APD)
St. Paul, MN 55144-1000
Medical information 800-328-0255

Medical information local 612-736-4930
Customer service 800-423-5197
Outside CA 800-423-5146
In CA 818-341-1300
and:
Allergy Control Products, Inc.
96 Danbury Rd. (APD)
PO Box 793 (APD)
Ridgefield, CT 06877
800-422-DUST (3878)
203-438-9580
Fax 203-431-8963
and:
Allergy Solutions
4909 W. Park Blvd. #169 (APD)
Plano, TX 75093
800-380-SNEEZ (7633)
214-612-4188
Fax 214-985-5573
and:
Allergy-Asthma Shopper™
PO Box 239 (APD)
Fate, TX 75132
800-447-1100
Fax 903-883-4513
and:
E.L. Foust Co., Inc.
PO Box 105 (APD)
Elmhurst, IL 60126
800-225-9549
708-834-4952
Fax 708-834-5341
and:
Lifestyle Fascination
55 Progress Pl. (APD)
Jackson, NJ 08527-3002
800-669-0987
908-928-1800
Fax 908-928-1107

Aeropleat® II

Disposable, medium efficiency (30%) pleated air filter; used alone or as prefilter; (fits most holding frames and side access housings); lofted, non-woven, reinforced cotton and synthetic media bonded to a welded wire grid to minimize air bypass; average efficiency of 25 to 30% on ASHRAE Test

Controlling Your Environment

For the Air

Standard of 72 to 76; average arrestance of 90%; various sizes
Available from:
Farr Co.
PO Box 92187 (APD)
Airport Station
Los Angeles, CA 90009
800-333-7320
Fax 800-441-0003
and
Farr Co.
500 S. Main Street (APD)
Crystal Lake, IL 60014
800-777-5260
Fax 800-441-0103

AirMedic+

Replaces standard furnace filter; electrostatically-charged fibers attract and hold dust, pollen, mold, smoke, and dander; pleated for greater surface area; replaceable
Available from
Hardware stores, home improvement stores, warehouse stores

Aller-Tech™ Furnace Filters

Series of layers trap particles; soft wide edges of filter fill in gaps and do not allow air to pass unfiltered; 99% efficiency; replaceable; various sizes, no custom fitting necessary
Available from:
Allergy Asthma Technology
4151 N. Kedzie (APD)
PO Box 18398 (APD)
Chicago, IL 60618
800-621-5545
312-465-8020
Fax 312-465-7619

Allergen™ Filter

Disposable, pleated panel, aluminum frame filter made with unblended Filtrete™; filters pollen tobacco smoke, dust, spores, dander, mildew; various sizes
Available from:
Allergen™ Air Filter Corp.

5205 Ashbrook (APD)
Houston, TX 77081
800-333-8880
In TX 713-668-2371

Allerx 84 Electrostatic Air Filter

Aluminum frame; electrostatic prefilter fits in window air conditioning unit or use as prefilter in electronic air cleaners; traps dust, pollen, mold, lint; washable; standard and custom sizes
Available from:
Allergy-Asthma Shopper™
PO Box 239 (APD)
Fate, TX 75132
800-447-1100
Fax 903-883-4513

Allerx Deluxe Filter

Washable, electrostatic air filter replaces standard heating or central air conditioning filter; traps up to 93% of dust, pollen, mold, lint; captures 21% of particles down to 0.3-6 micron; ASHRAE 52-76 standard test; standard and custom sizes
Available from:
Allergy-Asthma Shopper™
PO Box 239 (APD)
Fate, TX 75132
800-447-1100
Fax 903-883-4513

Allerx Disposable Charcoal Filter

Replaceable, activated charcoal filter adsorbs odors and fumes; polyester filter adsorbs smoke and household odors; 89.3% effective with allergens; CADR=300; aluminum frame with 3 carbon pads; standard and custom sizes
Available from:
Allergy-Asthma Shopper™
PO Box 239 (APD)
Fate, TX 75132
800-447-1100
Fax 903-883-4513

Controlling Your Environment

For the Air

Allerx Electrostatic Air Filter

Washable filter removes up to 90% of allergens; replaces standard heating filter; standard and custom sizes
Available from:
Allergy-Asthma Shopper™
PO Box 239 (APD)
Fate, TX 75132
800-447-1100
Fax 903-883-4513

Allerx Vent Filter Kit

Washable 8"x12" covers made of high efficiency polyester material cover central air system vents to catch dust; velcro attachments; use on only one vent at a time to avoid damage to system
Available from:
Allergy-Asthma Shopper™
PO Box 239 (APD)
Fate, TX 75132
800-447-1100
Fax 903-883-4513
and:
National Allergy Supply, Inc.
4400 Georgia Hwy. 120 (APD)
PO Box 1658 (APD)
Duluth, GA 30136
800-522-1448
In Atlanta 404-623-8077
Fax 404-623-5568

BioKontrol

Replaces standard furnace filter; electrostatically-charged fibers attract and hold dust, pollen, mold, smoke, and dander; pleated for greater surface area; replaceable
Available from
Hardware stores, home improvement stores, warehouse stores

Contractors Choice

Static-prone materials accept static charge to attract airborne pollutants; washable; average peak dust arrestance of 86% by weight on particles .001 to 80 micron; ozone-free; helps control bacteria, mold spores,

and mildew on filter surface; standard and custom sizes
Available from:
Newtron Products
PO Box 27175 (APD)
3874 Virginia Ave. (APD)
Cincinnati, OH 45227-0175
800-543-9149
In OH 800-544-3753
513-561-7373
Fax 513-561-3673

Dust Arrestor II®

Washable, self-charging electrostatic air filter replaces standard furnace filter; traps dust, pollen, mold spores, dander; ozone-free
Available from:
Absolute Environmental's Allergy Store
2615 S. University Dr. (APD)
Davie, FL 33328
Nationwide 800-771-ACHOO (2246)
In FL 800-329-3773
Broward 305-472-3773
Fax 305-474-0133

Dust Eater®

Permatron® washable filter removes pollen, dust, and airborne pollutants up to 93% arrestance efficiency; filter material creates electrostatic charge; ozone-free; replaces standard heating filter; standard and custom sizes
Available from:
AAir Purification Systems
7340 Trade St. #C (APD)
San Diego, CA 92121-2457
800-776-6746
619-578-2825
Fax 619-578-3762
and:
National Allergy Supply, Inc.
4400 Georgia Hwy. 120 (APD)
PO Box 1658 (APD)
Duluth, GA 30136
800-522-1448
In Atlanta 404-623-8077
Fax 404-623-5568
and:

Controlling Your Environment

For the Air

Permatron Corp.
11400 Melrose St. (APD)
Franklin Park, IL 60131-1325
800-882-8012
708-451-0999

Dust Plus®

Permatron filter with washable front panel is a woven, electrostatic fabric for dust and pollen; replaceable back panel is charcoal or zeolite for odors and fumes; removes odors (tobacco smoke, fuel, cleaning solutions) and non-toxic fumes; fits furnace or air conditioning system
Available from:
National Allergy Supply, Inc.
4400 Georgia Hwy. 120 (APD)
PO Box 1658 (APD)
Duluth, GA 30136
800-522-1448
In Atlanta 404-623-8077
Fax 404-623-5568
and:
Permatron Corp.
11400 Melrose St. (APD)
Franklin Park, IL 60131-1325
800-882-8012
708-451-0999

DUST-Magnet 90

Washable, electrostatic air filter; removes 90% of air-borne particles and 90 to 99% of most pollen and plant spores; fits into heating or air conditioning unit; standard, custom sizes
Available from:
Allergy Supply Co.
11994 Star Court (APD)
Herndon, VA 22071
800-323-6744
Metropolitan DC 703-391-2011
Fax 703-391-2014
BBS 703-521-0638

Electronic Air Cleaner Filters

Layers of electrostatic fabric media trap airborne particles like dust, pollen, and dirt; arrestance efficiency of 72%; washable with either flexible vinyl or stainless steel edge; standard and custom sizes; optional, disposable odor removal filters
Model H for heating/cooling systems
Model R prefilter for electronic air cleaners

Temperature and Humidity Recorder

Self-contained, battery powered unit measures and records temperature variations from 0 degreesto 100 degrees F for one week on a chart; metal case; charts and cartridge pens
Available from:
Permatron Corp.
11400 Melrose St. (APD)
Franklin Park, IL 60131-1325
800-882-8012
708-451-0999

Electrostatic Air Filter

Removes 90% to 99% airborne particles; washable; for furnace or air conditioner systems; standard and custom sizes
Available from:
Allergy Clean Environments
501 Station Ave. (APD)
Haddon Heights, NJ 08035
800-882-4110
In NJ 609-546-1101
Fax 609-546-1466
URL:
http:\\WWW.infomall.com\allergy.html

EZ-2000

Replaces disposable filter in wall grille, self-contained unit, or window unit; ozone-free; low air flow resistance; filters up to 96% of pollen, dust, allergens, smoke and other irritants
Available from:
Clean Air Services
2402 Elm St. (APD)
Allentown, PA 18104

Controlling Your Environment

For the Air

215-435-4355
Fax 215-435-4295

Filta-Air 4000 Turbo Air Cleaner

Prefilter for dust, large particles; electrostatic filter fibers for smoke and pollen; carbon layer for odors and gases; wall or ceiling mount, freestanding; adjustable vents
Available from:
Artform Int'l, Inc.
89 Taylor Ave. (APD)
Norwalk, CT 06854
203-854-9902
FAX 203-854-9952

Guardian™ Air Cleaner

Filter made of static prone polylmers with permanent electric charge to trap particles; pleated chambers trap dust particles in combination with a grid of positively charged co-polymer rods; ozone-free; washable
Available from:
Allergy Relief Distributors
Div. of E.C.Environmental Control, Inc.
177 Telegraph Rd. #365 (APD)
Bellingham, WA 98226
206-734-1646
Fax 206-734-3696
Canadian office in Vancouver, BC

Hi-Tech Filter

Washable filter replaces standard filter in furnace and air conditioner; ozone-free, creates own electrostatic charge; low air flow resistance; traps dust, pollen, mold, airborne irritants; 99.9% efficient to 10 micron; can be used as prefilter for HEPA filter; various standard sizes and custom sizes
Available from:
Aller-Guard,® Inc.
Southgate Office Park
1645 S.W. 41st St. (APD)
Topeka, KS 66609-1250
800-234-0816
913-267-9333

Fax 913-267-0072
and:
Allergy Control Products, Inc.
96 Danbury Rd. (APD)
PO Box 793 (APD)
Ridgefield, CT 06877
800-422-DUST (3878)
203-438-9580
Fax 203-431-8963
and:
Allergy Solutions
4909 W. Park Blvd. #169 (APD)
Plano, TX 75093
800-380-SNEEZ (7633)
214-612-4188
Fax 214-985-5573
and:
Environtrol® Corporation
PO Box 31313 (APD)
St. Louis, MO 63131
800-423-1982
In St. Louis 314-966-6886
and:
Hi-Tech Filter Corp. of America
80 Myrtle St. (APD)
N. Quincy, MA 02171
800-448-3249
In MA 617-328-7756
Fax 617-773-4192
and:
Skin & Allergy Shop,™ The
310 E. Broadway (APD)
Louisville, KY 40202
800-366-6483
In KY 502-585-4824
Fax 502-589-3429

Honeywell Media Air Filter

Pleated, nonwoven, reinforced cotton fabric traps pollen, dust, dander; cabinet installs in gas, oil, or electric forced air system; filters replaceable; various air flow ratings; various sizes
Available locally in various department and home center stores and
Available from:
Honeywell, Inc.
Home and Building Control
Honeywell Plaza

Controlling Your Environment

For the Air

PO Box 524 (APD)
Minneapolis, MN 55440-0524
612-951-1000
and
Honeywell, Inc.
740 Ellesmere Rd. (APD)
Scarborough, ON, M1P 2V9
Canada

King-Aire® Pro Pak

Woven polyester fiber furnace filters; reduces dust; replaces standard furnace filter; various sizes
Available from:
King-Aire®
1121 S.R. 32 E. (APD)
Noblesville, IN 46060
Mail to PO Box 398 (APD)
Noblesville, IN 46060-0398
800-999-KING (5464)
317-776-1600

Koch Multi-Pleat Air Filter

Pleated design for greater surface area and absorption; use in heating and cooling units; replaces standard filters; various sizes
Available from:
Environtrol® Corporation
PO Box 31313 (APD)
St. Louis, MO 63131
800-423-1982
In St. Louis 314-966-6886
and:
Skin & Allergy Shop,™ The
310 E. Broadway (APD)
Louisville, KY 40202
800-366-6483
In KY 502-585-4824
Fax 502-589-3429

Newtron Whistle Air

Washable electrostatic air filter whistles when cleaning is required; standard and custom sizes
Available from:
Allergy Clean Environments
501 Station Ave. (APD)
Haddon Heights, NJ 08035
800-882-4110

In NJ 609-546-1101
Fax 609-546-1466
URL:
http:\\WWW.infomall.com\allergy.html
and:
Newtron Products
PO Box 27175 (APD)
3874 Virginia Ave. (APD)
Cincinnati, OH 45227-0175
800-543-9149
In OH 800-544-3753
513-561-7373
Fax 513-561-3673

Newtron® Air Cleaner

Static-prone materials accept static charge to attract airborne pollutants; washable; removes up to 88.3% of particulates in the 0 to 5 micron range; ozone-free; helps control bacteria, mold spores, and mildew on filter surface; replaces furnace filter; standard and custom sizes
Available from:
Newtron Products
PO Box 27175 (APD)
3874 Virginia Ave. (APD)
Cincinnati, OH 45227-0175
800-543-9149
In OH 800-544-3753
513-561-7373
Fax 513-561-3673

Permastatic II Filter

Filters pollen, dust, particulates; replaces existing disposable filter; washable; standard and custom filter sizes
Available from:
Allergy Relief Shop,™ Inc.
3371 Whittle Springs Rd. (APD)
Knoxville, TN 37917
Orders 800-626-2810
Questions 615-522-2795
and:
Allergy Resources
Mail: PO Box 888 (APD)
UPS: 264 Brookridge Ave. (APD)
Palmer Lake, CO 80133
Orders 800-USE-FLAX (873-3529)

Controlling Your Environment

For the Air

Company plans to move; use 800 #
and:
AllerMed Corp.
31 Steel Rd. (APD)
Wylie, TX 75098
214-442-4898
Fax 214-442-4897
and:
Flowright Int'l Products
1495 N.W. Gilman Blvd. #4 (APD)
Issaquah, WA 98027
206-392-8357
and:
N.E.E.D.S.
527 Charles Ave. 12A (APD)
Syracuse, NY 13209
800-634-1380
Fax 800-295-NEED (6333)

Pro-Pak Furnace Filter

Replaceable, woven polyester fiber filters replace standard furnace filters for dust filtration; various sizes
Available from:
King-Aire®
1121 S.R. 32 E. (APD)
Noblesville, IN 46060
Mail to PO Box 398 (APD)
Noblesville, IN 46060-0398
800-999-KING (5464)
317-776-1600

Purity® Air Filter

Replaces furnace filter; removes 97% of pollen, 70% of dust, 20% of smoke; replaceable
Available from:
Skin & Allergy Shop,™ The
310 E. Broadway (APD)
Louisville, KY 40202
800-366-6483
In KY 502-585-4824
Fax 502-589-3429

Purolator® Puro Pleat

Replaces standard furnace filter; electrostatically-charged fibers attract and hold dust, pollen, mold, smoke, and dander; pleated for greater surface area; replaceable

Available from
Hardware stores, home improvement stores, warehouse stores

REMIND-AIR

Independent filter screens accumulate dust, pollen, and mold; washable; average peak dust arrestance of 86% by weight on particles .001 to 80 micron; ozone-free; helps control baacteria, mold spores, and mildew on filter surface; standard and custom sizes
Available from:
Newtron Products
PO Box 27175 (APD)
3874 Virginia Ave. (APD)
Cincinnati, OH 45227-0175
800-543-9149
In OH 800-544-3753
513-561-7373
Fax 513-561-3673

Riga-Flo®/100PH Filters

Replaceable filter; all-metal enclosing frame, diagonal support braces, pleated stabilizers, welded wire grid, rigid construction for variable volume systems up to 500 fpm; average efficiency of 80 to 85% on ASHRAE Test Standard 52 to 76; average arrestance of 98%; media filter is a high density icrofine glass fiber, forming a lofted filter blanket laminated to a reinforced backing; commercial and industrial uses
Available from:
Farr Co.
PO Box 92187 (APD)
Airport Station
Los Angeles, CA 90009
800-333-7320
Fax 800-441-0003
and
Farr Co.
500 S. Main Street (APD)
Crystal Lake, IL 60014
800-777-5260
Fax 800-441-0103

Controlling Your Environment

For the Air

Riga-Flo®/10PH Filters

Replaceable filter; all-metal enclosing frame, diagonal support braces, pleated stabilizers, welded wire grid, rigid construction for variable volume systems up to 500 fpm; average efficiency of 40 to 45% on ASHRAE Test Standard 52 to 76; average arrestance of 90%; media filter is a cotton/polyester with a non-woven microfiber on the air exiting side
Available from:
Farr Co.
PO Box 92187 (APD)
Airport Station
Los Angeles, CA 90009
800-333-7320
Fax 800-441-0003
and
Farr Co.
500 S. Main Street (APD)
Crystal Lake, IL 60014
800-777-5260
Fax 800-441-0103

Riga-Flo®/15PH Filters

Replaceable filter; all-metal enclosing frame, diagonal support braces, pleated stabilizers, welded wire grid, rigid construction for variable volume systems up to 500 fpm; average efficiency of 60 to 65% on ASHRAE Test Standard 52 to 76; average arrestance of 97%; media filter is a high density microfine glass fiber, forming a lofted filter blanket laminated to a reinforced backing; commercial and industrial uses
Available from:
Farr Co.
PO Box 92187 (APD)
Airport Station
Los Angeles, CA 90009
800-333-7320
Fax 800-441-0003
and
Farr Co.
500 S. Main Street (APD)
Crystal Lake, IL 60014
800-777-5260

Fax 800-441-0103

Riga-Flo®/200PH Filters

Replaceable filter; all-metal enclosing frame, diagonal support braces, pleated stabilizers, welded wire grid, rigid construction for variable volume systems up to 500 fpm; average efficiency of 90 to 95% on ASHRAE Test Standard 52 to 76; average arrestance of 99%; media filter is a high density icrofine glass fiber, forming a lofted filter blanket laminated to a reinforced backing; commercial and industrial uses
Available from:
Farr Co.
PO Box 92187 (APD)
Airport Station
Los Angeles, CA 90009
800-333-7320
Fax 800-441-0003
and
Farr Co.
500 S. Main Street (APD)
Crystal Lake, IL 60014
800-777-5260
Fax 800-441-0103

Riga-Flo®/XLPH Filters

Replaceable filter; all-metal enclosing frame, diagonal support braces, pleated stabilizers, welded wire grid, rigid construction for variable volume systems up to 500 fpm; average efficiency of 40 to 45% on ASHRAE Test Standard 52 to 76; average arrestance of 96%; media filter is a high density icrofine glass fiber, forming a lofted filter blanket laminated to a reinforced backing; commercial and industrial uses
Available from:
Farr Co.
PO Box 92187 (APD)
Airport Station
Los Angeles, CA 90009
800-333-7320
Fax 800-441-0003
and

Controlling Your Environment

For the Air

Farr Co.
500 S. Main Street (APD)
Crystal Lake, IL 60014
800-777-5260
Fax 800-441-0103

Safeguard Window Ventilator

Filtering screen for dirt, dust, pollen fits on double-hung windows; aluminum frame; washable; various sizes, adjustable
Available from:
Allergy Clean Environments
501 Station Ave. (APD)
Haddon Heights, NJ 08035
800-882-4110
In NJ 609-546-1101
Fax 609-546-1466
URL:
http:\\WWW.infomall.com\allergy.html

SERV-Aire

Disposable filter rated at 30 to 35% efficiency and 93% average arrestance; pleated; custom, standard sizes
Available from:
Allergy Supply Co.
11994 Star Court (APD)
Herndon, VA 22071
800-323-6744
Metropolitan DC 703-391-2011
Fax 703-391-2014
BBS 703-521-0638

Space-Gard® 2200

Traps dust, tobacco smoke, polllen, spores, pet dander, hair and dust larger than 1 micron; installs in forced air heating/cooling system; average efficiency of 65% at 1,200 CFM; particles from 0.01 to 30 micron; ozone-free; replaceable filter media; filtering area 78.6 sq. ft.; capacity 600 to 2,000 CFM; under 28 lbs.
Available from:
Allergy Supply Co.
11994 Star Court (APD)
Herndon, VA 22071
800-323-6744

Metropolitan DC 703-391-2011
Fax 703-391-2014
BBS 703-521-0638
and:
Research Products Corp.
1015 E. Washington Ave. (APD)
PO Box 1467 (APD)
Madison, WI 53701-1467
800-545-2219
608-257-8801
Fax 608-257-4357

Space-Gard® 2250

Replaces the return air grille of the central heating/cooling system; wall or ceiling; residential capacity 600 to 2,000 CFM; filtering area 78.6 sq. ft.; under 32 lbs.
Available from:
Research Products Corp.
1015 E. Washington Ave. (APD)
PO Box 1467 (APD)
Madison, WI 53701-1467
800-545-2219
608-257-8801
Fax 608-257-4357

Space-Gard® 2275

Filters pollen and mold; 99% efficiency for pollen and spores; two-speed fan; up to 140 cu. ft. of air per minute; ozone-free; removes particulates up to four times per hour in an average room; 10.8 sq. ft. of filtering surface; replaceable filter media; portable, 12lbs. 6 oz.; air flow 100 to 140 CFM
Available from:
Allergy Supply Co.
11994 Star Court (APD)
Herndon, VA 22071
800-323-6744
Metropolitan DC 703-391-2011
Fax 703-391-2014
BBS 703-521-0638
and:
Research Products Corp.
1015 E. Washington Ave. (APD)
PO Box 1467 (APD)
Madison, WI 53701-1467

Controlling Your Environment

For the Air

800-545-2219
608-257-8801
Fax 608-257-4357

Space-Gard® 2600

High efficiency filter removes up to 98% of pollutant particles; ozone-free; filters up to 15,000 cu. ft.; replaceable filter media; three-speed blower; average efficiency of 90% at 1,000 CFM; particles to 0.3 micron
Available from:
Research Products Corp.
1015 E. Washington Ave. (APD)
PO Box 1467 (APD)
Madison, WI 53701-1467
800-545-2219
608-257-8801
Fax 608-257-4357

Vent and Grille Filter

Non-rigid, 1/4" thick Hi-Tech filter fits behind air supply vent or outlet grille in walls and floors and window air conditioner units
Available from:
Environtrol® Corporation
PO Box 31313 (APD)
St. Louis, MO 63131
800-423-1982
In St. Louis 314-966-6886
and:
Hi-Tech Filter Corp. of America
80 Myrtle St. (APD)
N. Quincy, MA 02171
800-448-3249
In MA 617-328-7756
Fax 617-773-4192

Vent-Pro™

Disposable heating vent filter; electrostatically enhanced media filters air wth low air flow resistance; cut to size and place behind vent cover; 20"x24" sheet;
Available from:
Allergy Control Products, Inc.
96 Danbury Rd. (APD)
PO Box 793 (APD)
Ridgefield, CT 06877

800-422-DUST (3878)
203-438-9580
Fax 203-431-8963

Web, The

Electret filter traps up to 99% of pollen and up to 94% of dust and dander; ozone-free; adjustable to various filter sizes; washable; optional carbon pad for smoke and odors
Available from:
A-Plus Allergy Equipment & Supply
8325 Regis Way (APD)
Los Angeles, CA 90045-2646
Orders 800-86-ALLER (862-5537)
310-337-7468
Fax 310-337-1971

AUTOMOBILE FILTERS

160 AN Auto Air Purifier

Replaceable combination filter for dust, particulates, formaldehyde; plugs into cigarette lighter; filter should be replaced every six months regardless of actual use because it is absorbent; 9"x7"x16"
Available from:
E.L. Foust Co., Inc.
PO Box 105 (APD)
Elmhurst, IL 60126
800-225-9549
708-834-4952
Fax 708-834-5341

160 ANFC Auto Air Purifier

Replaceable combination filter for dust, particulates, formaldehyde; this filter has a different filter media for individuals sensitive to the 160 AN media; plugs into cigarette lighter; filter should be replaced every six months regardless of actual use because it is absorbent; 9"x7"x16"
Available from:
E.L. Foust Co., Inc.
PO Box 105 (APD)
Elmhurst, IL 60126
800-225-9549

Controlling Your Environment

For the Air

708-834-4952
Fax 708-834-5341

AIREOX Car Air Purifier 22

Plugs into cigarette lighter in cars, trucks, motor homes, and boats with 12 volt DC; optional converter for travel; two-speed fan; 2 lbs. activated carbon; one micron particle filter, optional 0.5 micron particle filter; 75 CFM; 6" tall by 11" diameter; replaceable cartridges
Available from:
A-Plus Allergy Equipment & Supply
8325 Regis Way (APD)
Los Angeles, CA 90045-2646
Orders 800-86-ALLER (862-5537)
310-337-7468
Fax 310-337-1971
and:
AAir Purification Systems
7340 Trade St. #C (APD)
San Diego, CA 92121-2457
800-776-6746
619-578-2825
Fax 619-578-3762
and:
Aireox Research Corp.
11015 Whitford Ave. (APD)
Riverside, CA 92505
909-689-2781
and:
Allergy-Asthma Shopper™
PO Box 239 (APD)
Fate, TX 75132
800-447-1100
Fax 903-883-4513
and:
N.E.E.D.S.
527 Charles Ave. 12A (APD)
Syracuse, NY 13209
800-634-1380
Fax 800-295-NEED (6333)
and:
National Heart, Lung/Blood Inst.
NIH Asthma Project
Bldg. 31 Rm. 4A-21
9000 Rockville Pike
Bethesda, MD 20892
301-496-4236

301-496-2411

Allergy Traveler™

Traps particulates and smog particulates; plugs into cigarette lighter; 4 lbs; 10"x7-1/4"x7-3/4"
Available from:
Allergy-Asthma Shopper™
PO Box 239 (APD)
Fate, TX 75132
800-447-1100
Fax 903-883-4513

AutoAire II

Works on 12 volt power; filters automotive pollutants, pollen, dust, smoke; removes 98% of particles to 1 micron; 115 CFM; 2-speed motor; two 3-stage filters; complete air exchange every 30 seconds; 10"x10"x8-1/2"; 10 lbs.
Available from:
Allergy Relief Shop,™ Inc.
3371 Whittle Springs Rd. (APD)
Knoxville, TN 37917
Orders 800-626-2810
Questions 615-522-2795
and:
Allergy Resources
Mail: PO Box 888 (APD)
UPS: 264 Brookridge Ave. (APD)
Palmer Lake, CO 80133
Orders 800-USE-FLAX (873-3529)
Company plans to move; use 800 #
and:
AllerMed Corp.
31 Steel Rd. (APD)
Wylie, TX 75098
214-442-4898
Fax 214-442-4897
and:
Flowright Int'l Products
1495 N.W. Gilman Blvd. #4 (APD)
Issaquah, WA 98027
206-392-8357
and:
N.E.E.D.S.
527 Charles Ave. 12A (APD)
Syracuse, NY 13209
800-634-1380

Controlling Your Environment

For the Air

Fax 800-295-NEED (6333)
and:
Priorities®
70 Walnut St. (APD)
Wellesley, MA 02181
800-553-5398
and:
Wheaton Regional Library
Health Information Center
11701 Georgia Ave. (APD)
Wheaton, MD 20902
301-929-5520
TDD 301-929-5524

HUMIDIFIERS

Aprilaire® 350

Independent of heating system; basement or utility room installation; installed with or without duct work; humidistat; 0.5 gals. per hour, operates at 150 CFM; humidifies up to 4,500 sq. ft.; uses hot water tank; 21 lbs.
Locally available and
Available from:
Research Products Corp.
1015 E. Washington Ave. (APD)
PO Box 1467 (APD)
Madison, WI 53701-1467
800-545-2219
608-257-8801
Fax 608-257-4357

Aprilaire® 360

Independent of heating system; installed without ductwork; humidistat; 0.5 gals. per hour, operates at 150 CFM; humidifies up to 4,5000 sq. ft.; uses hot water tank; 21 lbs.
Locally available and
Available from:
Research Products Corp.
1015 E. Washington Ave. (APD)
PO Box 1467 (APD)
Madison, WI 53701-1467
800-545-2219
608-257-8801

Fax 608-257-4357

Aprilaire® 440

Bypass humidifier; humidistat; humidifies up to 4,000 sq. ft. in an average home; drain; 15 lbs.
Locally available and
Available from:
Research Products Corp.
1015 E. Washington Ave. (APD)
PO Box 1467 (APD)
Madison, WI 53701-1467
800-545-2219
608-257-8801
Fax 608-257-4357

Aprilaire® 445

Bypass humidifier; water circulating system if no drain; humidistat; humidifies up to 4,200 sq. ft.; 0.7 gals. per hour; 19 lbs.
Locally available and
Available from:
Research Products Corp.
1015 E. Washington Ave. (APD)
PO Box 1467 (APD)
Madison, WI 53701-1467
800-545-2219
608-257-8801
Fax 608-257-4357

Aprilaire® 550

Bypass humidifier; installs at furnace; humidifies up to 3,000 sq. ft. in an average home; humidistat; 0.5 gals. per hour; 10 lbs.
Locally available and
Available from:
Research Products Corp.
1015 E. Washington Ave. (APD)
PO Box 1467 (APD)
Madison, WI 53701-1467
800-545-2219
608-257-8801
Fax 608-257-4357

Aprilaire® 760

Whole house humidifier; humidifies up to 4,200 sq. ft.; 18 gals.

Controlling Your Environment

For the Air

per day; humidistat; distributes
through heating ducts
Locally available and
Available from:
Research Products Corp.
1015 E. Washington Ave. (APD)
PO Box 1467 (APD)
Madison, WI 53701-1467
800-545-2219
608-257-8801
Fax 608-257-4357

Bemis Waterwick® 4161

One-speed fan; removable power
pak for ease to cleaning; refillable
water caddy; evaporative humidifier,
no white dust; automatic humidistat;
humidifies 2,0000 sq. ft.; grey
Available from:
Bemis Mfg. Co.
300 Mill St. (APD)
PO Box 901 (APD)
Sheboygan Falls, WI 53085-0901
800-558-7651
414-467-4621
Fax 414-467-8573

Bemis Waterwick® 4261 & 4262

Two-speed fan; removable power
pak for ease to cleaning; refillable
water caddy; evaporative humidifier,
no white dust; automatic humidistat
and automatic shut-off; humidifies
2,500 sq. ft.; 4261 is grey, 4262 dark
oak woodgrain
Available from:
Bemis Mfg. Co.
300 Mill St. (APD)
PO Box 901 (APD)
Sheboygan Falls, WI 53085-0901
800-558-7651
414-467-4621
Fax 414-467-8573

Bemis Waterwick® 4363

Three-speed fan; removable power
pak for ease to cleaning; refillable
water caddy; evaporative humidifier,
no white dust; automatic humidistat
and automatic shut-off; humidifies
2,750 sq. ft.; light oak woodgrain
Available from:
Bemis Mfg. Co.
300 Mill St. (APD)
PO Box 901 (APD)
Sheboygan Falls, WI 53085-0901
800-558-7651
414-467-4621
Fax 414-467-8573

Bemis Waterwick® 4973 & 4963

Variable speed fan; removable
power pak for ease to cleaning;
refillable water caddy; air filter for
4973; evaporative humidifier, no white
dust; automatic humidistat and
automatic shut-off; humidifies 3,0000
sq. ft.; light oak woodgrain
Available from:
Bemis Mfg. Co.
300 Mill St. (APD)
PO Box 901 (APD)
Sheboygan Falls, WI 53085-0901
800-558-7651
414-467-4621
Fax 414-467-8573

Bemis Waterwick® 5273 & 5271

System wicks water into filter,
traps minerals and dissolved solids;
evaporative humidifier, no white dust;
replaceable filter composed of Filtrete™
for dust, pollen, and airborne
pollutants and activated charcoal filter
for odors; removable powerpack for
ease of cleaning; 3 gals. per 24 hrs; 2-
speed control; model 5273 is light oak
woodgrain; model 5271 is grey
Available from:
Bemis Mfg. Co.
300 Mill St. (APD)
PO Box 901 (APD)
Sheboygan Falls, WI 53085-0901
800-558-7651
414-467-4621
Fax 414-467-8573

Controlling Your Environment

For the Air

Bemis Waterwick® 6974 & 6964

Variable speed fan; removable power pak for ease to cleaning; refillable water caddy; combination filtrete and carbon air filter for 6974; evaporative humidifier, no white dust; automatic humidistat and automatic shut-off; humidifies 2,750 sq. ft.; credenza, casters
Available from:
Bemis Mfg. Co.
300 Mill St. (APD)
PO Box 901 (APD)
Sheboygan Falls, WI 53085-0901
800-558-7651
414-467-4621
Fax 414-467-8573

Bemis Waterwick® 7260

Holds 1.75 gals. water for 28 hr. operation, output is 2 gals. per 24 hours; evaporative humidifier, no white dust; traps minerals and solids in the water; humidifies 800 sq. ft.; 2-speed fan; optional air cleaning filter; portable, 7.5 lbs.
Available from:
Bemis Mfg. Co.
300 Mill St. (APD)
PO Box 901 (APD)
Sheboygan Falls, WI 53085-0901
800-558-7651
414-467-4621
Fax 414-467-8573

Bemis Waterwick® 7370

Holds 1.75 gals. water for 28 hr. operation, output is 2.5 gals. per 24 hours without filter; evaporative humidifier, no white dust; traps minerals and solids in the water; humidifies 900 sq. ft.; 3-speed fat; replaceable air filter with polyester to trap dust, pollen, and smoke and activated carbon filter for odors; portable, 7.5 lb
Available from:
Bemis Mfg. Co.
300 Mill St. (APD)
PO Box 901 (APD)

Sheboygan Falls, WI 53085-0901
800-558-7651
414-467-4621
Fax 414-467-8573

Bionaire® Clear-Mist CM-1

Enclosed chamber with heating element; thermostatic protection against overheating; medication cup; on/off switch with power-on light; humidifies up to 1,000 sq. ft.; .6 gallon tank with built-in carry handle; 10.05"x4"x9.63"; 3 lbs.
Available from:
Absolute Environmental's Allergy Store
2615 S. University Dr. (APD)
Davie, FL 33328
Nationwide 800-771-ACHOO (2246)
In FL 800-329-3773
Broward 305-472-3773
Fax 305-474-0133
and:
Allergy Asthma Technology
4151 N. Kedzie (APD)
PO Box 18398 (APD)
Chicago, IL 60618
800-621-5545
312-465-8020
Fax 312-465-7619
and:
Bionaire Corp.
90 Boroline Rd. (APD)
Allendale, NJ 07401
80-253-2764
201-934-0755

Bionaire® Clear-Mist CM-2s

Enclosed chamber with steel element; thermostatic protection against overheating; medication cup; capacity of 2 gals. in transparent tank with cap; removable mineral collector tray; low and high output levels; humidifies up to 1,150 sq. ft.; 14.25"x8"x10.5"; 6.8 lbs.
Available from:
Absolute Environmental's Allergy Store
2615 S. University Dr. (APD)
Davie, FL 33328
Nationwide 800-771-ACHOO (2246)

Controlling Your Environment

For the Air

In FL 800-329-3773
Broward 305-472-3773
Fax 305-474-0133
and:
Appliance Sales & Service Co.
655 Mission St. (APD)
San Francisco, CA 94105
800-424-6783
In 415 area call 415-362-7195
and:
Bionaire Corp.
90 Boroline Rd. (APD)
Allendale, NJ 07401
80-253-2764
201-934-0755

Bionaire® Clear-Mist CMP-5
Enclosed misting chamber with steel element; thermostatic protection against overheating; power-on and low water indicator lights; automatic humidistat control; removable mineral collector tray; humidifies up to 1,600 sq. ft.; 2 2.5-gallon tanks with caps; 20.4"x8.7"x12.75"; 11.9 lbs.
Available from:
Bionaire Corp.
90 Boroline Rd. (APD)
Allendale, NJ 07401
80-253-2764
201-934-0755

Bionaire® Clear-Mist CP-0310
Enclosed misting chamber with cast element; thermostatic protection against overheating; power-on and low water indicator lights; low and high output levels; removable mineral collector tray; humidifies up to 1,400 sq. ft.; 2 1.5-gallon tanks with caps; 16.2"x8.7"x12.75"; 10.1 lbs.
Available from:
Bionaire Corp.
90 Boroline Rd. (APD)
Allendale, NJ 07401
80-253-2764
201-934-0755

Bionaire® Clear-Mist CP-0470
Enclosed misting chamber with cast element; thermostatic protection against overheating; power-on and low water indicator lights; automatic humidistat control; removable mineral collector tray; humidifies up to 1,400 sq. ft.; 2 2-gallon tanks with caps; 18.4"x8.7"x12.75"; 12.2 lbs.
Available from:
Bionaire Corp.
90 Boroline Rd. (APD)
Allendale, NJ 07401
80-253-2764
201-934-0755

Bionaire® Clear-Mist W-0210
Replaceable wick retains most minerals, lessening white dust; 2-speed fan; water level indicator; 1.5 gallon capacity with 2 gallon per day output; humidifies up to 1,150 sq. ft.; 10.7"x11.6"x9.8"; 6 lbs.
Available from:
Bionaire Corp.
90 Boroline Rd. (APD)
Allendale, NJ 07401
80-253-2764
201-934-0755

Bionaire® Clear-Mist W-0310
Replaceable wick retains most minerals, lessening white dust; 2-speed fan; water level indicator; 2 gallon capacity with 3 gallon per day output; humidifies up to 1,400 sq. ft.; 14.4"x10"x10.4"; 5.7 lbs.
Available from:
Bionaire Corp.
90 Boroline Rd. (APD)
Allendale, NJ 07401
80-253-2764
201-934-0755

Bionaire® Clear-Mist W-6/W-6s
Replaceable dual wicks retain most minerals, lessening white dust; wick replacer indicator; automatic humidity control; 3-speed fan; power-on and low water indicator lights; air

Controlling Your Environment

For the Air

filter of exhausting air removes up to 99% of airborne particulates; 2 3-gallon tanks; tank caps; humidifies up to 2,900 sq. ft.; casters; 23"x10"x21.75"; 23 lbs.

W-6s: without casters: air filter; 23:x10:x20"; 22.5 lbs.
Available from:
Bionaire Corp.
90 Boroline Rd. (APD)
Allendale, NJ 07401
80-253-2764
201-934-0755

Bionaire® Clear-Mist W-9

Replaceable dual wicks retain most minerals, lessening white dust; wick replacer indicator; automatic humidity control; 3-speed fan; power-on and low water indicator lights; air filter of exhausting air removes up to 99% of airborne particulates; 3 3-gallon tanks; tank caps; humidifies up to 3,500 sq. ft.; casters; 29"x10"x21.4"; 27.5 lbs.
Available from:
Absolute Environmental's Allergy Store
2615 S. University Dr. (APD)
Davie, FL 33328
Nationwide 800-771-ACHOO (2246)
In FL 800-329-3773
Broward 305-472-3773
Fax 305-474-0133
and:
Appliance Sales & Service Co.
655 Mission St. (APD)
San Francisco, CA 94105
800-424-6783
In 415 area call 415-362-7195
and:
Bionaire Corp.
90 Boroline Rd. (APD)
Allendale, NJ 07401
80-253-2764
201-934-0755
and:
Brookstone Co.
5 Vose Farm Road (APD)
Peterborough, NH 03458
800-926-7000

Fax 603-924-0093

Bionaire® Clear-Mist W-9s

Replaceable dual wicks retain most minerals, lessening white dust; wick replacer indicator; automatic humidity control; 3-speed fan; power-on and low water indicator lights; air filter; 3 3-gallon tanks; humidifies up to 2,900 sq. ft.; casters; 29"x10"x21.4"; 25.9 lbs.
Available from:
Absolute Environmental's Allergy Store
2615 S. University Dr. (APD)
Davie, FL 33328
Nationwide 800-771-ACHOO (2246)
In FL 800-329-3773
Broward 305-472-3773
Fax 305-474-0133
and:
Appliance Sales & Service Co.
655 Mission St. (APD)
San Francisco, CA 94105
800-424-6783
In 415 area call 415-362-7195
and:
Bionaire Corp.
90 Boroline Rd. (APD)
Allendale, NJ 07401
80-253-2764
201-934-0755

Bionaire® CP-0305/CP-0306

Enclosed misting chamber with cast element; no fan blade or motor; low and high output levels; thermostatic protection against overheating; power-on and low water indicator lights; removable mineral collector tray; humidifies up to 1,400 sq. ft.; 2 1.5-gallon tanks with caps; 16.2"x8.7"x12.75"; 9.8 lbs.
Available from:
Bionaire Corp.
90 Boroline Rd. (APD)
Allendale, NJ 07401
80-253-2764
201-934-0755

Controlling Your Environment

For the Air

Bonaire® Clear-Mist CMP-3

Enclosed misting chamber with steel element; thermostatic protection against overheating; power-on and low water indicator lights; automatic humidistat control; removable mineral collector tray; humidifies up to 1,400 sq. ft.; 2 1.5-gallon tanks; 16.2"x8.7"x12.75"; 10.1 lbs.
Available from:
Absolute Environmental's Allergy Store
2615 S. University Dr. (APD)
Davie, FL 33328
Nationwide 800-771-ACHOO (2246)
In FL 800-329-3773
Broward 305-472-3773
Fax 305-474-0133
and:
Appliance Sales & Service Co.
655 Mission St. (APD)
San Francisco, CA 94105
800-424-6783
In 415 area call 415-362-7195
and:
Bionaire Corp.
90 Boroline Rd. (APD)
Allendale, NJ 07401
80-253-2764
201-934-0755
and:
Brookstone Co.
5 Vose Farm Road (APD)
Peterborough, NH 03458
800-926-7000
Fax 603-924-0093

DynaMist® 1800

Capacity of 2.1 gals.; 22 to 26 hours operational; filter; on/off switch; directional spout; 4.3 lbs.
Locally available
Available from:
Kaz, Inc.
10 Columbus Circle (APD)
New York, NY 10019
800-241-1131
Fax 212-265-9248

DynaMist® 2000

Capacity of 2.5 gals.; 28 to 32 hours operational; filter; on/off switch; directional spout; 4.83 lbs
Locally available and
Available from:
Comfortably Yours
2515 E. 43rd St. (APD)
Chattanooga, TN 37422
201-368-0400
and:
Kaz, Inc.
10 Columbus Circle (APD)
New York, NY 10019
800-241-1131
Fax 212-265-9248

DynaMist® 370-F

Capacity of 1.2 gals.; 10 to 12 hours operational; filter; 3.17 lbs.
Locally available and
Available from:
Kaz, Inc.
10 Columbus Circle (APD)
New York, NY 10019
800-241-1131
Fax 212-265-9248

DynaMist® 370

Capacity of 1.2 gals.; 10 to 12 hours operational; dust-trap filter; 3.17 lbs.
Locally available and
Available from:
Kaz, Inc.
10 Columbus Circle (APD)
New York, NY 10019
800-241-1131
Fax 212-265-9248

Hankscraft by Sunbeam Humidi-Clear™1 5910D

Capacity of 1.2 gals., runs up to 17 hours; directional air flow grille; UL listed; no white dust
Available from:
Allergy-Asthma Shopper™
PO Box 239 (APD)
Fate, TX 75132

Controlling Your Environment

For the Air

800-447-1100
Fax 903-883-4513

HolmesAir® Cool Mist™ HM-460

Humidity control; 2.6-gallon output per 24 hours; multi-directional mist outlet with Medi-Cup™; automatic shut-off; 2-speed fan; power light; refill light; re-set button; built-in handle; 2.81.3 gallon portable tank; UL listed; 7.38 lbs
Available from:
Holmes Products Corp.
233 Fortune Blvd. (APD)
Milford, MA 01757
508-634-8050
Fax 508-634-1211

HolmesAir® Cool Pure Mist™ Evaporative Humidifier HM-2000

Multi-directional moisture-vents; pilot light; on/off control; high/low output control; refill light; 2-speed motor; 3 gallon output per 24 hours; 2 gallon portable tank; replaceable, dual wick filters; 6.6 lbs.
Available from:
Holmes Products Corp.
233 Fortune Blvd. (APD)
Milford, MA 01757
508-634-8050
CFax 508-634-1211

HolmesAir® Cool Pure Mist™ Evaporative Humidifier HM-406

Replaceable, dual wicks with bacteria retardant; 4 gallon tank;3.5 gallon output per 24 hours; humidistat; 2-speed motor; power light; 2-speed fan; build-in handles; absorbs minerals; 9.5 lbs.
Available from:
Holmes Products Corp.
233 Fortune Blvd. (APD)
Milford, MA 01757
508-634-8050

Fax 508-634-1211

HolmesAir® Warm Pure Mist™ Humidifier HM-5100A

Humidity control; 2-gallon output per 24 hours; mist outlet with Medi-Cup™; automatic shut-off; power light; refill light; 1.3 gallon portable tank; no demineralization cartridge needed; UL listed; 5.17 lbs
Available from:
Holmes Products Corp.
233 Fortune Blvd. (APD)
Milford, MA 01757
508-634-8050
Fax 508-634-1211

HolmesAir® Warm Pure Mist™ Humidifier HM-5110A

Humidity control; 2.2-gallon output per 24 hours; mist outlet with Medi-Cup™; automatic shut-off; power light; refill light; reset button; night light; no demineralization cartridge needed; 1.3 gallon portable tank; UL listed; 5.17 lbs.
Available from:
Holmes Products Corp.
233 Fortune Blvd. (APD)
Milford, MA 01757
508-634-8050
Fax 508-634-1211

HolmesAir® Warm Pure Mist™ Humidifier HM-5150

Humidity control; 2.6-gallon output per 24 hours; multi-directional mist outlet with Medi-Cup™; automatic shut-off; power light; refill light; re-set button; built-in handle; no demineralization cartridge needed; 2.8 gallon portable tank; UL listed; 7.38 lbs
Available from:
Holmes Products Corp.
233 Fortune Blvd. (APD)
Milford, MA 01757
508-634-8050

Controlling Your Environment

For the Air

Fax 508-634-1211

Humidi-Clear™ 2 5920

Capacity of 2 gals., runs up to 28 hours.; directional air flow grille; UL listed; on/off switch; water level indicator
Available from
Hardware stores, home improvement stores, warehouse stores

Humidi-Clear™ 3 5950

Capacity of 3.5 gals., runs up to 66 hours; 3 filters: 2 for dust and odors, 1 with an antibacterial agent; no white dust; modified activity: more mist when room humidity is low and less when room humidity is high
Available from
Hardware stores, home improvement stores, warehouse stores

Humidifier Model 1200D

Capacity of 1.2 gals., 8-10 hours running time; automatic shut-lff; key opened steam chamber; carrying handles; medicine cup
Available from
Hardware stores, home improvement stores, warehouse stores

Humidifier Model 1400D

Capacity of 1.7 gals., 16 hours running time; automatic shut-off; key opened steam chamber; carrying handles; medicine cup
Available from
Hardware stores, home improvement stores, warehouse stores

Humidifier Model 1600D

Capacity of 3 gals.; 18-20 hours running time; automatic shut-off; key opened steam chamber, carrying handles; medicine cup
Available from
Hardware stores, home improvement stores, warehouse stores

Humidifier Model 240D

Capacity of 1.6 gals.; directional spout; 360 degrees directional spout; 3 regulator settings
Available from
Hardware stores, home improvement stores, warehouse stores

Humidifier Model 241H

Capacity of 1.2 gals., 360 degrees directional spout; 3 regulator settings
Available from
Hardware stores, home improvement stores, warehouse stores

Humidifier Model 2500D

Removable tube and disk; 1.25 gals. capacity, 15-17 hours running time
Available from
Hardware stores, home improvement stores, warehouse stores

Humidifier Model 2700D

Removable tube and disk; 2 gal. capacity, 18-20 hours running time; charcoal filter; on-off switch; directional spout
Available from
Hardware stores, home improvement stores, warehouse stores

Humidifier Model 3972H

Capacity of 1 gallon; air filter; 3-wire grounded cord
Available from
Hardware stores, home improvement stores, warehouse stores

Humidifier Model 39972D

Capacity of 1 gal., 18-20 hours running time; air filter; on-off switch
Available from
Hardware stores, home improvement stores, warehouse stores

168

Controlling Your Environment

For the Air

Humidifier Model 5590D

Capacity of 1 gallon; automatic shut-off; chamber for vaporizer fluid; twist-lock cover
Available from
Hardware stores, home improvement stores, warehouse stores

Humidifier Model 5596D

Capacity of 2 gals.; automatic shut-off; chamber for vaporizer fluid; twist lock cover
Available from
Hardware stores, home improvement stores, warehouse stores

Humidifier Model Thermo-Shield 1600

Capacity of 2-1/4 gals.; 16-18 hours running time; key opened steam chamber, carrying handles; medicine cup
Available from
Hardware stores, home improvement stores, warehouse stores

Skuttle Steam Humidifier 60-1

Installs in the return or supply of heating systems; up to 13 gals. per day for homes up to 2,900 ft.; stainless steel cabinet; safety cut-off switch
Available from:
E.L. Foust Co., Inc.
PO Box 105 (APD)
Elmhurst, IL 60126
800-225-9549
708-834-4952
Fax 708-834-5341

Skuttle Steam Humidifier 60-2

Installs in the return or supply of heating systems; up to 17 gals. per day for homes up to 3,700 ft.; stainless steel cabinet; safety cut-off switch
Available from:
E.L. Foust Co., Inc.
PO Box 105 (APD)
Elmhurst, IL 60126

800-225-9549
708-834-4952
Fax 708-834-5341

Sunbeam® Warm Steam Vaporizer

Capacity of 1.5 gals.; runs 18-20 hours; built-in medication well; autmatic shut-off
Available from:
Allergy-Asthma Shopper™
PO Box 239 (APD)
Fate, TX 75132
800-447-1100
Fax 903-883-4513
and:
Sunbeam Corp.
2001 S. York Rd. (APD)
Oak Brook, IL 60521
312-654-1900

DEHUMIDIFIERS

Damp Rid®

Moisture absorber tray draws humidity from the air; refillable container
Available from:
Allergy-Asthma Shopper™
PO Box 239 (APD)
Fate, TX 75132
800-447-1100
Fax 903-883-4513

Electric Dehumidifier

Plugs into household current; warms air from floor level; warm air rises and cooler air is forced down to be warmed; steel with baked enamel finish; no moving parts, continuous operation; Model 500 for boats, small closets, engine compartments, storage closets; Model 1000 for areas up to 1,000 cu. ft.
Available from:
Allergy Asthma Technology
4151 N. Kedzie (APD)
PO Box 18398 (APD)
Chicago, IL 60618

Controlling Your Environment

For the Air

800-621-5545
312-465-8020
Fax 312-465-7619
and:
Herrington
3 Symmes Dr. (APD)
Londonderry, NH 03053
800-622-5221
In NH 603-437-4939
603-437-4638
and:
Sporty's® Preferred Living
Clermont County Airport (APD)
Batavia, OH 45103-9747
800-543-8633
Fax 513-732-6560

Frigidaire® Dehumidifier

Adjustable humidistat; holds 24 pts.; 2-speed fan; automatic shut-off; steel, wood-grain cabinet with casters, hose connection
Locally available

HI-E Dry 100

Removes 7 pints of water per kilowatt hour; at 90 degrees F. and 90% humidity, removes 178 pints per day; commercial capacity
Available from:
Therma-Stor Products
Div. of DEC Int'l., Inc.
1919 S. Stoughton Rd. (APD)
PO Box 8050 (APD)
Madison, WI 53708
800-533-7533
608-222-5301
Fax 608-222-1447

HI-E Dry 200

Removes over 200 lbs. of water per day; standard outlet; at 90 degrees F. and 90% humidity, removes 297 pints per day; commercial capacity
Available from:
Therma-Stor Products
Div. of DEC Int'l., Inc.
1919 S. Stoughton Rd. (APD)
PO Box 8050 (APD)
Madison, WI 53708

800-533-7533
608-222-5301
Fax 608-222-1447

Quiet-Dry™

Constant drain hook-up or automatic turn-off when full; adjustable humidistat; for bedroom or basement; 57 lbs.
Available from:
Allergy Control Products, Inc.
96 Danbury Rd. (APD)
PO Box 793 (APD)
Ridgefield, CT 06877
800-422-DUST (3878)
203-438-9580
Fax 203-431-8963

Sahara Ultra Efficient

Uses refrigeration to cool incoming air to remove moisture; dehumidistat settings from 20 to 80%; blower switch; removes 85 to 104 lbs. of water or 100 pints per 24 hours; standard outlet; six-foot drain hose; 110 lbs. portable

Attaches to existing forced air system with filter for mold, mildew, and mite control
Available from:
Therma-Stor Products
Div. of DEC Int'l., Inc.
1919 S. Stoughton Rd. (APD)
PO Box 8050 (APD)
Madison, WI 53708
800-533-7533
608-222-5301
Fax 608-222-1447

HEAT EXCHANGERS
VENTILATORS

ALDES DHV

Ventilating dehumidifier filters 95% of particles 1 micron and larger. Supplies and filters up to 100 CFM fresh air, filters indoor air, dehumidifiers to control indoor humidity levels. Operates continuously

Controlling Your Environment

For the Air

for ventilation or by timer or in response to humidity level. Portable unit with casters or connect to forced air system
Available from:
American ALDES Ventilation Corp.
Northgate Center Business Park
4537 Northgate Ct. (APD)
Sarasota, FL 34234-2124
800-255-7749
In FL 813-351-3441
Fax 813-351-3442

ALDES VMP-H

Ventilation system with heat recovery; exhausts indoor air and excess humidity from kitchen, laundry, and up to 4 bathrooms and supplies outdoor air heated by the air being exhausted to the living, dining, family, and bedrooms; 2-speed motor, fan operates at 970 rpm or 1,700 rpm; heat exchange surface is 160 sq. ft.; core encased in painted, galvanized sheet metal case with drain system; eliminates ventilating fans in bathrooms
Available from:
American ALDES Ventilation Corp.
Northgate Center Business Park
4537 Northgate Ct. (APD)
Sarasota, FL 34234-2124
800-255-7749
In FL 813-351-3441
Fax 813-351-3442

Berner AQ Plus+™

Filters gases, dust, and pollen; pollen/dust efficiency 90% to 5 micron, 60% to 1.5 micron; balances humidity; installs with 6" diameter air duct, household current; CFM up to 165; 27-1/2"x11"x17"; 55 lbs.; Berner Air Products, Inc. no longer manufactures AQ Plus+; however replacement filters are still available
Available from:
Allergy Relief Shop,™ Inc.
3371 Whittle Springs Rd. (APD)
Knoxville, TN 37917

Orders 800-626-2810
Questions 615-522-2795

E-Z-AIRE® Light Commercial Models Series 70

Counterflow air-to-air plate type heat exchanger; deals with radon, formaldehyde, gas, particulate pollutants, ozone, cigarette smoke, and humidity; self-contained; air flow ranges 600-4000 CFM; 70% effectiveness; weight ranges 390 to 1,900 lbs.
Available from:
Des Champs Laboratories, Inc.
66 Okner Pkwy. (APD)
Livingston, NJ 07039
201-535-8300
Fax 201-535-0537

E-Z-AIRE® Light Commercial Models Series 85

Counterflow air-to-air plate type heat exchanger; deals with radon, formaldehyde, gas, particulate pollutants, ozone, cigarette smoke, and humidity; self-contained; air flow ranges 600-4000 CFM; 85% effectiveness; weight ranges 510 to 2,200 lbs.
Available from:
Des Champs Laboratories, Inc.
66 Okner Pkwy. (APD)
Livingston, NJ 07039
201-535-8300
Fax 201-535-0537

E-Z-Vent® EZV-II

Rated air flow 240; ventilation system for radon pollutants, odors, and humidity; condensate rain; dual, variable-speed motor controls; under 80 lbs.
Available from:
Des Champs Laboratories, Inc.
66 Okner Pkwy. (APD)
Livingston, NJ 07039
201-535-8300
Fax 201-535-0537

Controlling Your Environment

For the Air

E-Z-Vent® Series 300

Air-to-air plate type heat exchanger (heat recovery ventilator) for pollutants, odors, and high humidity; 2-speed blowers; two washable filters; insulated heat exchanger; optional remote switch, humidistat, time control. EZV-310: rated air flow 110-145; 115 lbs. EZV-320: rated air flow 165-220; 115 lbs. EZV-340: rated air flow 310-415; 150 lbs.
Available from:
Des Champs Laboratories, Inc.
66 Okner Pkwy. (APD)
Livingston, NJ 07039
201-535-8300
Fax 201-535-0537

ERV 3615

Moisture transferred in vapor phase, eliminating wet surfaces, condensate drain, bacterial growth; winter humidification requirements reduced; downflow or horizontal flow; rooftop or pad mount; 500 to 1,500 CFM for commercial, industrial, institutional applications
Available from:
Airxchange, Inc.
401 V.F.W. Dr. (APD)
Rockland, MA 02370
617-871-4816
Fax 617-871-3029

ERV 400/500

Moisture transferred in vapor phase, eliminating wet surfaces, condensate drain, bacterial growth; winter humidification requirements reduced; wall or ceiling mount; 150 to 500 CFM; small commercial use; provides 15 CFM/person for 33 occupants
Available from:
Airxchange, Inc.
401 V.F.W. Dr. (APD)
Rockland, MA 02370
617-871-4816
Fax 617-871-3029

ERV 5230 Series

Moisture transferred in vapor phase, eliminating wet surfaces, condensate drain, bacterial growth; winter humidification requirements reduced; downflow or horizontal flow; rooftop or pad mount; 1,500 to 3,000 CFM for commercial, industrial, institutional applications
Available from:
Airxchange, Inc.
401 V.F.W. Dr. (APD)
Rockland, MA 02370
617-871-4816
Fax 617-871-3029

EZV-AIRE®

Various models with rated air flows of 600-4000; weights vary 390-2200 lbs.
Available from:
Des Champs Laboratories, Inc.
66 Okner Pkwy. (APD)
Livingston, NJ 07039
201-535-8300
Fax 201-535-0537

Filter-Vent™

Fresh air ventilator pulls air through standard media, extended surface filter 90 to 95% efficient (ASHRAE 52-76 Dust spot test); carbon filter with non-woven polyester base; optional media filter of pleated glass fiber paper; seven-day timer with 2-hour intervals; floor or hanging joist installation; standard outlet
Available from:
Therma-Stor Products
Div. of DEC Int'l., Inc.
1919 S. Stoughton Rd. (APD)
PO Box 8050 (APD)
Madison, WI 53708
800-533-7533
608-222-5301
Fax 608-222-1447

Controlling Your Environment

For the Air

Honeywell Energy Recovery Ventilator ER100 Series

Mount in basement utility room, closet or suspend from outside wall or ceiling; dehumidistat, variable speed ventilation rate, 2 fan speeds; line voltage fresh air control; ER100-A1001 capacity of 70 to 185 cu. ft./min., handles .3 air changes per hour in 4,500 sq. ft., 80% efficiency; ER100-A1019 (available in Canada only) capacity of 70 to 130 cu. ft./min., handles .3 air changes per hour in 3,000 sq. ft., 80% efficiency, frost control; ER100-A1027 capacity of 70 to 185 cu. ft./min., handles .3 air changes per hour in 4,500 sq. ft., 80% efficiency, frost control; ER100-A1035 (available in U.S. only) capacity of 70 to 185 cu. ft./min., handles .3 air changes per hour in 4,500 sq. ft., 80% efficiency, frost control
Available locally in various department and home center stores and
Available from:
Honeywell, Inc.
Home and Building Control
Honeywell Plaza
PO Box 524 (APD)
Minneapolis, MN 55440-0524
612-951-1000
and
Honeywell, Inc.
740 Ellesmere Rd. (APD)
Scarborough, ON, M1P 2V9
Canada

Honeywell Energy Recovery Ventilator ER200 Series

Mount in basement utility room, closet or suspend from outside wall or ceiling; dehumidistat, variable speed ventilation rate, 2 fan speeds; line voltage fresh air control; ER200-A1000 capacity of 80 to 250 cu. ft./min., handles .3 air changes per hour in 6,200 sq. ft., 85% efficiency, no frost control; ER200-A1018 capacity of 80 to 250 cu. ft./min., handles .3 air changes per hour in 6,200 sq. ft., 85% efficiency, frost control
Available locally in various department and home center stores and
Available from:
Honeywell, Inc.
Home and Building Control
Honeywell Plaza
PO Box 524 (APD)
Minneapolis, MN 55440-0524
612-951-1000
and
Honeywell, Inc.
740 Ellesmere Rd. (APD)
Scarborough, ON, M1P 2V9
Canada

Honeywell Energy Recovery Ventilator ER90 Series

Mount in basement utility room, closet or suspend from outside wall or ceiling; optional dehumidistat, variable speed ventilation rate, 2 fan speeds; line voltage fresh air control; ER90-A1004 and A1012 (available in Canada only) capacity of 70 to 185 cu. ft./min., handles .3 air changes per hour in 4,500 sq. ft., 77% efficiency; A1020 has frost control
Available locally in various department and home center stores and
Available from:
Honeywell, Inc.
Home and Building Control
Honeywell Plaza
PO Box 524 (APD)
Minneapolis, MN 55440-0524
612-951-1000
and
Honeywell, Inc.
740 Ellesmere Rd. (APD)
Scarborough, ON, M1P 2V9
Canada

LIFEBREATH™ 100 DEF

Heat exchange core of thermally efficient aluminum has cleanable air filter in exhaust and fresh air streams; optional remote dehumidistat; 2 fans, 2 motors; 5 position speed control;

Controlling Your Environment

For the Air

82% maximum temperature recovery; damper defrost; Model 100ND as above without defrost
Available from:
Therma-Stor Products
Div. of DEC Int'l., Inc.
1919 S. Stoughton Rd. (APD)
PO Box 8050 (APD)
Madison, WI 53708
800-533-7533
608-222-5301
Fax 608-222-1447

LIFEBREATH™ 150 MAX

Heat exchange core of thermally efficient aluminum has cleanable air filter in exhaust and fresh air streams; optional remote dehumidistat; built-in humidistat; 5 position speed control; 80% maximum temperature recovery; damper defrost
Available from:
Therma-Stor Products
Div. of DEC Int'l., Inc.
1919 S. Stoughton Rd. (APD)
PO Box 8050 (APD)
Madison, WI 53708
800-533-7533
608-222-5301
Fax 608-222-1447

LIFEBREATH™ 150 SP

Heat exchange core of thermally efficient aluminum has cleanable air filter in exhaust and fresh air streams; optional remote dehumidistat; 3 position speed control; 80% maximum temperature recovery; electric defrost
Available from:
Therma-Stor Products
Div. of DEC Int'l., Inc.
1919 S. Stoughton Rd. (APD)
PO Box 8050 (APD)
Madison, WI 53708
800-533-7533
608-222-5301
Fax 608-222-1447

LIFEBREATH™ 195 DCS

Heat exchange core of thermally efficient aluminum has cleanable air filter in exhaust and fresh air streams; optional remote dehumidistat; built-in humidistat; 5 position speed control; 94% maximum temperature recovery; damper defrost
Available from:
Therma-Stor Products
Div. of DEC Int'l., Inc.
1919 S. Stoughton Rd. (APD)
PO Box 8050 (APD)
Madison, WI 53708
800-533-7533
608-222-5301
Fax 608-222-1447

LIFEBREATH™ 200 MAX

Heat exchange core of thermally efficient aluminum has cleanable air filter in exhaust and fresh air streams; optional remote dehumidistat; built-in humidistat; 5 position speed control; 80% maximum temperature recovery; damper defrost
Available from:
Therma-Stor Products
Div. of DEC Int'l., Inc.
1919 S. Stoughton Rd. (APD)
PO Box 8050 (APD)
Madison, WI 53708
800-533-7533
608-222-5301
Fax 608-222-1447

LIFEBREATH™ 200 STD

Heat exchange core of thermally efficient aluminum has cleanable air filter in exhaust and fresh air streams; optional remote dehumidistat; built-in humidistat; 3 position speed control; 80% maximum temperature recovery; electric preheat defrost
Available from:
Therma-Stor Products
Div. of DEC Int'l., Inc.
1919 S. Stoughton Rd. (APD)
PO Box 8050 (APD)
Madison, WI 53708

Controlling Your Environment

For the Air

800-533-7533
608-222-5301
Fax 608-222-1447

LIFEBREATH™ 300 DCS

Heat exchange dual core of thermally efficient aluminum has cleanable air filter in exhaust and fresh air streams; optional remote dehumidistat; built-in humidistat; 5 position speed control; 94% maximum temperature recovery; damper defrost
Available from:
Therma-Stor Products
Div. of DEC Int'l., Inc.
1919 S. Stoughton Rd. (APD)
PO Box 8050 (APD)
Madison, WI 53708
800-533-7533
608-222-5301
Fax 608-222-1447

LIFEBREATH™ Commercial Models

Models 700, 1200, 1000; heat exchange core of thermally efficient aluminum has cleanable air filter in exhaust and fresh air streams
Available from:
Therma-Stor Products
Div. of DEC Int'l., Inc.
1919 S. Stoughton Rd. (APD)
PO Box 8050 (APD)
Madison, WI 53708
800-533-7533
608-222-5301
Fax 608-222-1447

QDT SAE 150

Modular thermal recovery unit; built-in condensation; positive seal between exhaust and fresh air flows; automatic defrost cycle; 2-speed fans; casing is 24-gauge galvenized steel; heat recovery module is aluminum and alloys; air-flow partition is galvenized steel; exterior coating is industrial enamel; internally insulated; 94 lbs.
Available from:
QDT, Ltd.

1000 Singleton Blvd.
Dallas, TX 75212-5214
214-741-1993
Fax 214-747-3614

Quiet-Vent®

Programmable, central exhaust ventilation system; lowers humidity; 2-speed motor; remote control; cleanable filter
Available from:
Therma-Stor Products
Div. of DEC Int'l., Inc.
1919 S. Stoughton Rd. (APD)
PO Box 8050 (APD)
Madison, WI 53708
800-533-7533
608-222-5301
Fax 608-222-1447

RTU 1000 Series

Moisture transferred in vapor phase, eliminating wet surfaces, condensate drain, bacterial growth; winter humidification requirements reduced; rooftop ventilator supplies 500 to 1000 CFM; 15 CFM/person for 66 occupants
Available from:
Airxchange, Inc.
401 V.F.W. Dr. (APD)
Rockland, MA 02370
617-871-4816
Fax 617-871-3029

HEATERS

Ceramic Raidant Heater 1624

Stay-cool grille; high temperature handle; thermostat controls away from heated area; indicator light; stainless steel frame; optional wheels
Available from:
N.E.E.D.S.
527 Charles Ave. 12A (APD)
Syracuse, NY 13209
800-634-1380
Fax 800-295-NEED (6333)

Controlling Your Environment

For the Air

DeLonghi Radiator

Portable 1,500 watt electric heater; fan-forced convection heater, oil-filled radiator; heats 180 sq. ft. room; foot levers control functions; thermostat; 22 1/2"x13 1/2"x7;" 19.2 lbs.
Available from:
Hammacher Schlemmer
147 E. 57th St. (APD)
New York, NY 10022
800-543-3366
212-421-9000

Patton Compact Heater

Adjustable thermostat with automatic shut-off; back-up safety fuse; 3 settings from 500 to 1,500 watts; fan-only setting; special setting to keep unoccupied rooms between 34 and 39 degrees F
Available from:
Brookstone Co.
5 Vose Farm Road (APD)
Peterborough, NH 03458
800-926-7000
Fax 603-924-0093

Patton Wall Mount Heater

Ground fault protection shuts off upon conact with water; safe for bathrooms; 4 settings from 500 to 1,500 watts; 30 minute timer; electrostatically charged filter for dust; free standing or wall mount
Available from:
Brookstone Co.
5 Vose Farm Road (APD)
Peterborough, NH 03458
800-926-7000
Fax 603-924-0093

Pelonis Disc Furnace B2

Portable ceramic heater; 6" cube with built-in carrying case; 1500 watt, 110 volts; 6 lbs.
Available from:
Allergy Relief Shop,™ Inc.
3371 Whittle Springs Rd. (APD)
Knoxville, TN 37917
Orders 800-626-2810

Questions 615-522-2795

Plug-In Heater-Fan

Cord-free heater plugs into grounded outlet; automatic shut-off; cooling fan (not hot to the touch); night light; 4,100 BTU heater with thermostat; 2 lbs
Available from:
Solutions®
PO Box 6878 (APD)
Portland, OR 97228
800-342-9988
Fax 503-643-1973

Radiant Heater

Honeycombed lens of aluminum reflects heat; cycles down automaticaly; no fan; floor stand or wall mount; 1.250 watts
Available from:
Brookstone Co.
5 Vose Farm Road (APD)
Peterborough, NH 03458
800-926-7000
Fax 603-924-0093

Techno-Therm Room Heater

Vacuum sealed boiler filled with water and ethylene glycol, heating element; rigid metal cabinet; mixture boils in seconds, vaporizes in vertical tubes, transferring heat to fins; fans directs heat to floor and in 3 directions; 2 safety switches and tip switch; no Fire Hazard Warning because does not initiate a flame; cabinet does not become hot; 12-1/2 lbs.
Available from:
Brookstone Co.
5 Vose Farm Road (APD)
Peterborough, NH 03458
800-926-7000
Fax 603-924-0093
and:
Hammacher Schlemmer
147 E. 57th St. (APD)
New York, NY 10022
800-543-3366

Controlling Your Environment

For the Air

212-421-9000
and:
Sporty's® Preferred Living
Clermont County Airport (APD)
Batavia, OH 45103-9747
800-543-8633
Fax 513-732-6560

Vornado™ Automatic Fan

Built-in temperature-sensing thermostat increases fan speed as temperature rises, slows as it cools
Available from:
Brookstone Co.
5 Vose Farm Road (APD)
Peterborough, NH 03458
800-926-7000
Fax 603-924-0093

Vornado™ Vortex Heater

Circuit breaker, over-heat sensor, tip-over switch; heated air exits at 120 degrees F. with cool surface; 1,000 to 1,500 watts; fan-only setting
Available from:
Brookstone Co.
5 Vose Farm Road (APD)
Peterborough, NH 03458
800-926-7000
Fax 603-924-0093

ASSOCIATED PRODUCTS HUMIDITY GAUGES

Airguide® Comfort Station

Dual digital display shows temperature and humidity; memory feature; acccuracy +-2 degrees F.; built-in stand or wall mount
Available from:
Allergy Asthma Technology
4151 N. Kedzie (APD)
PO Box 18398 (APD)
Chicago, IL 60618
800-621-5545
312-465-8020
Fax 312-465-7619
and:

Allergy-Asthma Shopper™
PO Box 239 (APD)
Fate, TX 75132
800-447-1100
Fax 903-883-4513

Airguide® Humidity Indicator

Indoor indicator 4 5/8" in diameter; gray metal case, chrome bezel, white dial
Available from:
Environtrol® Corporation
PO Box 31313 (APD)
St. Louis, MO 63131
800-423-1982
In St. Louis 314-966-6886

Airguide® Sensor 112

Calibrates from 30% to 80% with a plus or minus 3% accuracy; Farenheit and Centrigrade thermometer; metal die cast case, chrome-plated brass bezel; 5-1/4" in diameter
Available from:
Environtrol® Corporation
PO Box 31313 (APD)
St. Louis, MO 63131
800-423-1982
In St. Louis 314-966-6886

Bionaire® Climate Check BT-254C/BT-254F

Solid-state, digital humidity gauge and temperature gauge
Available from:
Bionaire Corp.
90 Boroline Rd. (APD)
Allendale, NJ 07401
80-253-2764
201-934-0755
and:
Priorities®
70 Walnut St. (APD)
Wellesley, MA 02181
800-553-5398

Bionaire® Digital Hygrometer

Digital display hyrometer and thermometer for desktop or wall

Controlling Your Environment

For the Air

mount; one AAA battery; 6-1/4"x4 3/4"
Available from:
Allergy Control Products, Inc.
96 Danbury Rd. (APD)
PO Box 793 (APD)
Ridgefield, CT 06877
800-422-DUST (3878)
203-438-9580
Fax 203-431-8963

Dial Gauge Humidity Indicator
Grey metal case with white dial and black numbers; range 0 to 100% in 1% increments; wall mount
Available from:
Edmund Scientific Co.
101 E. Gloucester Pike (APD)
Barrington, NJ 08007-1380
609-573-6250
Fax 609-573-6295

Dial Temperature/Humidity
Indicates relative humidity level in large numbers and temperature in Fahrenheit and Celsius on a separate scale; wall mount
Available from:
Edmund Scientific Co.
101 E. Gloucester Pike (APD)
Barrington, NJ 08007-1380
609-573-6250
Fax 609-573-6295

Digital Hygrometer
Flush mounted on panel or built-in, battery powered unit updates digital display every second; polystyrene panel
Available from:
Edmund Scientific Co.
101 E. Gloucester Pike (APD)
Barrington, NJ 08007-1380
609-573-6250
Fax 609-573-6295

Digital Thermometer/Hygrometer
Battery powered unit with LCD display; low battery warning
Available from:

Edmund Scientific Co.
101 E. Gloucester Pike (APD)
Barrington, NJ 08007-1380
609-573-6250
Fax 609-573-6295

Huger Hygrometer/Thermometer
Measures relative humidity by the coating on a metal spiral connected to a pointer; black metal frame, white face with black markings; outside diameter 4-7/8"
Available from:
Edmund Scientific Co.
101 E. Gloucester Pike (APD)
Barrington, NJ 08007-1380
609-573-6250
Fax 609-573-6295

Huger Hygrometer
Measures relative humidity from 20 to 100%, calibrated every 1%; wall mount, brass frame; white dial with black markings; outside diameter 4.5"
Available from:
Edmund Scientific Co.
101 E. Gloucester Pike (APD)
Barrington, NJ 08007-1380
609-573-6250
Fax 609-573-6295

Taylor Hygro-Thermometer 5502
Measures indoor humidity and temperature; 3-1/4" gauge
Available from:
Allergy Supply Co.
11994 Star Court (APD)
Herndon, VA 22071
800-323-6744
Metropolitan DC 703-391-2011
Fax 703-391-2014
BBS 703-521-0638
and:

Taylor Precision Hygro-Thermometer 5565
Measures indoor humidity and temperature; 5" gauge
Available from:
Allergy Supply Co.

Controlling Your Environment

For the Air

11994 Star Court (APD)
Herndon, VA 22071
800-323-6744
Metropolitan DC 703-391-2011
Fax 703-391-2014
BBS 703-521-0638

Thermo-Hygro
Digital readout displays temperature; puts highs and lows in Fahrenheit or Centigrade into memory for review; monitors indoor humidity; outside temperature probe on 10 ft. cable; battery
Available from:
Brookstone Co.
5 Vose Farm Road (APD)
Peterborough, NH 03458
800-926-7000
Fax 603-924-0093

Wall Humidity Gauge
Accurate within 3%; round gauge, white face with black markings
Available from:
Asthma Outreach Library
37 Pillsbury Rd. (APD)
Sandown, NH 03873
603-329-5301

Wall Mount Hygrometer
Wet and dry bulb thermometer with mahogany finish; range of 60 degrees to 220 degrees F; includes wick and tables
Available from:
Edmund Scientific Co.
101 E. Gloucester Pike (APD)
Barrington, NJ 08007-1380
609-573-6250
Fax 609-573-6295

MOLD, MINERAL, RESIDUE CONTROL FOR HUMIDIFIERS

Clean-Away DMS-215
Cleaning solution for scale, mineral deposits, and residue in humidifiers
Available from:
Appliance Sales & Service Co.
655 Mission St. (APD)
San Francisco, CA 94105
800-424-6783
In 415 area call 415-362-7195
and:
Bionaire Corp.
90 Boroline Rd. (APD)
Allendale, NJ 07401
80-253-2764
201-934-0755

Demineralization Cartridge
Cleans water in Bionaire ultrasonic humidifiers
Available from:
Appliance Sales & Service Co.
655 Mission St. (APD)
San Francisco, CA 94105
800-424-6783
In 415 area call 415-362-7195
and:
Bionaire Corp.
90 Boroline Rd. (APD)
Allendale, NJ 07401
80-253-2764
201-934-0755

DynaFilter® K14
Replacement cartridge filter for Kaz humidifiers
Locally available and
Available from:
Kaz, Inc.
10 Columbus Circle (APD)
New York, NY 10019
800-241-1131
Fax 212-265-9248

Controlling Your Environment

For the Air

Humidifier Bacteria Treatment

Scented liquid. For bacteria and algae buildup in wicking humidifiers
Available from:
Bemis Mfg. Co.
300 Mill St. (APD)
PO Box 901 (APD)
Sheboygan Falls, WI 53085-0901
800-558-7651
414-467-4621
Fax 414-467-8573

Impregon Bacteriostat

Concentrated liquid that prevents mold growth in humidifiers and air conditioners; does not kill existing mold; "non-allergenic"
Available from:
Allergy Asthma Technology
4151 N. Kedzie (APD)
PO Box 18398 (APD)
Chicago, IL 60618
800-621-5545
312-465-8020
Fax 312-465-7619
and:
Allergy Supply Co.
11994 Star Court (APD)
Herndon, VA 22071
800-323-6744
Metropolitan DC 703-391-2011
Fax 703-391-2014
BBS 703-521-0638

Pre-Filter

Demineralizes water to eliminate white dust in humidifiers
Available from:
Appliance Sales & Service Co.
655 Mission St. (APD)
San Francisco, CA 94105
800-424-6783
In 415 area call 415-362-7195
and:
Bionaire Corp.
90 Boroline Rd. (APD)
Allendale, NJ 07401
80-253-2764
201-934-0755

Smokemaster® Liquid Detergent

Concentrated detergent for washable electronic filters
Available from:
Air Quality Engineering, Inc.
3340 Winpark Dr. (APD)
Minneapolis, MN 55427-2083
800-328-0787
612-544-4426
Fax 612-544-4013

Ultrasonic Humidifier Replacement Pack

Model 6515-500: Canister and resin pack for most ultrasonic humidifiers
Available from:
Northern Electric Co.
Highway 49 North (APD)
PO Box 70 (APD)
Hattiesburg, MS 39402-0070
601-268-2880

Water Filter/Demineralizing Cartridge

For ultrasonic humidifier; reduces white dust from high mineral content in tap water; prefilters water
Available from:
Kaz, Inc.
10 Columbus Circle (APD)
New York, NY 10019
800-241-1131
Fax 212-265-9248

Water Hardness Analysis Kit

Assesses need for demineralization cartridges
Available from:
Bionaire Corp.
90 Boroline Rd. (APD)
Allendale, NJ 07401
80-253-2764
201-934-0755

Controlling Your Environment

For the Air

HOUSEHOLD AIDS

Aller-Tech™ Vent Guard

Cut to fit air supply vents; 85% efficient at 10 micron; in warm weather used over screens and window air conditioners to trap pollen and mold spores; installs with magnetic velcro strips; installation kit
Available from:
Allergy Asthma Technology
4151 N. Kedzie (APD)
PO Box 18398 (APD)
Chicago, IL 60618
800-621-5545
312-465-8020
Fax 312-465-7619

Allerx® Vent Filter Kit

Washable 8"x12" cover of high efficiency polyester material; covers central air system vent to trap dust; velcro attachments; used on only one vent at a time to avoid damage to system
Available from:
Allergy-Asthma Shopper(TM)
PO Box 239 (APD)
Fate, TX 75132
800-447-1100
Fax 903-883-4513

Basket Guard Furnace Filter

For Lennox style furnaces, cut to size and place in filter basket; replaceable; 3'x6'
Available from:
Allergy Asthma Technology
4151 N. Kedzie (APD)
PO Box 18398 (APD)
Chicago, IL 60618
800-621-5545
312-465-8020
Fax 312-465-7619

Dennyfoil® Vapor Barrier

Aluminum reflective insulation vapor barrier; meets FHA requirements for vapor protection; aluminum foil glue; mounted to Kraft® paper

Available from:
E.L. Foust Co., Inc.
PO Box 105 (APD)
Elmhurst, IL 60126
800-225-9549
708-834-4952
Fax 708-834-5341

Register Cover

Blend of small and large fibers in a 16"x60" roll; cut with scissors to fit room register; optional velcro® mounting kit
Available from:
Allergy Supply Co.
11994 Star Court (APD)
Herndon, VA 22071
800-323-6744
Metropolitan DC 703-391-2011
Fax 703-391-2014
BBS 703-521-0638

VACU-FILT™

Vacuum exhaust filter with imbedded electrostatic charges placed in vacuum canister over the exhaust grille; 8"x10" sheets cut to size with scissors; used for canister style orhard encased uprights
Available from:
Allergy Control Products, Inc.
96 Danbury Rd. (APD)
PO Box 793 (APD)
Ridgefield, CT 06877
800-422-DUST (3878)
203-438-9580
Fax 203-431-8963
and:
Allergy Relief Products
9 Renata Ct. (APD)
Dundas, ON L9H 6X1
Canada
905-628-5324 ?416
Fax 416-628-1734
and:
N.E.E.D.S.
527 Charles Ave. 12A (APD)
Syracuse, NY 13209
800-634-1380
Fax 800-295-NEED (6333)

Controlling Your Environment

For the Air

Vent and Grille Filter

Non-rigid, 1/4" thick Hi-Tech filter fits behind air supply vent and outlet grille in walls and floors and window air conditioner units
Available from:
Environtrol(R) Corporation
PO Box 31313 (APD)
St. Louis, MO 63131
800-423-1982
In St. Louis 314-966-6886
and:
Hi-Tech Filter Corp. of America
80 Myrtle St. (APD)
N. Quincy, MA 02171
800-448-3249
In MA 617-328-7756
Fax 617-773-4192

Vent-Pro™

Disposable heating vent filter; electrostatically enhanced media filters with low air flow resistance; cut to size and place behind vent cover; 20"x24" sheet
Available from:
Allergy Control Products, Inc.
96 Danbury Rd. (APD)
PO Box 793 (APD)
Ridgefield, CT 06877
800-422-DUST (3878)
203-438-9580
Fax 203-431-8963

AUTOMOBILE AIDS

Kasco TURBO 1

Air filtration unit for tractor, truck; installation through roof, kit included; runs on vehicle's electrical system; 2 fans; 585 CFM; dust particle filter and organic vapor filter (when spraying); 28 lbs.
Available from:
St. George Co., Ltd.
20 Consolidated Dr. (APD)
PO Box 430 (APD)
Paris, ON N3L 3T5
Canada
519-442-2046
Fax 519-442-7191
U.S. 800-461-4299

Power Pack C2 Converter

Allows you to operate Auto Air Purifier 160A on 110v current while traveling or visiting; 6 lbs.
Available from:
E.L. Foust Co., Inc.
PO Box 105 (APD)
Elmhurst, IL 60126
800-225-9549
708-834-4952
Fax 708-834-5341

HELP US TO HELP YOU

When writing to the companies and organizations listed here, be sure to use the initials (APD) as part of the address and tell them you saw them listed in *Allergy Products Directory.*

If you call, be sure to tell them you found them in *Allergy Products Directory.*

This is important to you because:

1. Lets the company know that its listings have helped you.

2. Encourages the company to keep *Allergy Products Directory* informed of its new products so that we can keep you informed.

3. Enables us to keep our listings accurate and up-to-date for you on the latest products, services, and innovations.

4. Enables us to keep the Directory price low for you.

INSECTS AND ARACHNIDS

STINGING INSECTS

The group of social, stinging insects, called Hymenoptera (like bees, hornets, yellow jackets, and wasps) can cause major problems. Hornets, yellow jackets, and wasps are known as Vespids and the treatment for their stings is different from that of the bee.

The stings of Harvester and fire-ants can produce allergic reactions that can be severe, but fire-ants seem to be the real problem. Fire-ants have a sting that can destroy skin tissue and thousands of them can overwhelm a victim.

Hornets, yellow jackets, and wasps are known as Vespids and the treatment for their stings is different from that of the bee.

Where they are prevalent, fire-ants can heavily populate an area with mounds reaching three feet across. Fire-ants do not keep to uninhabited fields, but can be found in lawns, parks, and playing fields.

TYPES OF REACTIONS

NORMAL REACTION

Most people have a normal reaction to a sting. This would involve localized pain, redness, swelling, and itchiness that ease by the next couple of days. Symptoms remain local and are caused by irritating chemicals in the venom itself.

TOXIC REACTION

If you were to disturb a nest, you could suffer a toxic reaction from multiple stings. A toxic reaction could cause some serious medical problems and even be life-threatening.

ALLERGIC REACTION

About one million Americans have the potential for a serious reaction to an insect sting, which may be life-threatening. Allergic reactions can occur from just one sting.

Controlling Your Environment

Insects and Arachnids

MILD ALLERGIC REACTION

A mild allergic reaction would involve hives, itching, a feeling of unease and fatigue.

MODERATE ALLERGIC REACTION

A more severe reaction could involve hives all over the body, a general swelling of the body, a feeling of tightness around the chest, swelling of the lips, face, or extremities, dizziness, cramps, nausea and sometimes vomiting.

SEVERE ALLERGIC REACTION

Severe reactions include the above symptoms and also confusion or shock, breathing difficulty because the tongue or throat is swelling, or asthma or lower respiratory symptoms.

LIFE-THREATENING, ALLERGIC REACTION

The symptoms of a severe, life-threatening, allergic reaction usually appear within 15 minutes of a sting. These symptoms may include flushing, a rapid drop in blood pressure, swelling, respiratory arrest, and/or loss of consciousness. These reactions develop almost immediately after the sting. This is a medical emergency and victims need emergency care as soon as possible.

DELAYED REACTION

Delayed reactions can occur as long as two weeks after a sting. Symptoms are pains in the body's joints, hives or other rashes, swollen lymph nodes.

WHAT TO DO IF YOU ARE STUNG

NON-ALLERGIC REACTION

✔ The honeybee leaves its stinger with venom sac in your body. Remove it as quickly as possible by scraping it with your fingernail. Don't try to pick it up or pinch it to remove it because you may squeeze out more venom.

✔ Yellow jackets, wasps, and hornets do not leave the venom sac in you when they sting, but the stinger can be broken off if you swat at them.

✔ It is important to note if the stinger is present or not. Is there a venom sac? Doctors must know if you were stung by a honeybee or by a Vespid in order to begin the proper therapy, if you need it.

✔ Brush off other stinging insects and leave the area.

Controlling Your Environment

Insects and Arachnids

✔ Place ice over the sting or wash with soap and cold water if no ice is available. Look for more serious symptoms, particularly extensive swelling.

✔ Take an antihistamine

✔ If you are stung by a fire-ant, try to avoid a secondary infection by keeping the wound clean and not scratching.

ALLERGIC REACTION

✔ If there is a stinger, remove it by scraping it with your nail. Note if there is a venom sac.

✔ Doctors must know if you were stung by a honeybee or by a Vespid or by a fire-ant in order to begin the proper therapy. Yellow jackets, wasps, and hornets do not leave the venom sac in you when they sting, but the stinger can be broken off if you swat at them.

✔ Know how to use your emergency kit or pen, available with pre-measured epinephrine in a syringe or be sure that someone you are with knows how to use it. These are available with a prescription. These pens and kits and other means of emergency communication (cards, pendants, or bracelets) are described in the listings that follow.

✔ If no pen or kit is available, try giving an antihistamine.

✔ Call the paramedics. This is a medical emergency. The victim must be taken to the nearest emergency room. If the victim is away from home, also call parents or family members.

PROTECT YOURSELF IF YOU HAVE BEEN STUNG

> ### *If you have suffered a severe reaction in the past. . .*
>
> • Protection can be obtained with pure venom therapy.
>
> • Carry a pen or bee sting kit with you at all times, especially if you have not been taking venom therapy for an adequate period of time.
>
> • Wear a pendant or bracelet or carry a warning card.
>
> • If you are taking any medications, especially heart or blood pressure medication, be sure to ask your doctor if you are at increased risk for a worse reaction from a bee sting. Beta blockers may make it more difficult to treat a severe reaction.

Controlling Your Environment

Insects and Arachnids

STEPS TO TAKE TO AVOID BEING STUNG

The major attractions for stinging insects are considered to be related to body odor, to be how much you sweat, your skin temperature, the level of carbon dioxide in the air around you, perfumes, aftershave, movement, and colorful clothing. Your emotional state and environmental factors influence body odor. While it is difficult to control your emotional levels, you may be able to control some environmental factors.

When outdoors, do not use perfume, cologne, suntan lotions, hair preparations, hair spray, deodorants, soaps, powders, or cosmetics — especially floral scents.

- Do not use perfume, cologne, hair preparations, hair spray, deodorants, soaps, powders, or cosmetics — especially floral scents— when outdoors. Suntan lotions should not be perfumed. This is an important caveat since many dermatologists are now recommending you use sunblock lotions all the time to avoid damage to the skin by the sun's ultraviolet rays.

- Do not wear brightly colored clothing, especially floral prints. The safest colors for outdoor clothing are khaki, tan, or light green.

- Stay away from open garbage cans, odor-producing flowers, open fields with clover or flowers, orchards, or plants.

- Stay away from anthills and antmounds.

- Wear clothes with long sleeves, long pants, and closed shoes. Don't go barefoot. At the beach, wear sneakers because there are wasps that live in the sand.

At the beach, wear sneakers.

There are wasps that live in the sand.

- Cover up in the garden. Wear gloves when gardening. Yellow jackets nest on the ground and will become angered by damage done to their nests by mowers or clippers. Wear a scarf to prevent bees from being tangled in your hair. Mowing the lawn or pruning flowers or flowering trees can be dangerous when insects are active. Consider having someone else do these chores.

- Be careful when reaching for a beach towel or other folded clothing. A stinging insect could be inside its folds.

- Keep garbage cans tightly covered and be sure cans have no holes in them. Try to keep them clean on the

Controlling Your Environment

Insects and Arachnids

outside. Trash containers are very attractive to stinging insects.

- Try to avoid eating outdoors. If you do picnic, keep foods covered except what you are eating. Never drink from an uncovered cup without first looking inside. There may be a wasp present.

- Feed your pets indoors. Their food is an attractant.

- Don't try to shoo a stinging insect away. It can become annoyed or frightened and sting. Move slowly away from the area without abrupt movement.

Never drink from an uncovered cup without first looking inside.

A wasp may be inside.

- If a yellow jacket, hornet, or wasp is a close to you, try to walk away very slowly without abrupt movement. Don't try to kill it by crushing it. There is a chemical in its venom sack that can attract other vespids up to 15 feet away.

- Vespids are attracted by odors from foods, soft drinks, fruit juices, leather, perspiration, bright colors, and water from a swimming pool or bird bath. If you are eating outdoors and attract wasps, you must leave the area. Don't leave food about after you have finished.

- Keep the swimming pool covered when not in use and keep your bird bath at the far end of the garden.

- Have a professional remove nests or swarms of stinging insects from your property.

- Keep your garden area free of pet excretia. It is an attractant.

Keep the swimming pool covered when not in use.

Keep your bird bath at the far end of the garden.

Vespids are attracted by water.

- There are other situations that have the potential to cause problems. Most of the time such activities can be enjoyed with safety so don't avoid everything, just be aware. Potential problems include. . .

- Driving the car with the windows open or a convertible with the top down

- Being on things that move: bicycles, motorcycles, horses, skates, lawn mowers or backhoes. You can collide with stinging insects.

Controlling Your Environment

Insects and Arachnids

Riding on things that move like horses or backhoes can be hazardous.

An insect can become trapped between your eyes and your glasses.

- Running, playing tennis, basketball, baseball, field hockey, or soccer can also be a problem. Even a rapid turn of your head can trap an insect between your eyes and your eyewear.

- If you live in a suburban or rural area, where there are many flowering and odor-producing plants, where there are many stinging insects anyway, consider growing an 'insect trap' in a far corner of your garden, away from your seating area. In this far corner, plant several flowering shrubs that are strong insect attractants.

Being on things that move like bicycles or skates can be hazardous

If you provide the power and are breathing with your mouth open, an insect can be impelled into your mouth or throat.

- If you are providing the moving power on a bicycle or roller skates, and breathing through your mouth, an insect can be pulled into your mouth or throat.

- There are also commercial insect traps which are listed below. Try making a trap of your own. Combine a small can of tuna with 2 tablespoons of chlorine powder and a little oil to mix. Place the can in a far corner and allow the stinging insects to feed. Be sure children and pets cannot reach. Keep the rest of your garden area uninteresting to stinging insects and use the avoidance techniques suggested above.

BITING INSECTS
TYPES OF REACTIONS

NORMAL REACTION

Biting insects like the various types of flies, midges, and mosquitoes cause small, localized swellings that become red and itchy. After an hour or so, symptoms disappear. Most of us consider these bites the penalty for being where we are and doing what we enjoy doing. We apply some Calamine lotion or zinc oxide, complain a little, and continue on. Others, however, suffer allergic reactions.

Controlling Your Environment

Insects and Arachnids

ALLERGIC REACTION

Stronger reactions involve the antibodies in your immune system which cause local itching, redness, and swelling; the red, swollen area becomes larger and does not ease for a couple of days. Sometimes a secondary infection can develop. You should see your doctor.

GENERALIZED REACTION

The most severe reaction is a generalized one, similar to that which is caused by stinging insects. This generalized reaction is not at all a common reaction to biting insects. Symptoms experienced with this reaction are shortness of breath, dizziness, nausea, general swelling.

DELAYED REACTION

If you suffer a delayed reaction, you will also note local itching, redness, and swelling, but not until two or three days have gone by. This delayed reaction can take as long as one to three weeks to ease. The bite can blister and you may feel sick, as though you had the flu. Sometimes a secondary infection can develop. See your doctor.

STEPS TO TAKE TO AVOID BEING BITTEN

Unfortunately, mosquitoes are attracted by carbon dioxide which we exhale during the normal breathing process, but there are steps you can take to minimize your exposure to biting insects, if their bites cause you problems:

• Wear long-sleeve clothing, long pants, and closed shoes; no open toes.

• There seems to be an area of disagreement regarding color. Some sources say to wear light colors, others say that dark, solid colors are attractive. Avoid spandex. It's too shiny a material even though fashionable.

Avoid spandex when you are outdoors.

Its shine makes it attractive to insects.

• Try to remain indoors in the evening and late afternoon if you are avoiding mosquitoes and blackflies; they swarm at these hours. Deerflies and horseflies are more active during the day and in specific areas.

• Be sure that house screens fit well. Patch holes.

Controlling Your Environment

Insects and Arachnids

- Don't wear perfumes or scented lotions, soaps, sprays, deodorants, or cosmetics. As odor chemicals, they are an attractant.

- Sweat can attract insects. Towel off if you can.

- Use an insect repellent, but test it to be sure that it does not irritate your lungs or skin. Diethyl-met-toluamide (DEET) and Ethyl hexanediol are generic ingredients to look for. Both must be used with care. Avoid products more than 30% DEET.

- Look for products regulated by the Environmental Protection Agency.

- Apply repellent to clothing rather than to skin whenever possible. When you apply the repellent, try to avoid your eyes and lip areas, and any broken skin. Look for a waterproof lotion since insect repellents are less effective if you are active and sweat a lot or if it is raining or you are swimming. Use it sparingly and wash with soap and water when the need for protection is over.

- You must take extra care with children because they are more vulnerable to DEET and should only use formulations with small percentages of DEET. Ask your doctor about Off!Skintastic, a lotion with 7% DEET that may be helpful for children. It is manufactured by S.C. Johnson Entomology Research Center.

Mosquitoes can breed wherever there is a small amount of water—birdbaths, saucers under flowerpots, dips in asphalt driveways.

- Permethrin spray kills ticks. Spray lightly on fabrics and let dry. Look for this spray in garden-supply stores.

- Avoid wet, marshy areas, swamps, stagnant pools where insects breed.

- If you camp, use mosquito netting. Bee keepers use fine mesh nets over their hats to protect their faces; you may prefer this.

Be sure your own home does not provide an attractive environment for breeding. Mosquitoes can breed wherever there is a small amount of water: birdbaths, saucers under flowerpots, dips in asphalt driveways.

For reliable information on handling insects in the garden, write to:

National Pest Control Association
8100 Oak St. (APD)
Dunn Loring, VA 22027

ARACHNIDS

Arachnids are spiders (like house dust mites), not insects. Spiders have eight legs and no antennae. Most do not bite and their venom varies in strength. The two spiders with the strongest venom are the black widow and the brown recluse.

The black widow (The hourglass marks the female.) prefers dark corners, nooks, crannies, log piles, piles of bedding, boxes, shoes, dark corners of barns. It lives throughout the United States.

The brown recluse likes the southern United States. This spider has a dark v-stripe on the top of its head. It prefers to be indoors in dark, quiet corners, attics, and basements.

STEPS TO TAKE TO AVOID BEING BITTEN

- Wear gloves, long sleeves, and long pants tucked into your socks, shoes when working on rock piles and barn areas.

- If you are cleaning out a closet, don't reach into a pile of shoes or sweaters. Lift items up, hold them away from your body and shake them.

- Avoid keeping unused collections of magazines or newspapers.

- Keep barns, basements, attics clear of rubbish.

- Black widow egg sacs are poisonous.

- Be very careful when cleaning out areas that have been undisturbed whether indoors or outdoors.

- Keep children's play areas free of rubbish and undisturbed piles of toys.

WHAT TO DO IF YOU ARE BITTEN

- ✔ Get to a doctor as quickly as possible.

- ✔ Wash a spider bite.

- ✔ Take an antiseptic and ice the area to relieve swelling.

- ✔ Be alert for allergic reactions like redness, itching, and swelling, hives, wheezing, nausea, dizziness, or pain.

- ✔ Try to bring the spider with you to the doctor for identification.

IRRITANT-FREE PEST CONTROL

PLANT PESTS IN THE GARDEN

PHYSICAL BARRIERS

Physical barriers can work well. Vegetable gum-based sticky barriers come in tubes. If you squeeze them on the ground around the trunk of bushes or trees, they can prevent garden ants from climbing up to tend aphids. When sticky barriers are squeezed around bedding plants, they can prevent snails and beetles from climbing up. These barriers are also available as sprays. Be sure they are vegetable-based.

Vegetable-based sticky barriers squeezed around bedding plants can keep snails and beetles away.

You will need to renew the barriers periodically. Try not to step in these gums and wear protective gloves because they are very sticky. For the same reason, keep children and pets away from these barriers.

If you put a barrier on the ground around the trunk of a tree that has a stake holding up the trunk, the ants will climb up the stake, transfer to the tree branches and tend the aphids. Squeeze the barrier around or on the stake as well.

Copper bands around the trunks of shrubs and trees also block snails. Surround a clump of plants with a raised border; generally, snails cannot climb over this barrier.

Remove the top and bottom of a used tin can and place the can over a seedling to protect it from cutworms and snails.

WASHING PLANTS

Directing a strong stream of water over plants to wash the leaves lowers somewhat populations of aphids, mealybugs, and spider mites. Do this early in the day and if you do it early in the season, you may keep the populations lower because all those removed insects would be unable to reproduce.

Washing also raises the humidity somewhat in the area and insects like spider mites prefer dusty, dirty plants and low humidity. Try weekly washings.

Controlling Your Environment
Irritant-free Pest Control

SUGGESTIONS FOR PLANT PESTS

The following possible solutions have been gathered over the years from varying sources; you will find some more effective than others and many of them probably ineffective. We haven't tested these approaches and so cannot vouch for any of them.

- Weed Killer: 3- or 4-inch layer of mulch or several layers of newspaper, held down with stone, dirt or leaves

- Dandelions: baking soda and water or salt and water

- Weeds: hand weeding is the safest and most effective; be sure to remove the entire root system

- Weeds and Insects: in the fall, turn the soil over so that you expose wintering seeds and insect eggs and larvae to the drying air

- Slugs: beer in shallow dishes or newspaper rolls placed among plants that snails are damaging

- Snails: ginger or beer in shallow dishes or newspaper rolls placed among plants that snails are damaging

- Oil Spray for over-wintering insects: combine 1 cup cooking oil with 1 tablespoon liquid dish washing detergent or 1 1/2 teaspoons in 1 cup of water for aphids, beet armyworms, spider mites, and whiteflies. Do not use on cauliflower, red cabbage, or squash.

OUTDOOR PESTS

The most important part of controlling pests without irritating chemicals is to be sure that your environment is not attracting them. Garbage should be wrapped in air tight containers. Glass, metal, and paper should be rinsed

Be sure your environment is not attracting pests!

before disposal. Garbage cans should have tightly fitting lids. Garbage cans should not have holes in them and should be placed or fenced so that they cannot be moved or broken into by pets or other animals.

FLIES

Remember that traps attract flies to an area. Place your traps where flies are already a problem: near garbage, near pet areas, or in a far corner of your lot.

Controlling Your Environment

Irritant-free Pest Control

There are several kinds of fly traps:

✔ Dehydrator traps simply keep flies imprisoned until they die.

✔ Jar traps, baited with raw meat for blow flies, have deflectors to prevent flies from escaping.

✔ Larger jar traps can be baited with a water-soluble pheromone (an attractant); you need to be sure you do not find this solution irritating.

✔ Traps with ultraviolet lights attract flies to electrically charged wire; these must be used in outbuildings like stables, barns, or kennels or in covered porches because flies cannot see ultraviolet in daylight.

There are many baits that seem to be attractive to flies. You want to be sure that you can tolerate them before using them. Also, most baits need to be moist in order to be effective. Try beer, beer with molasses, or ammonium carbonate and yeast for blow flies and stable flies

YELLOW JACKETS

Ground-nesting yellow jackets become problems if you are enjoying a barbecue, a picnic, are camping or swimming in a pool. They are attracted by food protein (barbecued food, drinks, and pet food) from about the time they become active as the weather warms until August. At that time, the population has grown considerably and sugar seems to attract them more: fruit trees, sodas, and juices.

Look for wasps inside a glass before drinking.

Move away from wasps if they are in the area. They will sting if you frighten them. Be careful when picking up a drink in a cup or glass without a lid; look inside to be sure no wasp is there.

Cleanliness is a good approach to making your home or camping area less attractive.

✔ Don't leave food or drinks uncovered outdoors.

✔ Rinse your food containers, papers, and packages before throwing them away.

✔ Garbage cans should not have holes in them; lids should be secure and fit tightly.

Place wasp traps downwind from seating areas.

Controlling Your Environment
Irritant-free Pest Control

If you have cats and dogs, feed them indoors.

Although there are aerosol sprays designed to destroy wasps in their nests, the spray may be irritating and even if you are not sensitive to stings, you should probably have the nest handled by a professional.

Place traps downwind from where you will be eating outdoors. There are chemical and synthetic baits, but if you want to avoid possible irritation, you can use bologna, chicken, or pet food; in August use overripe fruit, jams, or sodas.

Send $1 to Bio-Integral Resource Center, PO Box 7414, (ARD) Berkeley 94707. Ask for their list of publications on safe controls of yellow jackets and other insects.

FOR FURTHER INFORMATION...

Natural Pest Control
Bruce Chapman, David Penman, and Phillip Hicks
Nelson Publications, Port Chester, NY

The Garden Pest Book
Bruce Chapman, David Penman, and Phillip Hicks
Nelson Publications, Port Chester, NY

Pests, Predators, and Pesticides
Jeanette Conacher
Available from Organic Growers' Association of Washington
Wembley, WA

Common Sense Pest Control Quarterly
Bio-Integral Resource Center, Berkeley, CA

Pests of Lanscape Trees and Shrubs
Univ. Of California, Agriculture/Natural Resources
Oakland, CA

Pests of the Garden and Small Farm: A Grower's Guide to Using Less Pesticide
Univ. Of California, Agriculture/Natural Resources
Oakland, CA

Natural Enemies Are Your Allies
Univ. Of California, Agriculture/Natural Resources
Oakland, CA

Biological Control in the Western United States
Univ. Of California, Agriculture/Natural Resources
Oakland, CA

Controlling Your Environment

Irritant-free Pest Control

INDOOR ENVIRONMENT

PETS

Many doctors who work with allergic and asthmatic patients recommend giving dogs and cats away, or at least letting them go on vacation while families see how their asthma or allergy symptoms respond to the absence of their pet.

Since it may take several months for your home to clear of pet allergens, most families decide too early that their pet is not causing any problem. Another difficulty is that other changes should be made to your home environment as well before symptom changes would be noted.

Pet saliva, dander, and urine are allergens.

Your pet's saliva can be a major cause of problems. If you are very sensitive, your skin may turn red and itch where your pet licks you, and cat saliva on fur aerosolizes and is found in the air.

Pet dander is another allergic problem. Although your pet's dander or skin flakes are an allergic component of house dust, they are also an allergen by themselves. Dander is a long-lasting problem. It can remain in a home that has not had a pet for months, even years.

FLEAS

If your doctor agrees that your pet can stay, you may still have problems from your pet's fleas.

Entomologist Ricahrd J. Brenner of the Agriculture Department's Medical and veterinary Entomology Research Lab in Gainesville, FL identified two flea-related proteins that can elicit allergic responses. Both come from flea debris: feces, eggshells, molted skin, and body parts. The researchers harvested these allergens from house dust vacuumed from the bedding, furniture, and carpeting of homes with fleas.

Many people are allergic to the proteins in the saliva of fleas and that's why a flea bite can trigger a runny nose and watery eyes.

SUGGESTONS FOR FLEAS

The SPCA recommends non toxic flea repellents for dogs made from herbal distillates. SPCA says they can also repel mosquitoes. These repellents are available in health food stores. Be careful because these herbs have odors of their own and can be irritating, so you may not be able to use them. If you have an allergy to spices, you also may not be

Herbs have odors of their own and can be irritating.

Some people have allergies to spices.

able to use them. These potential repellents include citronella, cedar wood, eucalyptus, pennyroyal, peppermint, orange, sassafras, lavender, geranium, clove, rue, mint. The oil is applied to your dog's fur or collar or added in small quantities to its regular shampoo. Don't use too much or your pet will end up with a dermatitis.

You can dust your dog with powdered sage, wormwood, sassafras, bay leaf, or vetiver. Wear a mask and gloves to try to prevent these powders from irritating your lungs or your skin. Remember, it is possible that these can also irritate you.

Nothing takes the place of regular washing of your pet's bedding and frequent vacuuming. Spraying sleeping areas and areas where your pet spends a lot of time like the car or the yard is usually recommended, but you should use caution and common sense before considering use of a spray and discuss such a move with your doctor.

Nothing takes the place of regular washing of your pet's bedding and frequent vacuuming.

We've been reading more and more that washing your cat either once a week in distilled water or twice a month in warm water or once a month in warm tap water or once a week in a special solution will stop or diminish your cat's production of skin protein.

Our first thought is exactly how are you going to set up a routine of washing your cat? Remember that your cat's saliva is a problem that isn't solved by a washing routine, and pet urine is another identified allergen.

INDOOR PESTS

Select your pest-control solution with care because of your own and your family's sensitivities, especially if you have young children or pets. Keep countertops and floor clean. Ants are attracted by grease and sugar; cockroaches and flies by food crumbs.

The following possible solutions have been gathered over the years from varying sources; you will find some more effective than others and many of them probably ineffective. We haven't tested these approaches and so cannot vouch for any of them.

Controlling Your Environment

Irritant-free Pest Control

Most importantly, your choice should depend upon your own sensitivities.

✔ Ants: mixtures of sugar with Epsom salts or sugar and boric acid or mint or spearmint or whole cloves or talcum powder or chalk lines or damp coffee grounds or salt and pepper or red chili pepper or paprika or borax or white rice and salt or honey and boric acid

✔ Beetles: store grains with a bay leaf or store them in the refrigerator in an airtight container

✔ Cockroaches: baking soda and powdered sugar or a mixture of flour, coca powder, and borax or cucumber rinds or bay leaves or a mixture of oatmeal and plaster of Paris or Epson salts with boric acid or plain baking soda or boric acid sprinkled along baseboards or oil of peppermint or eucalyptus or a mixture of flour, borax, cocoa and plaster of Paris

---

Most importantly, your choice of pest control should depend upon your own sensitivities.

✔ Fleas: Brewer's yeast added to pet food or salt in crevices of the dog house or sleeping area

✔ Flies: fly swatter or flypaper made from brown paper coated with a boiled mixture of corn syrup, sugar, and water or window and door screens or orange peels (no citrus allergy is present) or beer or beer with molasses or ammonium carbonate and yeast or fruit

✔ Moths: store clothes (clean and stain-free) in containers sealed with tape to make them airtight or lavender or whole peppercorns or Epsom salts or wrap in paper, freeze for one week and then store in tightly fitting bags or newspapers

✔ Rodents: clean counters and floors and seal holes; mousetraps or mixture of plaster of Paris, cocoa, powder and flour or garlic

✔ Silverfish: boric acid mixed with flour, sugar, and placed on strips of paper

INSECT AND RODENT REPELLENTS

Pest control has been a problem over the centuries. This chapter presents possible methods of control that may be less likely to irritate lungs and skin. As always, what works for someone else may not work for you and what does not irritate you may not irritate pests either.

Catalogue companies may rotate their stock seasonally. If you see product here that is not in the current catalogue it may become available again during a more appropriate time of year for its use. You can always call the company to request the product. Catalogues generally like to stock for demand or they may be able to give you the name of the supplier.

Do not use hanging pest strips. They supply a constant release of pesticide into your air.

Electronic Flea Trap

Special light projecting onto a sticky surface lures adult fleas; attracts fleas from carpeting, not from pets; UL listed
Available from:
Home Trends
1450 Lyell Ave. (APD)
Rochester, NY 14606-2184
716-254-6520
Fax 716-458-9245

Gopher, Mole Eliminator

Aluminum stake vibrates, repells tunneling rodents (moles, gophers, voles); batteries
Available from:
Brookstone Co.
5 Vose Farm Road (APD)
Peterborough, NH 03458
800-926-7000
Fax 603-924-0093
and:
Home Trends
1450 Lyell Ave. (APD)
Rochester, NY 14606-2184
716-254-6520
Fax 716-458-9245

Insect Disposal System

Rechargeable vacuum-powered, hand-held tube sucks insects into nozzle and sealed, disposable cartridge; includes recharger; household current; on/off switch; unit made of ABS plastic
Available from:
Hammacher Schlemmer
147 E. 57th St. (APD)
New York, NY 10022
800-543-3366
212-421-9000
and:
Home Trends
1450 Lyell Ave. (APD)
Rochester, NY 14606-2184
716-254-6520
Fax 716-458-9245

Insect Eliminator

Fan-forced suction trap for mosquitoes, flies, moths, flying nsects; attractant ultraviolet light; water-filled retention tray; effective up to 1/2 acre; indoors, outdoors; household current
Available from:
Hammacher Schlemmer
147 E. 57th St. (APD)

Asthma Resources Directory

Insect, Rodent Repellents

New York, NY 10022
800-543-3366
212-421-9000

Insectigone®
Odor-free diatomaceous earth
Available from:
Home Trends
1450 Lyell Ave. (APD)
Rochester, NY 14606-2184
716-254-6520
Fax 716-458-9245

Mosquito Hawk
Imitates sound of a dragonfly's wings; range of 50 ft.; 9 volt battery
Available from:
Lifestyle Fascination
55 Progress Pl. (APD)
Jackson, NJ 08527-3002
800-669-0987
908-928-1800
Fax 908-928-1107

Over Nite® Flea Trap
Automatic, photo cell-operated night light draws fleas to a disposble, sticky surface; UL listed; does not remove fleas from pets
Available from:
Home Trends
1450 Lyell Ave. (APD)
Rochester, NY 14606-2184
716-254-6520
Fax 716-458-9245

Pest Trap
Box with a natural lure attracts insects that infest grains, flours, nuts, pet foods; sticky surface traps insects; for use in cabinets
Available from:
Vermont Country Store,® The
PO Box 3000 (APD)
Manchester Center, VT 05255-3000
802-362-2400
Fax 802-362-0285

PestChaser
High frequency tones repell rodents and insects; internal transformer; household current; UL listed
Available from:
Home Trends
1450 Lyell Ave. (APD)
Rochester, NY 14606-2184
716-254-6520
Fax 716-458-9245
and:
Plow & Hearth
301 Madison Rd. (APD)
PO Box 830 (APD)
Orange, VA 22960
800-627-1712
Fax 800-843-2509

PestContro™
Uses magnetic pulses and sonic waves; for ants, spiders, roaches, mice, rats; plugs into electric outlet
Available from:
Lifestyle Fascination
55 Progress Pl. (APD)
Jackson, NJ 08527-3002
800-669-0987
908-928-1800
Fax 908-928-1107

Protector, The™
Electronic pulse kills flies, other flying insects; FDA-permitted use in food preparation areas; emits attractant light with wavelength and flicker detected by insects; disposble adhesive pad trap; indoors
Available from:
Frontgate
4850 Smith Rd. (APD)
PO Box 0613 (APD)
Cincinnati, OH 45264-0613
800-626-6488
Fax 800-436-2105

Stainless Steel Bug Light
Black lights attract insects, house flies; electric charge protected by safety

shield; protects 1-1/2 acres; 11-3/8"x11-3/8"x30;" 30 lbs.
Available from:
Sporty's® Preferred Living
Clermont County Airport (APD)
Batavia, OH 45103-9747
800-543-8633
Fax 513-732-6560

Stinger Laser
Attracts light-sensitive flying insects to electrically charged grid; UV 40; rust-proof; UL listed
Available from:
Stinger Environmental Products
Div. of Dejaz® Corp.
Rt. 3, Box 46 (APD)
Greeneville, TN 37743

SureFire Yellow Jacket Trap
Hang near gathering area, but away from people; bright yellow color and partially cooked piece of meat are attractants; to reuse, unfold bottom and empty
Available from:
Brookstone Co.
5 Vose Farm Road (APD)
Peterborough, NH 03458
800-926-7000
Fax 603-924-0093
and:
Solutions®
PO Box 6878 (APD)
Portland, OR 97228
800-342-9988
Fax 503-643-1973

Terra Fly Catchers
Composed of mineral oil and rubber; four ribbons per package
Available from:
Allergy Relief Shop,™Inc.
3371 Whittle Springs Rd. (APD)
Knoxville, TN 37917
Orders 800-626-2810
Questions 615-522-2795

Terra Fly Swatters
Wire with cloth blade and wire handles
Available from:
Allergy Relief Shop,™Inc.
3371 Whittle Springs Rd. (APD)
Knoxville, TN 37917
Orders 800-626-2810
Questions 615-522-2795

Transonic ESP
Electronic, ultrasonic emitter; covers up to 10,000 sq. ft.
Available from:
Lifestyle Fascination
55 Progress Pl. (APD)
Jackson, NJ 08527-3002
800-669-0987
908-928-1800
Fax 908-928-1107

Transonic® IXL Pest Repeller
High-intensity sound higher than human perception reaches to 2,000 sq. ft.; rats, mice, bats, moquitoes, spiders, fleas; household current
Available from:
Solutions®
PO Box 6878 (APD)
Portland, OR 97228
800-342-9988
Fax 503-643-1973

Ultrasonic Flea Collar
Ultrasonic sound repells fleas, ticks; nylon collar for cats (elastic to prevent choking), dogs; replaceable lithium battery
Available from:
Hammacher Schlemmer
147 E. 57th St. (APD)
New York, NY 10022
800-543-3366
212-421-9000

Wasp/Yellow Jacket Trap
Hang near gathering area, but away from people; odorless sugar water attracts and traps stinging wasps and yellow jackets

Asthma Resources Directory

Insect, Rodent Repellents

Available from:
Brookstone Co.
5 Vose Farm Road (APD)
Peterborough, NH 03458
800-926-7000
Fax 603-924-0093

Whitefly Traps
Vegetable-based, sticky film on yellow card attracts whiteflies and gnats
Available from:
Home Trends
1450 Lyell Ave. (APD)
Rochester, NY 14606-2184
716-254-6520
Fax 716-458-9245

Yard Gard
Ultrasonic waves repell unwanted animals; various frequencies cover area up to 80'x50'
Available from:
Home Trends
1450 Lyell Ave. (APD)
Rochester, NY 14606-2184
716-254-6520
Fax 716-458-9245
and:
Plow & Hearth
301 Madison Rd. (APD)
PO Box 830 (APD)
Orange, VA 22960
800-627-1712
Fax 800-843-2509

VENOMOUS MARINE LIFE

If you have not experienced a marine sting before, but you enjoy being in the ocean, snorkeling, or diving, you should familiarize yourself with the hazards of venomous marine life.

The more adventurous your underwater activities are, the more important it is that you be prepared. Never go without a partner. Know where there is a facility that has antivenin (anti-venom).

Jolie Bookspan, Ph.D. writes that venomous marine life sting for food or for protection. When they sting for protection, it is usually because they are stepped on, or cornered, or, in the case of jellyfish, you make contact with them while they drift by.

In the same way it reacts to pollen and other allergens,
your body reacts to venoms by producing antibodies to protect itself.

This is an allergic reaction.

Jellyfish stinging cells will continue to release venom as long as they are touching your skin until their venom is exhuasted. Keep away from jellyfish washed on shore. They may still be potent even if they have been dead for a while.

Venoms are proteins and enzymes. They are foreign invaders in your body in the same way that pollen is. And in the same way it reacts to pollen and other allergens, your body reacts to venoms by producing antibodies to protect itself. This is the allergic reaction that causes your body to release histamine, one of the mediators of the allergic reaction.

Stinging marine life have chemical differences in their venoms
so first aid treatment differs.

Dr. Bookspan notes that pain is a result of the injury. Depending upon what has stung you, the pain can be severe, ranging from nausea to paralysis, respiratory difficulty, and even death.

Marine life, both animal and plant life, that stings have chemical differences in their venoms and so first aid treatment differs. Unfortunately, there is disagreement about what should be done.

Controlling Your Environment

Venomous Marine Life

According to Joseph W. Burnett, MD, University of Maryland, it is important to identify the source of the venom, but if you can't, stay quiet to prevent the venom from circulating and take a pain killer.

Jellyfish leave stinging capsules on your skin which break and sting when they are rubbed. These capsules must be removed or the venom counteracted, but don't try to brush them off and don't use bare hands.

Jellyfish's stinging capsules break and sting when they are rubbed.

Dr. Burnett writes that in Gulf waters and Atlantic waters south of the Chesapeake Bay, you should use vinegar to neutralize the venom, but in Pacific waters and north of the Chesapeake Bay, use water and baking soda in equal amounts. Try a topical anesthetic, an antaihistamine, or a corticosteroid.

Marine life that stings have chemical differences in their venoms and so first aid treatment differs.

Unfortunately, there is no standard or basic treatment.

Advice is confusing because observations differ. In one instance, cold water made sting symptoms worse. In another, pain was relieved with rubbing alcohol. In another, pain was not affected by rubbing alcohol, but was helped by vinegar. And, a final observation indicated that some jellyfish stings were helped with a freshwater shower, which made the stings of other jellyfish worse.

JELLYFISH

Dr. Paul Auerbach (*A Medical Guide to Hazardous Marine Life*) suggests the following when stung by jellyfish:

✔ Rinse with seawater.

✔ Soak with vinegar. Sometimes baking soda will work.

✔ Remove large tentacles with some tool such as a forceps. Don't touch them with your hands.

✔ Remove the remaining stinging cells by shaving with shaving cream.

✔ Soak with vinegar.

✔ Apply hydrocortisone if there is no sign of infection.

✔ Keep clean and dry.

✔ Apply antiseptic ointment

Controlling Your Environment
Venomous Marine Life

Dr. Bookspan reviews various stinging animals:

HYDROIDS, FIRE CORAL

These hydroid "plants" are really animals and fire coral is a group of hydroids. They are related to jellyfish and their stings should be handled in the same way.

Although corals can sting, they can also cut and infection can enter through bacteria in the water. Cuts should be cleaned with soap and fresh water and covered with an antibacterial ointment.

SPONGES

Sponges' spicules puncture and allow bacteria to enter the skin. Treat these punctures similarly to jellyfish stings, but don't shave them. Apply tape and pull the spicules out. Skin irritation may continue for some time and may need medical care.

VENOMOUS FISH

Stingrays, lionfish, stonefish, and catfish are the most common problems and of these, the most dangerous is the stingray.

Their tail spines are covered with a membrane that allows a continuous venom release as long as the membrane touches the skin. The skin turns blue from swelling and venom. The spine has sharp teeth and when it

---

The most dangerous of the venomous fish is the stingray.

---

is pulled out, the backward-slanting teeth tear the skin while venom continues to be injected. Even after the spine is out, fragments of the membrane sheath remain in the wound, causing further problems and infection.

Dr. Brookspan suggests:

✔ Remain quiet. Have someone else do the following

✔ Flush wound with fresh water.

✔ Soak in water as hot as you can tolerate for as long as 90 minutes.

✔ Try to remove the barb carefully, although it may break. Do not remove it if it is in the chest or neck.

✔ See a doctor as soon as possible. Recovery is slow.

Controlling Your Environment

Venomous Marine Life

SPINY FISH

Fish with spines are dangerous as well. Ratfish, catfish, and weeverfish have spines that inflict painful stings and cause inflammatory responses. Zebra fish inhabit coral reefs while scorpionfish and stonefish generally swim along sandy bottoms or rocks. The latter are camouflaged and very hard to see and the stonefish's spine is powerful enough to pierce your boot.

Never go without a partner.

You may be incapable of helping yourself.

Many other fish use spines for defense, but the wounds have commonalities. First there is the puncture as the spine penetrates. Foreign matter is introduced into the wound along with the venom and bacteria. As the spine is removed, those with recurved teeth damage the skin further. Sometimes some of the spiny material along with bits of sand remains in the wound, creasing chances of infection.

AAA RECOMMENDS THE FOLLOWING PRECAUTIONS

- Never go without a partner. If you are stung, you are the patient and you will need help. If you suffer a strong reaction, you may be incapable of doing anything to help yourself. If your partner is stung, you should know the emergency procedures. Do not underestimate either situation.

- Bring a bee-sting kit with an antihistamine for use in case of sting. Be sure you are familiar with the instructions for use. You'll need a doctor's prescription so plan ahead. Dr. G. Yancey Mebane, Duke University, does not recommend epinephrine for spiny wounds.

- Bring a standard first aid kit plus vinegar, rubbing alcohol, baking soda, a razor and shaving cream, antiseptic ointment, anelgesic, and tape. Try to find out the kinds of fish that live where you will be diving and ask about other safety supplies you should have.

- If you are scuba diving, ask about the emergency equipment carried on board, including oxygen. If you will be near shore, try to discover the location of a nearby medical facility.

- Know where there is a facility that has antivenin (anti-venom).

- Be familiar with CPR.

Controlling Your Environment

Venomous Marine Life

- Wear protective clothing, but remember that it can be pierced, even if it is rubber.

- Don't touch anything. These animals are not aggressive and will not attack you unless frightened.

- Don't reach where you can't see.

- Look before you leap. Jellyfish tentacles are hard to see and so are fish hiding in dark crevices.

- When you wade, shuffle your feet to warn stingrays that are buried in the sand.

- Don't back into anything.

- Try to learn about the fish prevalent in the area in which you are diving.

Controlling Your Environment

Preparing for Emergencies

EMERGENCIES

If you or a member of your family are involved in an accident, you may have to give accurate, detailed medical information about your health status and medical needs. Problems arise when you are unconscious, are unable to speak, or if the victim is a child, or elderly, or very upset.

Paramedics, ambulance personnel, doctors, emergency room personnel all need to know what your special needs are, especially if you are allergic or asthmatic.

Emergency medical data cards, vials, bracelets, key rings, tags all serve that function. They can communicate for you, including telephone numbers of family, doctors, medical information providers, blood type, allergies. They can allow you to receive more immediate, more appropriate, and safer health care.

Printed cards summarize your medical data, but the card may not be noticed. Be sure to carry them front and center in wallets and be sure that they have an emergency telephone number that operates 24 hours. ID necklaces have room for only a few words. They should also have an emergency telephone number with full data access.

Microfiches carry all the information necessary, but need special readers otherwise the information cannot be retrieved. Our listing describes one card which incorporates its own microfiche reader.

PREPARE FOR EMERGENCIES

Ana-Guard™
Treatment for anaphylactic reactions from insect stings, food, drugs, and life-threatening asthma attacks; pre-filled syringe contains two 0.3 ml. doses of epinephrine; barrel marked with 0.1 ml graduations for infants and children under 12 years; prescription required
Available from:
Miles Inc. Pharmaceutical Div.
Miles Allergy Products
(Hollister-Stier)
PO Box 3145 (APD)
3525 N. Regal (APD)
Spokane, WA 99220-3145
800-992-1120
509-489-5656

Ana-Kit®
Contains pre-filled syringe with two 0.3 ml. doses of epinephrine for anaphylactic reactions from insect stings, food, drugs, and life-threatenng asthma attacks; syringe marked for infants and children under 12; chewable antihistamine tablets; 2 alcohol prep pads; tourniquet; carrying case; prescription required
Available from:
Miles Inc. Pharmaceutical Div.
Miles Allergy Products
(Hollister-Stier)
PO Box 3145 (APD)
3525 N. Regal (APD)
Spokane, WA 99220-3145
800-992-1120
509-489-5656

Controlling Your Environment

Preparing for Emergencies

Child's Medical Record

Booklet for entering drug sensitivities, allergies, immunizations (with recommended schedule), illnesses, medications, injuries, operations, dental examinations, and a record of height and weight
Available from:
Child's Medical Record
PO Box 17718
Memphis, TN 38187
901-767-0239

EpiPen Jr.®

Automatically injects correct epinephrine dosage for children; FDA approved for reactions to insect stings, foods, drugs, and exercise-induced anaphylaxis
Available from:
Center Laboratories
35 Channel Dr. (APD)
PO Box 70 (APD)
Port Washington, NY 11050
Customer service 800-223-6837

EpiPen®

Automatically injects correct epinephrine dosage; FDA approved for reactions to insect stings, foods, drugs, and exercised-induced anaphylaxis
Available from:
Center Laboratories
35 Channel Dr. (APD)
PO Box 70 (APD)
Port Washington, NY 11050
Customer service 800-223-6837

Parent Package

For school children with anaphylaxis; 32 page booklet with information about anaphylaxis, guidelines for emergency procedures, overhead transparencies for school personnel, forms for co-operative procedures; literature on adrenaline injection devices; non-functioning injection unit; paypable in Canadian funds
Available from:

Allergy/Asthma Information Assn.
30 Eglinton Ave. W. #750 (APD)
Mississauga, ON L5R 3E7
Canada
905-712-AAIA (2242)
Fax 905-712-2245

Portable Medical Record (MEDPASS)

Lists allergies, allergies to medications; EKG, medications being taken, emergency contact, past history; for corporate subscribers to Global Emergenecy Medical Services; information is maintained online by a 24-hour medical help desk staffed by registered nurses with emergency room experience.
Available from:
Global Emergency Medical Services
2001 Westside Dr. #120
Alpharetta, GA 30201
800-860-1111

COMMUNICATION DURING EMERGENCIES

AT&T Language Line

800-628-8486 fee
For assistance with health language problems

Emergency Identification Sticker

Sticker states name, address, blood type, allergies, emergency telephone contact and insurance carrier; for use on bicycle helmet or bicycle frame
Available from:
Specialized
15130 Concord Cir. (APD)
Morgan Hill, CA 95037
800-688-3883
800-245-3462
and
Specialized Canada
5782 Cypihot St. (APD)
Ville St. Laurent, PQ H4S 1V7
Canada

Controlling Your Environment

Preparing for Emergencies

and:
Specialized U.K.
Unit D3
Longmed Business Centre
Felstead Rd. (APD)
Eepsom, Surrey KT19 9QN
England

Emergency Medical ID

Laminated, wallet-sized card details medical history on microfilm; your photo can be laminated (and replaced as needed) or slipped into pocket on card for ease of replacement; height, weight, and hair color can be changed as needed
Available from:
EMID
23 Wensley Rd. (APD)
Plainview, NY 11803
516-935-5809

Information Card

Wallet-size card with your medical information; when calling, ask for information desk and then an answer center representative
Available from:
American Medical Assn.
515 N. State St. (APD)
Chicago, IL 60610
312-464-5000
Fax 312-464-4184

Laser Card

For group providers, hospitals, HMO's, group practices.
Laser card holds graphics, x-rays; magnetic stripe or IC chip; lists medical problems, medications and interactions, insurance information, person to notify;
Available from:
Smart Card Systems
15911 Forsythia Cir. (APD)
Del Ray Beach, FL 33484
407-495-2590
Fax 407-243-8740

Lens-Card™

Card with medical information on microfilm with built-in lens; stickers for car or wallet to alert others that you have the card
Available from:
LENSCARD® Systems
7300 Corporate Center Dr. #2C03 (APD)
Miami, FL 33126
PO Box 025491 (APD)
Miami, FL 33102-5491
800-322-3025
In Fl 305-715-3405

Life Alert

Stainless steel or gold fill case contains metal pages with medical data; pendant or bracelet available; up to 50 words for medications, allergies, drug allergy, emergency contact, contact lenses, emergency phone numbers
Available from:
Life Alert
Ste. 112, 7710 5th St SE (APD)
Calgary, AB T2H 2L9
Canada
403-258-0822
Fax 403-242-9132
and
13807 S.E. McLoughlin Blvd. #43 (APD)
Portland, OR 97222

Lifedata Systems

Medical history on microfilm readable by magnifying glass, microscope, or microfiche reader; includes tag for key ring
Available from:
Lifedata Systems, Inc.
PO Box 399 (APD)
Nevada City, CA 95959
800-345-3557

Medic Alert

Metal bracelet or pendant (stainless steel, sterling silver, gold fill)

Controlling Your Environment
Preparing for Emergencies

engraved with medical condition(s), ID number, Medic Alert's emergency hotline number for computerized records
Available from:
Canada Medic-Alert
Affiliate of Medic Alert Foundation
250 Ferrand Dr. (APD)
Don Mills, ON M2C 2T9
Canada
416-696-0267
80-668-1507
and:
Medic Alert Foundation
2323 N. Colorado Ave. (APD)
PO Box 1009 (APD)
Turlock, CA 95381-1009
800-344-3226
800-432-5378
AK, HI 209-668-3333

Medic-Alert

Sports fabric bracelet with medical condition(s), ID number, Medic Alert's emergency hotline number for computerized records
Available from:
Canada Medic-Alert
Affiliate of Medic Alert Foundation
250 Ferrand Dr. (APD)
Don Mills, ON M2C 2T9
Canada
416-696-0267
80-668-1507

Medic-Card

Folding card in plastic case with medical data, including medications, allergies, immunizations, history; emergency notification, insurance, glasses Rx; optional magnet to affix to refrigerator door
Available from:
National Medi-Card Systems
1070 Commerce St. #F (APD)
San Marcos, CA 92069
800-266-1787
In CA 619-744-1787

Medical Alert

Bracelet with wallet card, key tag with wallet card; wallet cards have room for personal identification, social security number, emergency notification, doctor number, blood type, insurance company and medical information
Available from:
Apex™Medical Corp.
800 S. Van Eps Ave. (APD)
Sioux Falls, SD 57104
PO Box 1235 (APD)
Sioux Falls, SD 57101
800-328-2935
In SD 605-332-6689
Fax 605-332-6818

Smart Card

For group providers, hospitals, HMO's, group practices.
Plastic, wallet size card with integrated computer microchip; lists medical problems in a 62-item profile, including medications and interactions, insurance information, personal information, person to notify
Available from:
Smart Card Systems
15911 Forsythia Cir. (APD)
Del Ray Beach, FL 33484
407-495-2590
Fax 407-243-8740

SmartCare™

Card listed medical information, allergies, emergency phone numbers; insurance
Available from:
SmartPractice™
3400 E. McDowell (APD)
Phoenix, AZ 85008-7899
800-522-0800
Fax 800-522-8329

SportID

Rip-proof, weather proof decal and label for outside of helmet and bicycle frame; room for name, address, phone,

Controlling Your Environment
Preparing for Emergencies

emergency contact, insurance
information, allergies, other medical
information
Availble from
CycleAware, Inc.
655 Skyway (APD)
San Carlos, CA 94070
415-508-0599

PREPARE FOR TRAVEL EMERGENCIES

Travelers Health Hotline
CDC Voice Information System
404-332-4555
404-332-4559
24-hour information line for
health advisories, vaccination
recommendations, food and water
safety; needs a touch-tone phone

Corporate Membership Program for Emergencies
Travelers and expatriates
subscribe to service. If a health
problem arises, there is a 24-hour help
desk staffed by registered nurses with
emergency room experience and
computer-based triage system. Nurse
assesses situation and refers to most
appropriate, English-speaking doctor,
clinic or hospital. If after hours, and
emergency or urgent care is needed,
Global calls to make arrangements.
Available from:
Global Emergency Medical Services
2001 Westside Dr. #120
Alpharetta, GA 30201
800-860-1111

Dept. of State Citizens Emergency Center
202-647-5225
Works with embassies to keep
families informed if you are
hospitalized overseas; refers to
emergency medical transport
companies; 8:15 am to 10:00 pm EST
M-F, 9:00 am to 3:00 pm EST Sat. For

afterhours emergency contact: 202-
634-3600 and ask for the duty officer
of the Citizens Emergency Center

Immunization Alert!
Database of health information for
travelers internationally
Available from
Immunization Alert!
PO Box 406 (APD)
Storrs, CT 06268
203-487-0002

TRAVAX
Subscription computer database
of travel health information for 229
countries includes health and safety
information. Itinerary check: enter
countries for specific recommendations
for immunizations, travel advisories.
Appropriate for hospitals, clinics,
corporate health departments, military
Available from:
Shoreland Medical Marketing, Inc.
10625 W. North Ave. #209 (APD)
Milwaukee, WI 53226
PO Box 13795 (APD)
Milwauakee, WI 53213-0795
414-774-4600

Traveller Clinical Record
Folder with personal information,
medications, alert for allergies,
electrocardiogram, schedule of dosages
for hyposensitization
Available from:
Int'l Assn. for Medical Assistance
to Travellers/(IAMAT)
736 Center St. (APD)
Lewiston, NY 14092
716-754-4883
and
40 Regal Rd. (APD)
Guelph, ON N1K 1B5
Canada
and
188 Nicklin Rd. (APD)
Guelph, ON N1H 7L5
Canada
and:

Controlling Your Environment
Preparing for Emergencies

Int'l Assn. for Medical Assistance
to Travellers/(IAMAT)
1287 St. Clair Ave. W. (APD)
Toronto, ON M6E 1B8
Canada
and
575 Bourke St. 12 Flr. (APD)
Melbourne 3000
Australia
and
57 Voirets (APD)
1212 Grand-Lancy, Geneva
Switzerland
and:
Int'l Assn. for Medical Assistance
to Travellers/(IAMAT)
PO Box 5049 (APD)
Christchurch 5

New Zealand

U.S.Public Health

Travel advisor gives specific
information
Chicago: 312-894-2960; 12:00 pm to
8:00 pm
Honolulu: 808-541-2552; 6:00 am to
3:00 pm
Los Angeles: 310-215-2365 8:00 am to
5:00 pm
Miami: 305-526-2910; 8:00 am to 5:00
pm
New York: 718-553-1685; 8:00 am to
10:00 pm
San Francisco: 415-876-2872; 8:00 am
to 4:30 pm

SUPPORT AND INFORMATION PROGRAMS

ALLERGY PROGRAMS FOR INDIVIDUALS AND FAMILIES

AAFA Support Groups
Call for information for a support group in your area
Available from:
Asthma & Allergy Foundation of America
1125 15th St. N.W. #502 (APD)
Washington, DC 20005
202-466-7643
Fax 202-466-8940

"Allergies: Medicine for the Public"
Available from:
Allergy & Asthma Network/
Mothers of Asthmatics, Inc.
3554 Chain Bridge Rd. Ste 200 (APD)
Fairfax, VA 22030-2709
Orders 800-878-4403
703-385-4403
Fax 703-352-4354

"Bee's Knees, The"
Video explains allergy to Hymenoptera and treatment
Available from:
American Academy Allergy/Imm.
611 E. Wells St. 4th Flr. (APD)
Milwaukee, WI 53202-3816
800-822-ASMA (2762)
414-272-6071
Fax 414-276-3349

"Controlling Allergens in Your Environment"
Video addresses how to control allergens in the home environment such as mites and dander
Available from:
American Academy Allergy/Imm.
611 E. Wells St. 4th Flr. (APD)
Milwaukee, WI 53202-3816
800-822-ASMA (2762)
414-272-6071

Fax 414-276-3349

"Environment, Allergies, and You, The"
Video discusses various house pollutants' affecting allergy
Available from:
American Academy Allergy/Imm.
611 E. Wells St. 4th Flr. (APD)
Milwaukee, WI 53202-3816
800-822-ASMA (2762)
414-272-6071
Fax 414-276-3349

"IgA and the Immune System"
William Brown, MD
Audtiotape
Available from:
Celiac Sprue Assn./
United States of America
PO Box 31700 (APD)
Omaha, NE 68131-0700
402-558-0600

"Immunotherapy - Old Fashioned or Futuristic"
Orientation video discusses technique, reasons, and expectations
Available from:
American Academy Allergy/Imm.
611 E. Wells St. 4th Flr. (APD)
Milwaukee, WI 53202-3816
800-822-ASMA (2762)
414-272-6071
Fax 414-276-3349

Support Group Resource Kit
Nancy Sanker, OTR
Ideas for starting and sustaining support groups; includes audio tape
Available from:
Asthma & Allergy Foundation of America
1125 15th St. N.W. #502 (APD)
Washington, DC 20005
202-466-7643
Fax 202-466-8940

Controlling Your Environment
Support and Information Programs

"Visit to the Allergy Doctor, A"

Orientation video discusses syndromes, tests, and common questions
Available from:
American Academy Allergy/Imm.
611 E. Wells St. 4th Flr. (APD)
Milwaukee, WI 53202-3816
800-822-ASMA (2762)
414-272-6071
Fax 414-276-3349

ALLERGY PROGRAMS FOR SCHOOL AND COMMUNITY

"Anaphylaxis"

Color slides with script, bibliography
Available from:
American College of
Allergy/Asthma/Imm.
85 W. Algonquin Rd. #550 (APD)
Arlington Heights, IL 60005
800-842-7777 information packets
708-427-1200

"Approach to the Patient with Suspected Immunodeficiency"

By William T. Shearer, MD, PhD; lecture slides for lay or professional audiences; includes types, diagnosis and treatment
Available from:
American Academy Allergy/Imm.
611 E. Wells St. 4th Flr. (APD)
Milwaukee, WI 53202-3816
800-822-ASMA (2762)
414-272-6071
Fax 414-276-3349

"Controversial Procedures in Allergy"

Abba I. Terr, MD; lecture slides for lay or professional audiences
Available from:
American Academy Allergy/Imm.
611 E. Wells St. 4th Flr. (APD)
Milwaukee, WI 53202-3816
800-822-ASMA (2762)

414-272-6071
Fax 414-276-3349

"Current Concepts in Asthma Diagnosis/Management"

Color slides with script, bibliography
Available from:
American College of
Allergy/Asthma/Imm.
85 W. Algonquin Rd. #550 (APD)
Arlington Heights, IL 60005
800-842-7777 information packets
708-427-1200

"Diagnosis and Management of Drug Allergy"

By Paul Van Arsdel, MD; lecture slides for lay or professional audiences
Available from:
American Academy Allergy/Imm.
611 E. Wells St. 4th Flr. (APD)
Milwaukee, WI 53202-3816
800-822-ASMA (2762)
414-272-6071
Fax 414-276-3349

"Exercise-induced Bronchospasm"

Color slides with script, bibliography
Available from:
American College of
Allergy/Asthma/Imm.
85 W. Algonquin Rd. #550 (APD)
Arlington Heights, IL 60005
800-842-7777 information packets
708-427-1200

"Go Ahead; Ask Your Pharmacist"

Video program to educate patients about their medications
Available from:
American Soc. of Hospital Pharmacists (ASHP)
7272 Wisconsin Ave. (APD)
Bethesda, MD 20814
202-289-1700

Controlling Your Environment
Support and Information Programs

HCT
Health Check Test
Pharmacist-presented slide and tape program on keeping track of medications
Available from:
Transit Medica, Inc.
779 Susquehanna Ave. (APD)
Franklin Lakes, NJ 07417
201-891-8240

"New Directions in Allergen Immunotherapy"
Roy Patterson, MD, Leslie C. Grammer, MD, Martha A. Shaughnessy, BS; lecture slides for lay or professional audiences
Available from:
American Academy Allergy/Imm.
611 E. Wells St. 4th Flr. (APD)
Milwaukee, WI 53202-3816
800-822-ASMA (2762)
414-272-6071
Fax 414-276-3349

NMAT
National Medication Awareness Test
Pharmacist-presented slide and tape program on patient medications, interactions, side effects
Available from:
Transit Medica, Inc.
779 Susquehanna Ave. (APD)
Franklin Lakes, NJ 07417
201-891-8240

"Overview of Allergy, An"
Videotape answers questions about allergy
Available from:
American College of Allergy/Asthma/Imm.
85 W. Algonquin Rd. #550 (APD)
Arlington Heights, IL 60005
800-842-7777 information packets
708-427-1200

SMAT
Self-Medication Awareness Test

Pharmacist-presented slide and tape program educating individuals about over-the-counter medications
Available from:
Transit Medica, Inc.
779 Susquehanna Ave. (APD)
Franklin Lakes, NJ 07417
201-891-8240

Speakers Bureau
Information on prescription and non-prescription medications; health topics of interest
Available from:
Albany College of Pharmacy
Div. of Extension Services
106 New Scotland Ave. (APD)
Albany, NY 12208
518-445-7233

"Sting Hymenoptera"
Color slides with script, bibliography
Available from:
American College of Allergy/Asthma/Imm.
85 W. Algonquin Rd. #550 (APD)
Arlington Heights, IL 60005
800-842-7777 information packets
708-427-1200

"Update on Diagnosis & Management of Anaphylaxis"
Diana L. Marquardt, MD; lecture slides for lay or professional audiences
Available from:
American Academy Allergy/Imm.
611 E. Wells St. 4th Flr. (APD)
Milwaukee, WI 53202-3816
800-822-ASMA (2762)
414-272-6071
Fax 414-276-3349

Controlling Your Environment
Support and Information Programs

"Update on Immunotherapy"

Color slides with script, bibliography
Available from:
American College of
Allergy/Asthma/Imm.
85 W. Algonquin Rd. #550 (APD)
Arlington Heights, IL 60005
800-842-7777 information packets
708-427-1200

Using Your Medicines Wisely

Use of prescription medications; in conjunction with pharmacist or nurse to answer questions
Available from:
American Assn. of Retired Persons (AARP)
1909 K St. N.W. (APD)
Washington, DC 20049
202-728-4451

ALLERGY PROGRAMS FOR PROFESSIONALS

"Approach to the Patient with Suspected Immunodeficiency"

By William T. Shearer, MD, PhD; lecture slides for lay or professional audiences; includes types, diagnosis and treatment
Available from:
American Academy Allergy/Imm.
611 E. Wells St. 4th Flr. (APD)
Milwaukee, WI 53202-3816
800-822-ASMA (2762)
414-272-6071
Fax 414-276-3349

"Asthma and Allergy Support Groups: The Clinician's Role"

Available from:
Asthma & Allergy Foundation of America
1125 15th St. N.W. #502 (APD)
Washington, DC 20005
202-466-7643
Fax 202-466-8940

"Controversial Procedures in Allergy"

Abba I. Terr, MD; lecture slides for lay or professional audiences
Available from:
American Academy Allergy/Imm.
611 E. Wells St. 4th Flr. (APD)
Milwaukee, WI 53202-3816
800-822-ASMA (2762)
414-272-6071
Fax 414-276-3349

"Diagnosis and Management of Drug Allergy"

By Paul Van Arsdel, MD; lecture slides for lay or professional audiences
Available from:
American Academy Allergy/Imm.
611 E. Wells St. 4th Flr. (APD)
Milwaukee, WI 53202-3816
800-822-ASMA (2762)
414-272-6071
Fax 414-276-3349

"Exercise-induced Bronchospasm"

Color slides with script, bibliography
Available from:
American College of
Allergy/Asthma/Imm.
85 W. Algonquin Rd. #550 (APD)
Arlington Heights, IL 60005
800-842-7777 information packets
708-427-1200

"New Directions in Allergen Immunotherapy"

Roy Patterson, MD, Leslie C. Grammer, MD, Martha A. Shaughnessy, BS; lecture slides for lay or professional audiences
Available from:
American Academy Allergy/Imm.
611 E. Wells St. 4th Flr. (APD)
Milwaukee, WI 53202-3816
800-822-ASMA (2762)
414-272-6071
Fax 414-276-3349

Controlling Your Environment
Support and Information Programs

"Overview of Allergy, An"
Videotape answers questions about allergy
Available from:
American College of
Allergy/Asthma/Imm.
85 W. Algonquin Rd. #550 (APD)
Arlington Heights, IL 60005
800-842-7777 information packets
708-427-1200

"Sting Hymenoptera"
Color slides with script, bibliography
Available from:
American College of
Allergy/Asthma/Imm.
85 W. Algonquin Rd. #550 (APD)
Arlington Heights, IL 60005
800-842-7777 information packets
708-427-1200

"Update on Diagnosis & Management of Anaphylaxis"
Diana L. Marquardt, MD; lecture slides for lay or professional audiences
Available from:
American Academy Allergy/Imm.
611 E. Wells St. 4th Flr. (APD)
Milwaukee, WI 53202-3816
800-822-ASMA (2762)
414-272-6071
Fax 414-276-3349

"Update on Immunotherapy"
Color slides with script, bibliography
Available from:
American College of
Allergy/Asthma/Imm.
85 W. Algonquin Rd. #550 (APD)
Arlington Heights, IL 60005
800-842-7777 information packets
708-427-1200

Controlling Your Environment

Allergy/Asthma Stores

SUPPLIERS OF ALLERGY AND ASTHMA PRODUCTS

A-Plus Equipment & Supply

Products for the air; cotton products; products for the home; respiratory care
Available from:
A-Plus Allergy Equipment & Supply
8325 Regis Way (APD)
Los Angeles, CA 90045-2646
Orders 800-86-ALLER (862-5537)
310-337-7468
Fax 310-337-1971

Absolute Environmental's Allergy Store

Products for the air; products for the home; respiratory care
Available from:
Absolute Environmental's Allergy Store
2615 S. University Dr. (APD)
Davie, FL 33328
Nationwide 800-771-ACHOO (2246)
In FL 800-329-3773
Broward 305-472-3773
Fax 305-474-0133

Aller-Guard®

Products for the air; products for the home
Available from:
Aller-Guard,® Inc.
Southgate Office Park
1645 S.W. 41st St. (APD)
Topeka, KS 66609-1250
800-234-0816
913-267-9333
Fax 913-267-0072

Allergy Aide Centre

Products for the air; products for the home; respiratory care
Available from:
Allergy Aid Centre
1st Floor Pran Central Shop 56
325 Chapel St. (APD)
Prahran, Vic 3181

Australia
03-529-7348
03-529-8459

Allergy Asthma Technology

Products for the air; products for the home; respiratory care
Available from:
Allergy Asthma Technology
4151 N. Kedzie (APD)
PO Box 18398 (APD)
Chicago, IL 60618
800-621-5545
312-465-8020
Fax 312-465-7619

Allergy Clean Environments

Products for the air; products for the home
Available from:
Allergy Clean Environments
501 Station Ave. (APD)
Haddon Heights, NJ 08035
800-882-4110
In NJ 609-546-1101
Fax 609-546-1466
URL:
http:\\WWW.infomall.com\allergy.html

Allergy Control Products, Inc.

Products for the air; products for the home; respiratory care
Available from:
Allergy Control Products, Inc.
96 Danbury Rd. (APD)
PO Box 793 (APD)
Ridgefield, CT 06877
800-422-DUST (3878)
203-438-9580
Fax 203-431-8963

Allergy Relief Products

Products for the air; products for the home; publications
Available from:

Controlling Your Environment

Allergy/Asthma Stores

Allergy Relief Products
9 Renata Ct. (APD)
Dundas, ON L9H 6X1
Canada
905-628-5324 ?416
Fax 416-628-1734

Allergy Relief Shop, Inc.
Products for the air; products for the home
Available from:
Allergy Relief Shop,™ Inc.
3371 Whittle Springs Rd. (APD)
Knoxville, TN 37917
Orders 800-626-2810
Questions 615-522-2795

Allergy Resources
Products for the air; products for the home
Available from:
Allergy Resources
Mail: PO Box 888 (APD)
UPS: 264 Brookridge Ave. (APD)
Palmer Lake, CO 80133
Orders 800-USE-FLAX (873-3529)
Company plans to move; use 800 #

Allergy Shop, Ltd., The
Products for the air; products for the home;
Available from:
Allergy Shop, Ltd.
3420 Cardston Crescent N.W. (APD)
Calgary, AB T2L 0S6
Canada
403-289-9052

Allergy Supply Co., Inc., The
Products for the air; products for the home; respiratory care
Available from:
Allergy Supply Co.
11994 Star Court (APD)
Herndon, VA 22071
800-323-6744
Metropolitan DC 703-391-2011
Fax 703-391-2014
BBS 703-521-0638

Allergy-Asthma Shopper™
Products for the air; products for the home; respiratory care
Available from:
Allergy-Asthma Shopper™
PO Box 239 (APD)
Fate, TX 75132
800-447-1100
Fax 903-883-4513

American Allergy Supply
Products for the air; products for the home; respiratory care
Available from:
PO Box 722022 (APD)
Houston, TX 77272-2022
800-321-1096
713-995-6110

Bermuda Asthma & Allergy Relief Center
Caribbean Asthma & Allergy Relief Center
The Recorder Bldg.
63 Court St. (APD)
Hamilton HM 12
Bermuda
809-292-9258
Fax 809-292-4535

DeVilbiss, Inc.
Products for the air; products for the home; respiratory care
Available from:
Sunrise Medical/DeVilbiss, Inc.
PO Box 635 (APD)
Somerset, PA 15501-0635
800-DeV-1988 (338-1988)
814-443-4881
Fax 800-345-2202
In Canada 705-728-5522

E.L. Foust Company, Inc.
Products for the air; products for the home
Available from:
E.L. Foust Co., Inc.
PO Box 105 (APD)
Elmhurst, IL 60126
800-225-9549

Controlling Your Environment

Allergy/Asthma Stores

708-834-4952
Fax 708-834-5341

Environtrol®

Products for the air; products for
the home
Available from:
Environtrol® Corporation
PO Box 31313 (APD)
St. Louis, MO 63131
800-423-1982
In St. Louis 314-966-6886

Flowright International Products

Products for the air; products for
the home
Available from:
Flowright Int'l Products
1495 N.W. Gilman Blvd. #4 (APD)
Issaquah, WA 98027
206-392-8357

N.E.E.D.S.

Products for the air; products for
the home; respiratory care
Available from:
N.E.E.D.S.
527 Charles Ave. 12A (APD)
Syrcause, NY 13209
800-634-1380
Fax 800-295-NEED (6333)

National Allergy Supply, Inc.

Products for the air; products for
the home; respiratory care
Available from:
National Allergy Supply, Inc.
4400 Georgia Hwy. 120 (APD)
PO Box 1658 (APD)
Duluth, GA 30136
800-522-1448
In Atlanta 404-623-8077
Fax 404-623-5568

Priorities®

Products for personal use
70 Walnut St. (APD)
Wellesley, MA 02181
800-553-5398

Skin & Allergy™ Shop, Inc., The

Available from:
Skin & Allergy Shop,™The
310 E. Broadway (APD)
Louisville, KY 40202
800-366-6483
In KY 502-585-4824
Fax 502-589-3429

Controlling the Environment
Catalogues and Mail Order

CATALOGUES AND MAIL ORDER

AIR FILTERS AND MOLD CONTROL

3M Company
PO Box 33275 (APD)
St. Paul, MN 55133-3275
3M Center Bldg.(APD)
St. Paul, MN 55144-1000
Medical information 800-328-0255
Medical information local 612-736-4930
Customer service 800-423-5197
Outside CA 800-423-5146
In CA 818-341-1300

A-Plus Allergy Equipment & Supply
8325 Regis Way (APD)
Los Angeles, CA 90045-2646
Orders 800-86-ALLER (862-5537)
310-337-7468
Fax 310-337-1971

AAir Purification Systems
7340 Trade St. #C (APD)
San Diego, CA 92121-2457
800-776-6746
619-578-2825
Fax 619-578-3762

Absolute Environmental's Allergy Store
2615 S. University Dr. (APD)
Davie, FL 33328
Nationwide 800-771-ACHOO (2246)
In FL 800-329-3773
Broward 305-472-3773
Fax 305-474-0133

Air Quality Engineering, Inc.
3340 Winpark Dr. (APD)
Minneapolis, MN 55427-2083
800-328-0787
612-544-4426
Fax 612-544-4013

Aireox Research Corp.
11015 Whitford Ave. (APD)
Riverside, CA 92505
909-689-2781

Aller-Guard,® Inc.
Southgate Office Park
1645 S.W. 41st St. (APD)
Topeka, KS 66609-1250
800-234-0816
913-267-9333
Fax 913-267-0072

Allergen™ Air Filter Corp.
5205 Ashbrook (APD)
Houston, TX 77081
800-333-8880
In TX 713-668-2371

Allergy Aid Centre
1st Floor Pran Central Shop 56
325 Chapel St. (APD)
Prahran, Vic 3181
Australia
03-529-7348
03-529-8459

Allergy Asthma Technology
4151 N. Kedzie (APD)
PO Box 18398 (APD)
Chicago, IL 60618
800-621-5545
312-465-8020
Fax 312-465-7619

Allergy Clean Environments
501 Station Ave. (APD)
Haddon Heights, NJ 08035
800-882-4110
In NJ 609-546-1101
Fax 609-546-1466
URL:
http:\\WWW.infomall.com\allergy.html

Allergy Control Products, Inc.
96 Danbury Rd. (APD)
PO Box 793 (APD)

Controlling the Environment
Catalogues and Mail Order

Ridgefield, CT 06877
800-422-DUST (3878)
203-438-9580
Fax 203-431-8963

Allergy Relief Products
9 Renata Ct. (APD)
Dundas, ON L9H 6X1
Canada
905-628-5324 ?416
Fax 416-628-1734

Allergy Relief Shop,™ Inc.
3371 Whittle Springs Rd. (APD)
Knoxville, TN 37917
Orders 800-626-2810
Questions 615-522-2795

Allergy Resources
Mail: PO Box 888 (APD)
UPS: 264 Brookridge Ave. (APD)
Palmer Lake, CO 80133
Orders 800-USE-FLAX (873-3529)
Company plans to move; use 800 #

Allergy Supply Co., Inc., The
11994 Star Court (APD)
Herndon, VA 22071
800-323-6744
Metropolitan DC 703-391-2011
Fax 703-391-2014
BBS 703-521-0638

Allergy-Asthma Shopper™
PO Box 239 (APD)
Fate, TX 75132
800-447-1100
Fax 903-883-4513

Appliance Sales & Service Co.
655 Mission St. (APD)
San Francisco, CA 94105
800-424-6783
In 415 area call 415-362-7195

Brookstone Co.
5 Vose Farm Road (APD)
Peterborough, NH 03458
800-926-7000
Fax 603-924-0093

Cloud 9®
Div. of Mason Engineering Corp.
777 Edgewood Ave. (APD)
Wood Dale, IL 60191
708-595-5000

DeVilbiss
Available from:
Sunrise Medical/DeVilbiss, Inc.
PO Box 635 (APD)
Somerset, PA 15501-0635
800-DeV-1988 (338-1988)
814-443-4881
Fax 800-345-2202
In Canada 705-728-5522

E.L. Foust Co., Inc.
PO Box 105 (APD)
Elmhurst, IL 60126
800-225-9549
708-834-4952
Fax 708-834-5341

Edmund Scientific Co.
101 E. Gloucester Pike (APD)
Barrington, NJ 08007-1380
609-573-6250
Fax 609-573-6295

Honeywell/Enviracaire®
Honeywell Environmental Air Control
100 Jamison Ct. (APD)
Hagerstown, MD 21740-5185
800-332-1110

Environtrol® Corporation
PO Box 31313 (APD)
St. Louis, MO 63131
800-423-1982
In St. Louis 314-966-6886

Flowright Int'l Products
1495 N.W. Gilman Blvd. #4 (APD)
Issaquah, WA 98027
206-392-8357

Gempler's
211 Blue Mounds Rd. (APD)
PO Box 270 (APD)
Mt. Horeb, WI 53572

Controlling the Environment

Catalogues and Mail Order

800-382-8473
Fax 800-551-1128

Hammacher Schlemmer
Heaters, mold control, bedding
Available from:
Hammacher Schlemmer
147 E. 57th St. (APD)
New York, NY 10022
800-543-3366
212-421-9000

Herrington
3 Symmes Dr. (APD)
Londonderry, NH 03053
800-622-5221
In NH 603-437-4939
603-437-4638

Hi-Tech Filter Corp. of America
80 Myrtle St. (APD)
N. Quincy, MA 02171
800-448-3249
In MA 617-328-7756
Fax 617-773-4192

Holmes Products Corp.
233 Fortune Blvd. (APD)
Milford, MA 01757
508-634-8050
Fax 508-634-1211

King-Aire®
1121 S.R. 32 E. (APD)
Noblesville, IN 46060
Mail to PO Box 398 (APD)
Noblesville, IN 46060-0398
800-999-KING (5464)
317-776-1600

N.E.E.D.S.
527 Charles Ave. 12A (APD)
Syracuse, NY 13209
800-634-1380
Fax 800-295-NEED (6333)

National Allergy Supply, Inc.
4400 Georgia Hwy. 120 (APD)
PO Box 1658 (APD)
Duluth, GA 30136

800-522-1448
In Atlanta 404-623-8077
Fax 404-623-5568

Newtron Products
PO Box 27175 (APD)
3874 Virginia Ave. (APD)
Cincinnati, OH 45227-0175
800-543-9149
In OH 800-544-3753
513-561-7373
Fax 513-561-3673

Research Products, Corp.
1015 E. Washington Ave. (APD)
PO Box 1467 (APD)
Madison, WI 53701-1467
800-545-2219
608-257-8801
Fax 608-257-4357

Skin & Allergy Shop,™ The
310 E. Broadway (APD)
Louisville, KY 40202
800-366-6483
In KY 502-585-4824
Fax 502-589-3429

Sporty's® Preferred Living
Clermont County Airport (APD)
Batavia, OH 45103-9747
800-543-8633
Fax 513-732-6560

Tectronic Products Co., Inc.
PO Box 157 (APD)
6500 Badgley Rd. (APD)
E. Syracuse, NY 13057-0157
800-227-1375
315-463-0240
Fax 315-437-7290

HELP US TO HELP YOU
When writing to the companies
and organizations listed here, be sure
to use the initials (APD) as part of the
address and tell them you saw them
listed in *Allergy Products Directory.*

Controlling the Environment
Catalogues and Mail Order

COTTON CLOTHING AND HOUSEHOLD SUPPLY

A-Plus Allergy Equipment & Supply
8325 Regis Way (APD)
Los Angeles, CA 90045-2646
Orders 800-86-ALLER (862-5537)
310-337-7468
Fax 310-337-1971

Allergy Relief Shop,™ Inc.
3371 Whittle Springs Rd. (APD)
Knoxville, TN 37917
Orders 800-626-2810
Questions 615-522-2795

Allergy Resources
Mail: PO Box 888 (APD)
UPS: 264 Brookridge Ave. (APD)
Palmer Lake, CO 80133
Orders 800-USE-FLAX (873-3529)
Company plans to move; use 800 #

Allergy-Asthma Shopper™
PO Box 239 (APD)
Fate, TX 75132
800-447-1100
Fax 903-883-4513

Australian Conservation Foundation
340 Gore St. (APD)
Fitzroy Vic 3065
Australia
(03)-416-1166
008-332-510

Childcraft, Inc.
PO Box 29149 (APD)
Mission, KS 66201
800-631-5657
Fax 913-752-1095

Clothcrafters, Inc.
PO Box 176 (APD)
Elkhart Lake, WI 53020
414-876-2112
Fax 800-876-2009
Comfortably Yours

2515 E. 43rd St. (APD)
Chattanooga, TN 37422
201-368-0400

Cotton On Clothing Co., Ltd., The
Monmouth Place (APD)
Bath BA1 2NP
England
44-022-546-1155
Fax-44-022-546-1464

Domestications
PO Box 40 (APD)
Hanover, PA 17333-0040
800-746-2555

Dona Designs
1611 Bent Tree St. (APD)
Seagoville, TX 75159
214-287-7834
Don & Dona Shrier

French Creek
RD #1 (APD)
Elverson, PA 19520-0110
215-286-5700

Janice Corp.
198 US Hwy. 46 (APD)
Budd Lake, NJ 07828-3001
800-JANICES (526-4237)
Fax 201-691-5459

L.L. Bean, Inc.
Freeport, ME 04033
800-221-4221

Lands' End & Coming Home
1 Lands' End Ln. (APD)
Dodgeville, WI 53595
800-345-3696
TDD 800-541-3459

N.E.E.D.
527 Charles Ave 12A (APD)
Syracuase, NY 13209
800-634-1380
Fax 800-295-NEED (6333)

Controlling the Environment

Catalogues and Mail Order

PlayClothes, Inc.
PO Box 29137 (APD)
Overland Park, KS 66201-9137
800-362-PLAY (7529)
Fax 913-752-1095

Primary Layer, The
PO Box 6697 (APD)
Portland, OR 97228
800-282-8206

S&H® Uniform Corp.
200 Wiliam St. (APD)
Port Chester, NY 10573
914-937-6800
Fax 914-937-00741

HOUSEHOLD AND PERSONAL AIDS

A-Plus Allergy Equipment & Supply
8325 Regis Way (APD)
Los Angeles, CA 90045-2646
Orders 800-86-ALLER (862-5537)
310-337-7468
Fax 310-337-1971

Absolute Environmental's Allergy Store
2615 S. University Dr. (APD)
Davie, FL 33328
Nationwide 800-771-ACHOO (2246)
In FL 800-329-3773
Broward 305-472-3773
Fax 305-474-0133

Aller-Guard,® Inc.
Southgate Office Park
1645 S.W. 41st St. (APD)
Topeka, KS 66609-1250
800-234-0816
913-267-9333
Fax 913-267-0072

Allergy Aid Centre
1st Floor Pran Central Shop 56
325 Chapel St. (APD)
Prahran, Vic 3181

Australia
03-529-7348
03-529-8459

Allergy Clean Environments
501 Station Ave. (APD)
Haddon Heights, NJ 08035
800-882-4110
In NJ 609-546-1101
Fax 609-546-1466
URL:
http:\\WWW.infomall.com\allergy.html

Allergy Control Products, Inc.
96 Danbury Rd. (APD)
PO Box 793 (APD)
Ridgefield, CT 06877
800-422-DUST (3878)
203-438-9580
Fax 203-431-8963

Allergy Relief Distributors
Div. of E.C.Environmental Control, Inc.
177 Telegraph Rd. #365 (APD)
Bellingham, WA 98226
206-734-1646
Fax 206-734-3696
Canadian office in Vancouver, BC

Allergy Relief Products
9 Renata Ct. (APD)
Dundas, ON L9H 6X1
Canada
905-628-5324 ?416
Fax 416-628-1734

Allergy Relief Shop,™ Inc.
3371 Whittle Springs Rd. (APD)
Knoxville, TN 37917
Orders 800-626-2810
Questions 615-522-2795

Allergy Resources
Mail: PO Box 888 (APD)
UPS: 264 Brookridge Ave. (APD)
Palmer Lake, CO 80133
Orders 800-USE-FLAX (873-3529)
Company plans to move; use 800 #

Controlling the Environment

Catalogues and Mail Order

Allergy Supply Co.
11994 Star Court (APD)
Herndon, VA 22071
800-323-6744
Metropolitan DC 703-391-2011
Fax 703-391-2014
BBS 703-521-0638

Allergy-Asthma Shopper™
PO Box 239 (APD)
Fate, TX 75132
800-447-1100
Fax 903-883-4513

Apex™ Medical Corp.
800 S. Van Eps Ave. (APD)
Sioux Falls, SD 57104
PO Box 1235 (APD)
Sioux Falls, SD 57101
800-328-2935
In SD 605-332-6689
Fax 605-332-6818

Ar-Ex Ltd.
156 N. Jefferson St. #205 (APD)
Chicago, IL 60661
312-879-0017
Fax 312-879-0019

Aussie Wool Quilts & Pillows
RMB 2276 (APD)
Bullswamp Rd.
Warragul Sth. 3820
Australia
056-26-1242

Brookstone Co.
5 Vose Farm Road (APD)
Peterborough, NH 03458
800-926-7000
Fax 603-924-0093

Conney Safety Products
3203 Latham Dr. (APD)
PO Box 44190 (APD)
Madison, WI 53744-4190
800-356-9100
Fax 800-845-9095

Consolidated Plastics Co., Inc.
8181 Darrow Rd. (APD)
Twinsburg, OH 44087
800-362-1000
216-425-3900
Fax 216-425-3333

DeVilbiss
Available from:
Sunrise Medical/DeVilbiss, Inc.
PO Box 635 (APD)
Somerset, PA 15501-0635
800-DeV-1988 (338-1988)
814-443-4881
Fax 800-345-2202
In Canada 705-728-5522

Direct Safety Co.
7815 S. 46th St. (APD)
Phoenix, AZ 85044-5399
PO Box 50050 (APD)
Phoenix, AZ 85076-0050
800-528-7405
In AZ 602-968-7009
Fax 800-366-9662

Discount Safety
Available from:
Interex Safety & Industrial Supplies
176 Newington Rd. (APD)
W. Hartford, CT 06110
800-225-5910
Fax 800-334-2594

Dona Designs
1611 Bent Tree St. (APD)
Seagoville, TX 75159
214-287-7834
Don & Dona Shrier

E.L. Foust Co., Inc.
PO Box 105 (APD)
Elmhurst, IL 60126
800-225-9549
708-834-4952
Fax 708-834-5341

Environtrol® Corporation
PO Box 31313 (APD)
St. Louis, MO 63131

Controlling the Environment

Catalogues and Mail Order

800-423-1982
In St. Louis 314-966-6886

Flowright Int'l Products
1495 N.W. Gilman Blvd. #4 (APD)
Issaquah, WA 98027
206-392-8357

Gempler's
211 Blue Mounds Rd. (APD)
PO Box 270 (APD)
Mt. Horeb, WI 53572
800-382-8473
Fax 800-551-1128

Hammacher Schlemmer
147 E. 57th St. (APD)
New York, NY 10022
800-543-3366
212-421-9000

Industrial Safety Co.
1390 Neubrecht Rd. (APD)
Lima, OH 45801-3196
Orders 800-537-9721
Customer Service 419-227-6030
Fax 419-228-5034

Janice Corp.
198 US Hwy. 46 (APD)
Budd Lake, NJ 07828-3001
800-JANICES (526-4237)
Fax 201-691-5459

N.E.E.D.S.
527 Charles Ave. 12A (APD)
Syracuse, NY 13209
800-634-1380
Fax 800-295-NEED (6333)

National Allergy Supply, Inc.
4400 Georgia Hwy. 120 (APD)
PO Box 1658 (APD)
Duluth, GA 30136
800-522-1448
In Atlanta 404-623-8077
Fax 404-623-5568

Rx Systems, Inc.
#20 Point West Blvd. (APD)

St. Charles, MO 63301
800-922-9142
Fax 314-925-0041

Skin & Allergy Shop,™ The
310 E. Broadway (APD)
Louisville, KY 40202
800-366-6483
In KY 502-585-4824
Fax 502-589-3429

Solutions®
PO Box 6878 (APD)
Portland, OR 97228
800-342-9988
Fax 503-643-1973

Sun Precautions, Inc.
2815 Wetmore Ave. (APD)
Everett, WA 98201
800-882-7860
206-303-8585
Fax 206-303-0836

Touch of Class
1905 N. Van Buren St. (APD)
Huntingburg, IN 47542-9595
800-457-7456
Fax 812-683-5921

West Coast Shoe Co.
52828 N.W. Shoe Factory Ln. (APD)
PO Box 607 (APD)
Scappoose, OR 97056-0607
800-326-2711
503-543-7114
Fax 503-543-7110

HELP US TO HELP YOU
When writing to the companies and organizations listed here, be sure to use the initials (APD) as part of the address and tell them you saw them listed in *Allergy Products Directory*.

If you call, be sure to tell them you found them in *Allergy Products Directory*.

Controlling the Environment

Catalogues and Mail Order

RESPIRATORY TOOLS

Absolute Environmental's Allergy Store
2615 S. University Dr. (APD)
Davie, FL 33328
Nationwide 800-771-ACHOO (2246)
In FL 800-329-3773
Broward 305-472-3773
Fax 305-474-0133

Aller-Guard,® Inc.
Southgate Office Park
1645 S.W. 41st St. (APD)
Topeka, KS 66609-1250
800-234-0816
913-267-9333
Fax 913-267-0072

Allergy Aid Centre
1st Floor Pran Central Shop 56
325 Chapel St. (APD)
Prahran, Vic 3181
Australia
03-529-7348
03-529-8459

Allergy Control Products, Inc.
96 Danbury Rd. (APD)
PO Box 793 (APD)
Ridgefield, CT 06877
800-422-DUST (3878)
203-438-9580
Fax 203-431-8963

Allergy Supply Co.
11994 Star Court (APD)
Herndon, VA 22071
800-323-6744
Metropolitan DC 703-391-2011
Fax 703-391-2014
BBS 703-521-0638

Allergy-Asthma Shopper™
PO Box 239 (APD)
Fate, TX 75132
800-447-1100
Fax 903-883-4513

Conney Safety Products
3203 Latham Dr. (APD)
PO Box 44190 (APD)
Madison, WI 53744-4190
800-356-9100
Fax 800-845-9095

Consolidated Plastics Co., Inc.
8181 Darrow Rd. (APD)
Twinsburg, OH 44087
800-362-1000
216-425-3900
Fax 216-425-3333

DeVilbiss
Available from:
Sunrise Medical/DeVilbiss, Inc.
PO Box 635 (APD)
Somerset, PA 15501-0635
800-DeV-1988 (338-1988)
814-443-4881
Fax 800-345-2202
In Canada 705-728-5522

Direct Safety Co.
7815 S. 46th St. (APD)
Phoenix, AZ 85044-5399
PO Box 50050 (APD)
Phoenix, AZ 85076-0050
800-528-7405
In AZ 602-968-7009
Fax 800-366-9662

N.E.E.D.S.
527 Charles Ave. 12A (APD)
Syracuse, NY 13209
800-634-1380
Fax 800-295-NEED (6333)

National Allergy Supply, Inc.
4400 Georgia Hwy. 120 (APD)
PO Box 1658 (APD)
Duluth, GA 30136
800-522-1448
In Atlanta 404-623-8077
Fax 404-623-5568

Skin & Allergy Shop,™ The
310 E. Broadway (APD)
Louisville, KY 40202

Controlling the Environment
Catalogues and Mail Order

800-366-6483
In KY 502-585-4824
Fax 502-589-3429

WORK ENVIRONMENT

Airgard, Inc.
12601 Pleasant Grove #10 (APD)
Syracuse, IN 46567
219-457-5237

Allerderm Laboratories, Inc.
PO Box 2070 (APD)
Petaluma, CA 94953-2070
800-365-6868
707-765-6868
Fax 800-926-4568

Allied Glove & Safety Products Corp.
4711 W. Armitage Ave. (APD)
Chicago, IL 60639
800-621-3861
312-804-1800
Fax 312-804-1810

Conney Safety Products
3203 Latham Dr. (APD)
PO Box 44190 (APD)
Madison, WI 53744-4190
800-356-9100
Fax 800-845-9095

Gempler's
211 Blue Mounds Rd. (APD)
PO Box 270 (APD)
Mt. Horeb, WI 53572
800-382-8473
Fax 800-551-1128

Industrial Safety Co.
1390 Neubrecht Rd. (APD)
Lima, OH 45801-3196
Orders 800-537-9721
Customer Service 419-227-6030

Fax 419-228-5034

Interex Safety & Industrial Supplies
176 Newington Rd. (APD)
W. Hartford, CT 06110
800-225-5910
Fax 800-334-2594

Masuen™ Co.
490 Fillmore Ave. (A{D)
Tonawanda, NY 14150
800-831-0894
In IL 312-956-1255
Fax 800-222-1934

Medical Equipment Designs, Inc.
23461 Ridge Route Dr. #F (APD)
Laguna Hills, CA 92653
800-323-1674
714-859-7779

Pioneer Industrial Products
512 E. Tiffin St. (APD)
Willard, OH 44890
800-537-2897
In OH 419-933-2211
Fax 419-933-2710
Telex 210-498-2691

RH Hinchliffe & Sons, Ltd.
58 Bridge St. (APD)
Pershore
Worcestershire WR10 3AX
England

St. George Co., Ltd.
20 Consolidated Dr. (APD)
PO Box 430 (APD)
Paris, ON N3L 3T5
Canada
519-442-2046
Fax 519-442-7191
U.S. 800-461-4299

Controlling Your Environment

SPECIAL SERVICES

CONSULTING SERVICES

Allergy/Asthma DATASearch

American Allergy Assn. will search its database of thousands of listings for information on allergy, asthma, food allergy products, services, resources and where to find help. Donation requested.
AllergyAid@aol.com

Allergy Relief Shop Consulting Services

Phone consultation, product recommendation; on-site consultation and recommendations; considers mold, remodeling, duct work, heating systems, dust

Cotton mattresses in custom sizes; cotton futons in varying sizes
Available from:
Allergy Relief Shop,™ Inc.
3371 Whittle Springs Rd. (APD)
Knoxville, TN 37917
Orders 800-626-2810
Questions 615-522-2795

Camp Advisory Service

If you need a camp in a certain geographical area because of your child's allergy or asthma constraints, this service will let you know which camps are in that area and what they specialize in: music, sports, computer, etc.
Available from:
Camp Advisory Service
501 E. Boston Post Rd. (APD)
Mamaroneck, NY 10543
212-696-0499

Dietitian Referral in Spanish

Available from:
American Dietetic Assn.
216 W. Jackson Blvd. #800 (APD)
Chicago, IL 60606-6995
312-899-0040

Fax 312-899-1979

Footwear Industries of America

If you have an unusual shoe problem, this organization may be of help
Footwear Industries of America
1420 K St. NW, Ste. 600 (APD)
Washington, DC 20005-2505
202-789-1420
Fax 202-789-4058

Imperial Adhesives & Chemicals

If you have an unusual shoe problem relating to adhesives, this company may be of help
Imperial Adhesives & Chemicals
6315 Wiehe Rd. (APD)
Cincinnati, OH 45237-4277
800-365-1301
513-351-1300
Fax 513-351 1994

Insurance Liaison

800-423-8891 Ext. 1571
Discusses insurance coverage for clinic programs with your insurance carrier if there is a question about coverage
Available from:
National Jewish Center for Immunology
and Respiratory Medicine
1400 Jackson at ColFax (APD)
Denver, CO 80206-2762
800-222-LUNG (5864)
In CO 303-355-LUNG (5864)
303-398-1907

Product Specialist

800-537-8484
Discusses product function and appropriateness for your need (The Protector insect trap)

Controlling Your Environment

Special Services

United Shoe Machinery

If you have an unusual shoe problem relating to adhesives, this company may be of help
United Shoe Machinery Corp.
400 Research Dr. (APD)
Wilmington, MA 01887-1055
508-657-4700
Fax 508-658-7459

HOUSEHOLD SERVICES

ALK Indoor Allergen Analysis

Test measures cat and mice allergen levels in dust samples from living or working environment; repeat measurements monitor effectiveness.
Orders 800-326-9181 Ext. 222
Available from:
ALK Indoor Allergen Analysis
PO Box 200 (APD)
Spring Mills, PA 16875-9988
814-422-8165

Allergy Clean Environments

Custom size encasings for bedding; comforter encasings
Available from:
Allergy Clean Environments
501 Station Ave. (APD)
Haddon Heights, NJ 08035
800-882-4110
In NJ 609-546-1101
Fax 609-546-1466
URL:
http:\\WWW.infomall.com\allergy.html

Allergy Relief Products Ltd.

Dust-proof encasings made to size for cots, futons, cushions, bunkbeds
Available from:
Allergy Relief Products, Ltd.
39 Spring Crescent (APD)
Southampton SO2 1FZ
England
44-0703-586709
Fax 44-0703-676226

Allergy Relief Products, Ltd.

Custom size dust-proof mattress, pillow, duvet, encasings
Available from:
Allergy Relief Products
9 Renata Ct. (APD)
Dundas, ON L9H 6X1
Canada
905-628-5324 ?416
Fax 416-628-1734

Dona Designs

Custom size futons
Available from:
Dona Designs
1611 Bent Tree St. (APD)
Seagoville, TX 75159
214-287-7834
Don & Dona Shrier

Dust Analysis Test

Separate tests for your house dust; collector and instructions provided; test for dust mite allergen, cockroach, cat, cat allergen; mold spore count
Available from:
Allergy-Asthma Shopper™
PO Box 239 (APD)
Fate, TX 75132
800-447-1100
Fax 903-883-4513

Mold Test Plate

Kit allows you to collect samples at home in a U.S. Postal Service approved sample collection and shipping container with label; sample is mailed to EPA certified labaoratory for analysis and report
Available from:
Allergy Resources
Mail: PO Box 888 (APD)
UPS: 264 Brookridge Ave. (APD)
Palmer Lake, CO 80133
Orders 800-USE-FLAX (873-3529)
Company plans to move; use 800 #

Controlling Your Environment

Special Services

Touch of Class

Custom size envelopes made from sheets protect comforters; act as duvets
Available from:
Touch of Class
1905 N. Van Buren St. (APD)
Huntingburg, IN 47542-9595
800-457-7456
Fax 812-683-5921

AIR DUCT CLEANING SERVICES

Absolute Air Duct Cleaning

Cleans dust, molds, bacteria from central air conditioning systems and ventillation systems, dryer vents, building intakes; residential, commercial, industrial. Serves Dade, Broward, and Palm Beach counties in Florida
Available from:
Absolute Environmental's Allergy Store
2615 S. University Dr. (APD)
Davie, FL 33328
Nationwide 800-771-ACHOO (2246)
In FL 800-329-3773
Broward 305-472-3773
Fax 305-474-0133

Air Doctors, Inc.

Cleans bacteria and fungi from ducts and vents of heating, ventilating, and air conditioning systems; residential, commercial, industrial
Available from:
Air Doctors, Inc.
3632 Meadow Ln. (APD)
Jackson, MS 39212
PO Box 7147 (APD)
Jackson, MS 39282-7147
601-371-8928
Fax 601-373-2623

Clean Air Services

Cleans dust, molds, bacteria from central air conditioning systems and ventilation systems

Available from:
Clean Air Services
2402 Elm St. (APD)
Allentown, PA 18104
215-435-4355
Fax 215-435-4295

FILTER SERVICES

3M Company

PO Box 33275 (APD)
St. Paul, MN 55133-3275
3M Center Bldg.(APD)
St. Paul, MN 55144-1000
Medical information 800-328-0255
Medical information local 612-736-4930
Customer service 800-423-5197
Outside CA 800-423-5146
In CA 818-341-1300

AAir Purification Systems

7340 Trade St. #C (APD)
San Diego, CA 92121-2457
800-776-6746
619-578-2825
Fax 619-578-3762

Absolute Environmental's Allergy Store

2615 S. University Dr. (APD)
Davie, FL 33328
800-771-ACHOO (2246) nationwide
In FL 800-329-3773
Broward 305-472-3773
Fax 305-474-0133

Aller-Guard,® Inc.

Southgate Office Park
1645 S.W. 41st St. (APD)
Topeka, KS 66609-1250
800-234-0816
913-267-9333
Fax 913-267-0072

Allergy Control Products, Inc.

96 Danbury Rd. (APD)
PO Box 793 (APD)
Ridgefield, CT 06877

Controlling Your Environment

Special Services

800-422-DUST (3878)
203-438-9580
Fax 203-431-8963

Allergy Supply Co., Inc. The
11994 Star Court (APD)
Herndon, VA 22071
800-323-6744
Metropolitan DC 703-391-2011
Fax 703-391-2014
BBS 703-521-0638

Appliance Sales & Service Co.
655 Mission St. (APD)
San Francisco, CA 94105
800-424-6783
In 415 area call 415-362-7195

DeVilbiss
Sunrise Medical/DeVilbiss, Inc.
PO Box 635 (APD)
Somerset, PA 15501-0635
800-DeV-1988 (338-1988)
814-443-4881
Fax 800-345-2202
In Canada 705-728-5522

Environtrol® Corp.
PO Box 31313 (APD)
St. Louis, MO 63131
800-423-1982
In St. Louis 314-966-6886

Farr Co.
PO Box 92187 (APD)
Airport Station
Los Angeles, CA 90009
800-333-7320
Fax 800-441-0003
and
Farr Co.
500 S. Main Street (APD)
Crystal Lake, IL 60014
800-777-5260
Fax 800-441-0103

Hi-Tech Filter Corp. of America
80 Myrtle St. (APD)
N. Quincy, MA 02171
800-448-3249

In MA 617-328-7756
Fax 617-773-4192

National Allergy Supply, Inc.
4400 Georgia Hwy. 120 (APD)
PO Box 1658 (APD)
Duluth, GA 30136
800-522-1448
In Atlanta 404-623-8077
Fax 404-623-5568

Newtron Products
PO Box 27175 (APD)
3874 Virginia Ave. (APD)
Cincinnati, OH 45227-0175
800-543-9149
In OH 800-544-3753
513-561-7373
Fax 513-561-3673

Permatron Corp.
11400 Melrose St. (APD)
Franklin Park, IL 60131-1325
800-882-8012
708-451-0999

EQUIPMENT REPAIR, LEASING

Entech®
Repairs respiratory equipment in the continental U.S.; mail service
4411 S. 40th St., Ste. 6 (APD)
Phoenix, AZ 85040-2901
800-451-0591
In AZ: 602-437-9081

General Biomedical Service, Inc.
Repairs respiratory equipment in Alabama, Louisiana, Mississippi; sells in the continental U.S. to hospitals, industry, homes; mails with UPS
1000 Riverbend Blvd. #5 (APD)
St. Rose, LA 70087
800-558-9449
504-468-8597

Controlling Your Environment

Special Services

Med-Electronics

Leases, sells, and repairs parts for air filters, air cleaners, nebuilizers and spirometers in Maryland, Virginia, District of Columbia
9723 Baltimore Ave. #4 (APD)
College Park, MD 20740
301-345-8826
FAX 301-345-5686

Mediq/PRN

Repairs, leases, and sells parts for respiratory equipment for hospital use in the continental U.S.
1 Mediq Plaza (APD)
Pennsauken, NJ 08110
800-257-7477
In NJ: 800-232-6900

New Life Systems, Inc.

Leases, repairs, sells parts, and used respiratory equipment for hospital, industrial, and home use in the continental U.S.
PO Box 8767 (APD)
Coral Springs, FL 33075
Send repairs to:
1870 N. State Rd. 7 (APD)
Margate, FL 33063
305-972-4600
FAX 305-968-1990

Puritan-Bennett Corp.

Repairs and sells parts and respiratory equipment for hospitals, medical care dealers, and homes in the continental U.S. and Canada
Available from:
Puritan-Bennett
900 Springer Dr. (APD)
Lombard, IL 60148-6404
800-255-5444
Regional IL 800-255-6773
Regional GA 404-822-0700
For Home Care 800-248-0890
708-495-5444
Fax 800-755-8075
Fax 708-495-4433

Radiometer America, Inc.

Leases, repairs, and sells parts and used respiratory equipment for hospitals in the continental U.S.
811 Sharon Dr. (APD)
Westlake, OH 44145
800-377-7004
In OH: 216-871-8900

Respiratory Management Services, Inc.

Leases, repairs and sells parts and used respiratory equipment for hospitals, industry, and home in the continental U.S.; parts repaired by UPS
364 Adams St. (APD)
Bedford Hills, NJ 10507
800-431-2460
In NY: 914-666-2990

DIRECTORIES

"AAA Resource Handbook"

Covers services, products, and sources of information
Available from:
AROA/Allergy Assn. Australia
PO Box 298 (APD)
Ringwood, Vic 3134
Australia

"Allergy/Asthma Finding Help"

National and international sources of written, personal, and computerized help
Available from:
Allergy Publications
1259 El Camino #254 (APD)
Menlo Park, CA 94025
415-322-1663

"Controlling Your Environment"

Articles cover methods of environmental improvement with lists of products and where to buy them
Available from:
Allergy Publications
1254 El Camino 3254 (APD)
Menlo Park, CA 94025
415-322-1663

"Health Care Resource Directory

National sources of health care information
Available from:
Metro Publishing
5308 Elm St., Bldg C (APD)
Houston, TX 77081
800-473-5555
713-666-7841

IN RELATED AREAS

"Asthma Resources Directory"

Covers services, products, sources of information; includes articles and lsits of products and where to buy them
Available from:
Allergy Publications
1254 El Camino #254 (APD)
Menlo Park, CA 94025
415-322-1663

"Detweiler Directory of Medical Market Sources"

Available from:
S.M. Detweiler & Assoc., Inc.
PO Box 15308 (APD)
Ft. Wayne, IN 46885-5308
219-74-6534
Fax 219-493-6717
Internet 76670.221@compuserve.com

"Hospital School Programs: A Directory"

Available from:
Assn. for Care of Children's Health
7910 Woodmont Ave. #300 (APD)
Bethesda, MD 20814-3015
301-654-6549
Fax 301-986-4553

"New Jersey Self-Help Group Directory, The"

Includes national groups
Available from:
New Jersey Self-Help Clearinhouse (Regional)
St. Clares-Riverside Med. Center
Pocono Rd. (APD)
Denville, NJ 07834
NJ 800-FOR-MASH (367-6274)
201-625-9565
TDD 201-625-9053

NEWSLETTERS

FOR ALLERGY AND ASTHMA PATIENTS AND THEIR FAMILIES

"AAAR Times"
Available from:
American Assn. for Respiratory Care
11030 Ables Ln. (APD)
Dallas, TX 75229-4593
214-243-2272
Fax 214-484-2720

"Advance"
Available from:
Asthma & Allergy Foundation of
America
1125 15th St. N.W. #502 (APD)
Washington, DC 20005
202-466-7643
Fax 202-466-8940

"Air Currents"
Available from:
Allen & Hanburys™
Div. of Glaxo, Inc.
5 Moore Dr. (APD)
Research Triangle Park, NC 27709
919-248-2100
Medical services 919-248-2100

"Airways"
Quarterly
Available from:
Allergy & Asthma Center
2233-F Willamette (APD)
Eugene, OR 97401
503-485-0316

"Allergy Answers"
Available from:
Demos Publications
156 Fifth Ave. Ste 1018 (APD)
New York, NY 10010
212-255-8768

"Allergy Forum™"
(available through doctor's office)

"American Lung Association, Bulletin"
Available from:
American Lung Assn.
800-LUNG-USA (5864-872)
Refers to local ALA for information

"Asthma and Allergy Advocate"
Available from:
American Academy Allergy/Imm.
611 E. Wells St. 4th Flr. (APD)
Milwaukee, WI 53202-3816
800-822-ASMA (2762)
414-272-6071
Fax 414-276-3349

"Asthma Update"
Available from:
Asthma Update
123 Monticello Ave. (APD)
Annapolis, MD 21401
410-267-0309

"Healthlines"
(for and by teens)
Available from:
Asthma & Allergy Foundation of
America
1125 15th St. N.W. #502 (APD)
Washington, DC 20005
202-466-7643
Fax 202-466-8940

"LungLine Letter"
Available from:
National Jewish Center for
Immunology
and Respiratory Medicine
1400 Jackson at ColFax (APD)
Denver, CO 80206-2762
800-222-LUNG (5864)
In CO 303-355-LUNG (5864)
303-398-1907

"New Directions"
For donors
Available from:

Controlling Your Environment

Newsletters

National Jewish Center for
Immunology
and Respiratory Medicine
1400 Jackson at ColFax (APD)
Denver, CO 80206-2762
800-222-LUNG (5864)
In CO 303-355-LUNG (5864)
303-398-1907

"MA Report"
Available from:
Allergy & Asthma Network/
Mothers of Asthmatics, Inc.
3554 Chain Bridge Rd. Ste 200 (APD)
Fairfax, VA 22030-2709
Orders 800-878-4403
703-385-4403
Fax 703-352-4354

FOR PROFESSIONALS IN THE FIELD

"Medical/Scientific UPDATE"
Available from:
National Jewish Center for
Immunology
and Respiratory Medicine
1400 Jackson at ColFax (APD)
Denver, CO 80206-2762
800-222-LUNG (5864)
In CO 303-355-LUNG (5864)
303-398-1907

IN OTHER COUNTRIES

"Allergy Asthma Quarterly"
Available from:
Allergy/Asthma Information Assn.
30 Eglinton Ave. W. #750 (APD)
Mississauga, ON L5R 3E7
Canada
905-712-AAIA (2242)
Fax 905-712-2245

"Asthma Network"
Available from:
World Network of Asthma
Organizations
Canadian Secretariat

c/o Canadian Lung Assn.
1900 City Park Dr. #508 (APD)
Gloucester, ON K1J 1A3
Canada
613-747-6766
Fax 613-747-7430

"Easy Breathing"
Manitoba Lung Assn.
629 McDermot Ave. 2nd Flr. (APD)
Winnipeg, MB R3A 5P6
Canada

"Newsletter for People with Lung Problems, A"
Lung Assn. (Metro, Toronto, York
Region)
573 King St. E. Ste. 201 (APD)
Toronto, ON M5A 1M5
Canada

"Canadian Society for Immunology, Bulletin"
(for professionals in the field)
Canadian Society for Immunology
Dr. C. Ottaway
St. Michael's Univ. of Toronto
Toronto, ON M5S 1A8
Canada

OF RELATED INTEREST

"ACCH Network"
Available from:
Assn. for Care of Children's Health
7910 Woodmont Ave. #300 (APD)
Bethesda, MD 20814-3015
301-654-6549
Fax 301-986-4553

"Americans for Nonsmokers' Rights Update"
Available from:
Americans for Nonsmokers' Rights
2530 San Pablo Ave. #J (APD)
Berkeley, CA 94702
PO Box 668 (APD)
Berkeley, CA 94704
510-841-3032

Controlling Your Environment

Newsletters

"ASH Smoking and Health Review"
Available from:
Action on Smoking and Health
2013 H St. N.W. (APD)
Washington, DC 20006
202-659-4310

"Common Sense Pest Control"
Available from:
Bio-Integral Resource Center, The
PO Box 7414 (APD)
Berkeley, CA 94707
510-524-2567
Fax 510-524-1758

"Drugs & Therapeutics"
Available from:
Drug Information Center - Mercy
Mercy Hospital of Pittsburgh
1400 Locust St. (APD)
Pittsburgh , PA 15219-5166
412-232-7903 (APD)

"HealthFacts"
Consumer-oriented, general, medical information
Available from:
Comfortably Yours
2515 E. 43rd St. (APD)
Chattanooga, TN 37422
201-368-0400

"Health Gazette: A Digest of Medical Facts and News"
Available from:
Health Gazette®
PO Box 1786 (APD)
Indiannapolis, IN 46206
317-253-7104
Fax 317-253-8582

"Helping Ourselves"
Available from:
Michigan Self-Help Clearinghouse
(Regional)
106 W. Allegan #210 (APD)
Lansing, MI 48933-1706
MI 800-777-5556
Business line 517-484-7373

"Indoor Air Quality Updates"
(for Professionals)
Available from
Cutter Information Corp.
37 Broadway (APD)
Arlington, MA 02174-5539
800-964-5118
617-641-5118
Fax 800-888-1816
Fax 617-648-1950

"Lifeline"
Available from:
Celiac Sprue Assn./
United States of America
PO Box 31700 (APD)
Omaha, NE 68131-0700
402-558-0600

"Network"
(self-help clearinghouse)
Available from:
New Jersey Self-Help Clearinhouse
(Regional)
St. Clares-Riverside Med. Center
Pocono Rd. (APD)
Denville, NJ 07834
NJ 800-FOR-MASH (367-6274)
201-625-9565
TDD 201-625-9053

"NSHC Newsletter"
Available from:
National Self-Help Clearinghouse
25 W. 43rd St. Rm. 620 (APD)
New York, NY 10036
212-642-2944
NY City Referrals 212-586-5770
Fax 212-719-2488

"Pediatrics for Parents"
Available from:
Pediatrics for Parents
358 Broadway #105 (APD)
Bangor, ME 04401
207-942-6212

Controlling Your Environment
Information In Print

INFORMATION IN PRINT

Some books may not be readily available through a bookstore, even with a special order. Try your library. Ask about an inter-library loan or write the publisher.

Some books are out of print. Used book stores may be able to list the book you want in *A Bookman's Weekly* for a small fee. Be patient. A response can take months. Try *Guide to Out-of-Print Books*. It is a catalogue on microfiche and is available for free from UMI at PO Box 1467, Ann Arbor, MI 48106; 800-521-0600. You can most likely use your library's microfiche system to read it.

ALLERGY INFORMATION IN PRINT

"ABC's of Latex Allergy"
Available from:
Asthma & Allergy Foundation of America
1125 15th St. N.W. #502 (APD)
Washington, DC 20005
202-466-7643
Fax 202-466-8940

"Advice for the Patient"
(Available through doctors)
Available from:
U.S. Pharmacopeia, Inc.
12601 Twinbrook Pkwy (APD)
Rockville, MD 20852
800-227-8772
301-881-0666
Fax 301-816-8299

"Air Purifiers Part 1 Claims, Types"
Available from:
American Allergy Assn.
1259 El Camino #254 (APD)
Menlo Park, CA 94025
415-322-1663
Internet AllergyAid@aol.com

"Air Purifiers Part II Considerations, Testing, Questions"
Available from:
American Allergy Assn.
1259 El Camino #254 (APD)

Menlo Park, CA 94025
415-322-1663
Internet AllergyAid@aol.com

"Airborne Allergens"
USDHHS
Available from:
American Allergy Assn.
1259 El Camino #254 (APD)
Menlo Park, CA 94025
415-322-1663
Internet AllergyAid@aol.com

"Airborne and Allergenic Pollen of North America"
W. Lewis
P. Vinay
V. Zenger
Available from:
Johns Hopkins University Press
701 W. 40th St. #275 (APD)
Baltimore, MD 21211
800-537-5487
MD 301-338-6932

"Allergic Contact Dermatitis"
USDHHS
Available from:
American Allergy Assn.
1259 El Camino #254 (APD)
Menlo Park, CA 94025
415-322-1663
Internet AllergyAid@aol.com

"Allergic Pneumonia Hypersensitivity Pneumonitis"
USDHHS

Controlling Your Environment

Information In Print

Available from:
American Allergy Assn.
1259 El Camino #254 (APD)
Menlo Park, CA 94025
415-322-1663
Internet AllergyAid@aol.com

"Allergic Rhinitis Definition, Description, Importance"
USDHS
Available from:
American Allergy Assn.
1259 El Camino #254 (APD)
Menlo Park, CA 94025
415-322-1663
Internet AllergyAid@aol.com

"Allergic Traveler's Passport to Worry-Free Vacations"
Availble from
Life Sciences Press
PO Box 1174 (APD)
Tacoma, WA 98401
206-922-0442

"Allergies and You"
Available from:
American Lung Assn.
800-LUNG-USA (5864-872)
Refers to local ALA for information

"Allergies in the Desert"
Donald L. Unger, MD
Available from:
American Allergy Assn.
1259 El Camino #254 (APD)
Menlo Park, CA 94025
415-322-1663
Internet AllergyAid@aol.com

"Allergies"
Michael Kaliner, MD
Available from:
USDHHS - Public Health Service
National Institutes of Health
200 Independence Ave. SW Rm 716G (APD)
Washington, DC 20201-0001

"Allergies: Complete Guide to Diagnosis, Treatment, & Daily Management"
Young, MD
Available from:
Anderson Continuing Education
for Nursing Professionals
3268 Ramos Cir. (APD)
PO Box 276297 (APD)
Sacramento, CA 95827
800-532-2332
and:
Consumers Union
256 Washington St. (APD)
Mt. Vernon, NY 10553

"Allergies: Medicine for the Layman"
Available from:
National Institute of Allergy
& Infectious Diseases
NIH - Public Health Services
Bldg. 31 Rm. 72-32 (APD)
Public Health Services
9000 Rockville Pike
Bethesda, MD 20892-0001
301-496-5717
301-496-4000

"Allergy & Asthma '95"
Annually
Available from:
Healthline Publishing, Inc.
830 Menlo Ave. #100
Menlo Park, CA 94025
800-766-5566
325-6457

"Allergy Alerts from Living with Allergies"
Available from:
American Allergy Assn.
1259 El Camino #254 (APD)
Menlo Park, CA 94025
415-322-1663
Internet AllergyAid@aol.com

"Allergy and the Immune System"
Robert N. Hamburger, MD
Available from:

Controlling Your Environment

Information In Print

American Allergy Assn.
1259 El Camino #254 (APD)
Menlo Park, CA 94025
415-322-1663
Internet AllergyAid@aol.com

"Allergy Basics"
Available from:
Asthma & Allergy Foundation of
America
1125 15th St. N.W. #502 (APD)
Washington, DC 20005
202-466-7643
Fax 202-466-8940

"Allergy Encyclopedia"
Craig T. Norback, Editor
Available from:
C.V. Mosby Co.
Subs. of Times Mirror Co.
11830 Westline Industrial Dr. (APD)
PO Box 46908 (APD)
St. Louis, MO 63146-9988
800-325-4177
MO 314-872-8370
Orders 800-426-4545

"Allergy Environmental Control"
Available from:
Health Services Consultants
2670 Del Mar Heights Rd. #194 (APD)
Del Mar, CA 92014

"Allergy Relief Guide"
AAAI and Kimberly-Clark Corp.
Available from:
American Academy Allergy/Imm.
611 E. Wells St. 4th Flr. (APD)
Milwaukee, WI 53202-3816
800-822-ASMA (2762)
414-272-6071
Fax 414-276-3349

"Allergy under the Mistletoe"
Donald L. Unger, MD
Available from:
American Allergy Assn.
1259 El Camino #254 (APD)
Menlo Park, CA 94025

415-322-1663
Internet AllergyAid@aol.com

"Allergy: The Facts"
Robert Davies
Susan Ollier
Available from:
Oxford University Press
200 Madison Ave. (APD)
New York, NY 10016
800-334-4249
212-679-7300
Orders 800-451-7556

"Americans with Disabilities Act"
Available from:
Asthma & Allergy Foundation of
America
1125 15th St. N.W. #502 (APD)
Washington, DC 20005
202-466-7643
Fax 202-466-8940

"Antihistamines Part 1"
FDA
Available from:
American Allergy Assn.
1259 El Camino #254 (APD)
Menlo Park, CA 94025
415-322-1663
Internet AllergyAid@aol.com

"Antihistamines Part 2"
FDA
Available from:
American Allergy Assn.
1259 El Camino #254 (APD)
Menlo Park, CA 94025
415-322-1663
Internet AllergyAid@aol.com

"Asthma and Allergy Medicines: Side Effects"
Available from:
Asthma & Allergy Foundation of
America
1125 15th St. N.W. #502 (APD)
Washington, DC 20005
202-466-7643
Fax 202-466-8940

Controlling Your Environment

Information In Print

"Asthma: The Complete Guide to Self-Management of Asthma & Allergies for Patients & Their Families"
Allan M. Weinstein, MD
Available from:
Allergy & Asthma Network/
Mothers of Asthmatics, Inc.
3554 Chain Bridge Rd. Ste 200 (APD)
Fairfax, VA 22030-2709
Orders 800-878-4403
703-385-4403
Fax 703-352-4354
and:
Allergy Solutions
4909 W. Park Blvd. #169 (APD)
Plano, TX 75093
800-380-SNEEZ (7633)
214-612-4188
Fax 214-985-5573
and:
Asthma & Allergy Foundation of America
1125 15th St. N.W. #502 (APD)
Washington, DC 20005
202-466-7643
Fax 202-466-8940
and:
Asthma Outreach Library
37 Pillsbury Rd. (APD)
Sandown, NH 03873
603-329-5301
and:
McGraw-Hill Publishing Co.
1221 Avenue of the Americas (APD)
New York, NY 10020
in NY 212-512-2000
800-722-4726

"Bee Sting"
Available from:
American Allergy Assn.
1259 El Camino #254 (APD)
Menlo Park, CA 94025
415-322-1663
Internet AllergyAid@aol.com

"Best Guide to Allergies, The"
A. Giannini, MD, et. al.
Available from:

Consumers Union
256 Washington St. (APD)
Mt. Vernon, NY 10553

"Biological Pollutants in Your Home"
Available from:
American Lung Assn.
800-LUNG-USA (5864-872)
Refers to local ALA for information

"Care of the Skin with Eczema"
Dr. John English
Available from:
American Allergy Assn.
1259 El Camino #254 (APD)
Menlo Park, CA 94025
415-322-1663
Internet AllergyAid@aol.com

"Chemical Sensitivities"
Available from:
Asthma & Allergy Foundation of America
1125 15th St. N.W. #502 (APD)
Washington, DC 20005
202-466-7643
Fax 202-466-8940

"Common Allergies in Children"
NIH
Available from:
American Allergy Assn.
1259 El Camino #254 (APD)
Menlo Park, CA 94025
415-322-1663
Internet AllergyAid@aol.com

"Complete Book of Children's Allergies, The"
B.R. Feldman, MD
David Carroll
Times Books
Available from:
Asthma & Allergy Foundation of America
1125 15th St. N.W. #502 (APD)
Washington, DC 20005
202-466-7643
Fax 202-466-8940

Controlling Your Environment

Information In Print

and:
Asthma Outreach Library
37 Pillsbury Rd. (APD)
Sandown, NH 03873
603-329-5301
and:
Priorities®
70 Walnut St. (APD)
Wellesley, MA 02181
800-553-5398
and:
Random House, Inc.
201 E. 50th St. 31st Flr. (APD)
New York, NY 10022
212-751-2600
Orders 800-733-3000
Inquiries 800-726-0600

"Conquering Your Child's Allergies"
M. Eric Gershwin, MD
Edwin L. Klingelhofer, PhD
Available from:
Addison-Wesley Publishing Co.
Medical\Nursing Division
1 Jacob Way (APD)
Reading, MA 01867
617-944-3700
800-447-2227

"Consumer Guide for Room Air Cleaners"
Available from:
Assn. of Home Appliance
Manufacturers
AHAM
20 N. Wacker Dr. (APD)
Chicago, IL 60606
312-984-5800

"Coping and Living with Allergies"
Claude A. Frazier, MD
Available from:
Prentice Hall
Div. of Simon & Schuster, Inc.
15 Columbus Cir. (APD)
New York, NY 10023
800-922-0579
212-373-8500

"Cosmetic Allergies Part 1 Identification Problems"
Available from:
American Allergy Assn.
1259 El Camino #254 (APD)
Menlo Park, CA 94025
415-322-1663
Internet AllergyAid@aol.com

"Cosmetic Allergies Part 2 Testing Products and Ingredients"
Available from:
American Allergy Assn.
1259 El Camino #254 (APD)
Menlo Park, CA 94025
415-322-1663
Internet AllergyAid@aol.com

"Cosmetic Dermatology"
Available from
Knolls Publishing Group
PO Box 555 (APD)
Cedar Knolls, NJ 07927

"Cosmetics"
Available from:
American Allergy Assn.
1259 El Camino #254 (APD)
Menlo Park, CA 94025
415-322-1663
Internet AllergyAid@aol.com

"Development and Inheritance of IgE and Allergy"
Robert N. Hamburger, MD
Available from:
American Allergy Assn.
1259 El Camino #254 (APD)
Menlo Park, CA 94025
415-322-1663
Internet AllergyAid@aol.com

"Down with the Dust Mite"
Available from:
American Allergy Assn.
1259 El Camino #254 (APD)
Menlo Park, CA 94025
415-322-1663

Controlling Your Environment

Information In Print

Internet AllergyAid@aol.com

"Drug Allergy"
Available from:
National Institute of Allergy
& Infectious Diseases
NIH - Public Health Services
Bldg. 31 Rm. 72-32 (APD)
Public Health Services
9000 Rockville Pike
Bethesda, MD 20892-0001
301-496-5717
301-496-4000

"Dust 'n' Stuff"
Linda Alpert, RN, BSN
Available from:
Asthma Foundation of Southern
Arizona
National Foundation for Asthma
PO Box 30069 (APD)
Tucson, AZ 85751-0069
520-323-6046

"Dust Allergy"
Available from:
National Institute of Allergy
& Infectious Diseases
NIH - Public Health Services
Bldg. 31 Rm. 72-32 (APD)
Public Health Services
9000 Rockville Pike
Bethesda, MD 20892-0001
301-496-5717
301-496-4000

"Eczema During Pregnancy"
National Eczema Society London
Available from:
American Allergy Assn.
1259 El Camino #254 (APD)
Menlo Park, CA 94025
415-322-1663
Internet AllergyAid@aol.com

"Electronic Air Cleaners and HEPA Filters, Ion Machines, Portable Air Cleaners
J. Gordon King
Available from:

American Allergy Assn.
1259 El Camino #254 (APD)
Menlo Park, CA 94025
415-322-1663
Internet AllergyAid@aol.com

"Electronic Air Cleaners, HEPA Filters"
J. Gordon King
Available from:
American Allergy Assn.
1259 El Camino #254 (APD)
Menlo Park, CA 94025
415-322-1663
Internet AllergyAid@aol.com

"Empty Your Bucket: Practical Steps to Overcome Allergy and Allergic Asthma"
Stephen H. Astor, MD
Available from:
Priorities®
70 Walnut St. (APD)
Wellesley, MA 02181
800-553-5398
and:
Two A's Industries, Inc.
285 South Dr. (APD)
Mountain View, CA 94040-4318
415-968-3111

"Ensuring Clean Indoor Air"
Judy Lee Bachman, PhD
Available from:
Health Services Consultants
2670 Del Mar Heights Rd. #194 (APD)
Del Mar, CA 92014

"Environmental Allergens Part 1 House Dust, Control of House Dust"
Available from:
American Allergy Assn.
1259 El Camino #254 (APD)
Menlo Park, CA 94025
415-322-1663
Internet AllergyAid@aol.com

Controlling Your Environment

Information In Print

"Environmental Allergens Part 2 Dog and Cat Sensititivity"
Available from:
American Allergy Assn.
1259 El Camino #254 (APD)
Menlo Park, CA 94025
415-322-1663
Internet AllergyAid@aol.com

"Environmental Allergens Part 3 Pollen Allergy, Mold Spores, Other Offenders"
Available from:
American Allergy Assn.
1259 El Camino #254 (APD)
Menlo Park, CA 94025
415-322-1663
Internet AllergyAid@aol.com

"Facts About Asthma"
Available from:
National Asthma Education Program
Information Center
4733 Bethesda Ave. #530 (APD)
Bethesda, MD 20814
PO Box 30105 (APD)
Bethesda, MD 20824-0105
301-251-1222

"Family Medical Kit"
Available from:
Assn. for Care of Children's Health
7910 Woodmont Ave. #300 (APD)
Bethesda, MD 20814-3015
301-654-6549
Fax 301-986-4553

"Food Allergy"
Edited by D. Metcalfe
H. Sampson
R. Simon
Available from:
Blackwell Scientific Pubns., Inc.
238 Main St. (APD)
Cambridge, MA 02142
800-445-6638
617-225-0430

"Food Allergy: A Primer for People"
S. Allan Bock, MD
Available from:
Asthma & Allergy Foundation of America
1125 15th St. N.W. #502 (APD)
Washington, DC 20005
202-466-7643
Fax 202-466-8940

"Fragrance Dermatitis"
Available from:
American Allergy Assn.
1259 El Camino #254 (APD)
Menlo Park, CA 94025
415-322-1663
Internet AllergyAid@aol.com

"General Management of Eczema"
National Eczema Society London
Available from:
American Allergy Assn.
1259 El Camino #254 (APD)
Menlo Park, CA 94025
415-322-1663
Internet AllergyAid@aol.com

"Guide to Seasonal Allergens"
Available from:
Schering Corp.
2000 Galloping Hill Rd. (APD)
Kenilworth, NJ 07033
201-558-4000

"Headaches Part 1"
Oscar L. Frick, MD, Reviewed
Available from:
American Allergy Assn.
1259 El Camino #254 (APD)
Menlo Park, CA 94025
415-322-1663
Internet AllergyAid@aol.com

"Headaches Part 2
Oscar L. Frick, MD, Reviewed
Available from:
American Allergy Assn.
1259 El Camino #254 (APD)

Controlling Your Environment

Information In Print

Menlo Park, CA 94025
415-322-1663
Internet AllergyAid@aol.com

"Hints for Control of the Home Environment for the Allergic Person"

Available from:
American Lung Assn.
800-LUNG-USA (5864-872)
Refers to local ALA for information

"Holiday Allergies: 'Tis the Season!"

Available from:
Asthma & Allergy Foundation of
America
1125 15th St. N.W. #502 (APD)
Washington, DC 20005
202-466-7643
Fax 202-466-8940

"Household Allergies: Dust, Mold, Pets, and Cockroaches"

Available from:
Asthma & Allergy Foundation of
America
1125 15th St. N.W. #502 (APD)
Washington, DC 20005
202-466-7643
Fax 202-466-8940

"How to Avoid Stinging Insects"

Available from:
Miles Inc. Pharmaceutical Div.
Miles Allergy Products
(Hollister-Stier)
PO Box 3145 (APD)
3525 N. Regal (APD)
Spokane, WA 99220-3145
800-992-1120
509-489-5656

"How to Create a Clean Room"

Available from:
Summit Hill Laboratories
Ship to 429 Highway 36 (APD)
Mail to PO Box 535 (APD)
Navesink, NJ 07752
800-922-0722

201-291-3600

"Indoor Air Pollution"

Available from:
Summit Hill Laboratories
Ship to 429 Highway 36 (APD)
Mail to PO Box 535 (APD)
Navesink, NJ 07752
800-922-0722
201-291-3600

"Insect Allergy"

Available from:
National Institute of Allergy
& Infectious Diseases
NIH - Public Health Services
Bldg. 31 Rm. 72-32 (APD)
Public Health Services
9000 Rockville Pike
Bethesda, MD 20892-0001
301-496-5717
301-496-4000

"Insects and Allergy"

Univ. of Oklahoma Press
Oklahoma City, OK 73190
Claude A. Frazier, MD
F.K. Brown

"Is Your Child Allergic?"

Jan A. Kuzemko
Available from:
Borgo Press
PO Box 2845 (APD)
San Bernardino, CA 92406
909-884-5813

"Keys to Dealing with Childhood Allergies"

Judy Bachman
Available from:
Barron's Educational Series, Inc.
250 Wireless Blvd. (APD)
PO Box 8040 (APD)
Hauppauge, NY 11788
800-645-3476
In NY 800-257-5729

"Kinds of Eczema"

Available from:

Controlling Your Environment

Information In Print

American Allergy Assn.
1259 El Camino #254 (APD)
Menlo Park, CA 94025
415-322-1663
Internet AllergyAid@aol.com

"Leaflets Three: Poison Ivy and Oak"
Available from:
Asthma & Allergy Foundation of America
1125 15th St. N.W. #502 (APD)
Washington, DC 20005
202-466-7643
Fax 202-466-8940

"Living Allergy Free"
Eric M. Gershwin
Edwin L. Kingelhofer
Available from:
Humana Press
999 Riverview Dr. #208 (APD)
Totowa, NJ 07512
201-256-1699

"Living with Allergies"
Available from:
American Allergy Assn.
1259 El Camino #254 (APD)
Menlo Park, CA 94025
415-322-1663
Internet AllergyAid@aol.com

"Living with Your Allergies and Asthma"
Theodore Berland
Lucia Fischer-Pap
Available from:
St. Martin's Press, Inc.
175 Fifth Ave. (APD)
New York, NY 10010

"Living With Your Allergy"
Michael Bright
Available from:
Beekman Publishers, Inc.
PO Box 888 (APD)
Woodstock, NY 12498
914-679-2300

"Management of Allergy in the 1990's"
Michael A. Kaliner, MD
Available from:
Hogrefe & Huber, Publishers
PO Box 2487 (APD)
Kirkland, WA 98083-2487
800-228-3749-
206-820-1500

"Manual of Problems in Asthma, Allergy, and Related Disorders"
B. Bukstein, Editor
R. Strunk, Editor
Available from:
Little, Brown & Co.
Div. of Time, Inc.
34 Beacon St. (APD)
Boston, MA 02108
800-343-9204
MA 617-227-0730

"Moving or Traveling? Consider Your Hay Fever"
Available from:
American Allergy Assn.
1259 El Camino #254 (APD)
Menlo Park, CA 94025
415-322-1663
Internet AllergyAid@aol.com

"My Sinuses Are Killing Me!"
Available from:
Asthma & Allergy Foundation of America
1125 15th St. N.W. #502 (APD)
Washington, DC 20005
202-466-7643
Fax 202-466-8940

"On the Nature of the Allergic Reaction"
V. Marinkovich, MD
Available from:
American Allergy Assn.
1259 El Camino #254 (APD)
Menlo Park, CA 94025
415-322-1663
Internet AllergyAid@aol.com

Controlling Your Environment

Information In Print

"One Minute Asthma: What You Need to Know"

Thomas Plaut, MD
    English or Spanish
Available from:
Allergy & Asthma Network/
Mothers of Asthmatics, Inc.
3554 Chain Bridge Rd. Ste 200 (APD)
Fairfax, VA 22030-2709
Orders 800-878-4403
703-385-4403
Fax 703-352-4354
and:
Allergy Asthma Technology
4151 N. Kedzie (APD)
PO Box 18398 (APD)
Chicago, IL 60618
800-621-5545
312-465-8020
Fax 312-465-7619
and:
Allergy Clean Environments
501 Station Ave. (APD)
Haddon Heights, NJ 08035
800-882-4110
In NJ 609-546-1101
Fax 609-546-1466
URL:
http:\\WWW.infomall.com\allergy.html
and:
Asthma & Allergy Foundation of
America
1125 15th St. N.W. #502 (APD)
Washington, DC 20005
202-466-7643
Fax 202-466-8940
and:
Asthma Outreach Library
37 Pillsbury Rd. (APD)
Sandown, NH 03873
603-329-5301
and:
Pedipress, Inc.
125 Red Gate Lane (APD)
Amherst, MA 01002

" 'Over-the-Counter' Medications: Do They Work for Allergies?"

Available from:

Asthma & Allergy Foundation of
America
1125 15th St. N.W. #502 (APD)
Washington, DC 20005
202-466-7643
Fax 202-466-8940

"Parent's Guide to Allergies & Asthma, A"

Marion Steinmann
Available from:
Delta Delacorte
Div. of Bantam Doubleday Dell
666th Ave. (APD)
New York, NY 10103
800-221-4676
212-765-6500

"Parents Handbook of Childhood Allergies"

Richard Garber
Ballantine Books, Inc
Available from:
Random House, Inc.
201 E. 50th St. 31st Flr. (APD)
New York, NY 10022
212-751-2600
Orders 800-733-3000
Inquiries 800-726-0600

"Parents Handbook of Childhood Allergies"

Richard Garber
Available from:
Random House, Inc.
201 E. 50th St. 31st Flr. (APD)
New York, NY 10022
212-751-2600
Orders 800-733-3000
Inquiries 800-726-0600

"People's Handbook of Allergies and Allergens, The"

Ruth Wink
    In Canada: Beaverbooks, Ltd.
195 Allstate Parkway
Valleywood Business Park
Markham, ON L3R 4T8
Canada
Available from:

Controlling Your Environment

Information In Print

Contemporary Books, Inc.
180 N. Michigan Ave. (APD)
Chicago, IL 60601

"Perfumes"
Available from:
American Allergy Assn.
1259 El Camino #254 (APD)
Menlo Park, CA 94025
415-322-1663
Internet AllergyAid@aol.com

"Planning A Move?"
Available from:
Asthma & Allergy Foundation of
America
1125 15th St. N.W. #502 (APD)
Washington, DC 20005
202-466-7643
Fax 202-466-8940

"Poison Ivy Allergy"
USDHHA
Available from:
American Allergy Assn.
1259 El Camino #254 (APD)
Menlo Park, CA 94025
415-322-1663
Internet AllergyAid@aol.com

"Pollen Aeroallergens of the United States"
Available from:
Center Laboratories
35 Channel Dr. (APD)
PO Box 70 (APD)
Port Washington, NY 11050
Customer service 800-223-6837

"Pollen Allergy"
Available from:
National Institute of Allergy
& Infectious Diseases
NIH - Public Health Services
Bldg. 31 Rm. 72-32 (APD)
Public Health Services
9000 Rockville Pike
Bethesda, MD 20892-0001
301-496-5717
301-496-4000

"Pollen Guide for Allergy"
Available from:
Miles Inc. Pharmaceutical Div.
Miles Allergy Products
(Hollister-Stier)
PO Box 3145 (APD)
3525 N. Regal (APD)
Spokane, WA 99220-3145
800-992-1120
509-489-5656

"Preparation and Maintenance of a Dust-free Room"
Available from:
Miles Inc. Pharmaceutical Div.
Miles Allergy Products
(Hollister-Stier)
PO Box 3145 (APD)
3525 N. Regal (APD)
Spokane, WA 99220-3145
800-992-1120
509-489-5656

"Questions and Answers about Asthma and Allergy"
Available from:
National Institute of Allergy
& Infectious Diseases
NIH - Public Health Services
Bldg. 31 Rm. 72-32 (APD)
Public Health Services
9000 Rockville Pike
Bethesda, MD 20892-0001
301-496-5717
301-496-4000

"Remodeling, New Construction, and Allergies"
Available from:
Asthma & Allergy Foundation of
America
1125 15th St. N.W. #502 (APD)
Washington, DC 20005
202-466-7643
Fax 202-466-8940

"Seasonal Allergies: Pollens and Mold"
Available from:

Controlling Your Environment

Information In Print

Asthma & Allergy Foundation of
America
1125 15th St. N.W. #502 (APD)
Washington, DC 20005
202-466-7643
Fax 202-466-8940

"Sneezing Your Head Off?"
Peter B. Boggs, MD
Available from:
Allergy & Asthma Network/
Mothers of Asthmatics, Inc.
3554 Chain Bridge Rd. Ste 200 (APD)
Fairfax, VA 22030-2709
Orders 800-878-4403
703-385-4403
Fax 703-352-4354
and:
People Drug Stores, Inc.
6315 Bren Mar Dr. (APD)
Alexandria, VA 22312
703-750-6710

"Sunscreens"
Available from:
American Allergy Assn.
1259 El Camino #254 (APD)
Menlo Park, CA 94025
415-322-1663
Internet AllergyAid@aol.com

"Take Care of Yourself in an Emergency"
Available from:
American Allergy Assn.
1259 El Camino #254 (APD)
Menlo Park, CA 94025
415-322-1663
Internet AllergyAid@aol.com

"Taming Asthma and Allergy: Controlling Your Environent"
Robert A. Wood, MD
Available from:
Asthma & Allergy Foundation of
America
1125 15th St. N.W. #502 (APD)
Washington, DC 20005
202-466-7643
Fax 202-466-8940

"Tips on Mold Avoidance"
Available from:
Miles Inc. Pharmaceutical Div.
Miles Allergy Products
(Hollister-Stier)
PO Box 3145 (APD)
3525 N. Regal (APD)
Spokane, WA 99220-3145
800-992-1120
509-489-5656

"Treating Allergies"
Available from:
American Allergy Assn.
1259 El Camino #254 (APD)
Menlo Park, CA 94025
415-322-1663
Internet AllergyAid@aol.com

"Types of Allergic Reactions"
USDHHS
Available from:
American Allergy Assn.
1259 El Camino #254 (APD)
Menlo Park, CA 94025
415-322-1663
Internet AllergyAid@aol.com

"Understanding Allergy"
Available from:
National Jewish Center for
Immunology
and Respiratory Medicine
1400 Jackson at ColFax (APD)
Denver, CO 80206-2762
800-222-LUNG (5864)
In CO 303-355-LUNG (5864)
303-398-1907

"Understanding the Immune System"
Available from:
National Institute of Allergy
& Infectious Diseases
NIH - Public Health Services
Bldg. 31 Rm. 72-32 (APD)
Public Health Services
9000 Rockville Pike
Bethesda, MD 20892-0001

Controlling Your Environment

Information In Print

301-496-5717
301-496-4000

"Unproven Methods in Diagnosing and Treating Allergies"
Available from:
Asthma & Allergy Foundation of America
1125 15th St. N.W. #502 (APD)
Washington, DC 20005
202-466-7643
Fax 202-466-8940

"Venom Attack Force"
Available from:
Miles Inc. Pharmaceutical Div.
Miles Allergy Products
(Hollister-Stier)
PO Box 3145 (APD)
3525 N. Regal (APD)
Spokane, WA 99220-3145
800-992-1120
509-489-5656

"What's New in Allergy?"
S. Astor, MD
Available from:
Priorities®
70 Walnut St. (APD)
Wellesley, MA 02181
800-553-5398
and:
Two A's Industries, Inc.
285 South Dr. (APD)
Mountain View, CA 94040-4318
415-968-3111

"Your Allergic Nose"
Available from:
Demos Publications
156 Fifth Ave. Ste 1018 (APD)
New York, NY 10010
212-255-8768

"Your Indoor Environment"
Available from:
American Allergy Assn.
1259 El Camino #254 (APD)
Menlo Park, CA 94025

415-322-1663
Internet AllergyAid@aol.com

"Your Working Lungs Part 1: Description, Function, Problem Pollutants"
FDA
Available from:
American Allergy Assn.
1259 El Camino #254 (APD)
Menlo Park, CA 94025
415-322-1663
Internet AllergyAid@aol.com

"Your Working Lungs Part 2: Diseases, Examination, Treatment"
FDA
Available from:
American Allergy Assn.
1259 El Camino #254 (APD)
Menlo Park, CA 94025
415-322-1663
Internet AllergyAid@aol.com

"Allergy Products Directory"
Controlling Your Environment
Allergy/Asthma Finding Help
Asthma Resources Directory
Protecting Your Skin
Foods Resources Directory
Available from:
Allergy Publications
PO Box 640 (APD)
Menlo Park, CA 94025
415-322-1663

Medical Fact Sheets
Allergy: Rhinitis, Testing, Animals and Pets, Environmental Control
Available from:
National Jewish Center for Immunology
and Respiratory Medicine
1400 Jackson at ColFax (APD)
Denver, CO 80206-2762
800-222-LUNG (5864)
In CO 303-355-LUNG (5864)
303-398-1907

Controlling Your Environment

Information In Print

IN PRINT FOR CHILDREN

"Child Goes to the Hospital, A"
Available from:
Assn. for Care of Children's Health
7910 Woodmont Ave. #300 (APD)
Bethesda, MD 20814-3015
301-654-6549
Fax 301-986-4553

"I'll Never Love Anything Again"
Judy Dalton
Available from:
Albert Whitman & Co.
5747 W. Howard St. (APD)
Niles, IL 60648
708-647-1355

"Let's Talk About Going to the Hospital"
Available from:
Health Edco, Inc.
PO Box 21207 (APD)
Waco, TX 76702-1207
817-776-6461
800-433-2677

"Allergies: What They Are What They Do"
Available from:
Greenwillow Books
Div. of William Morrow & Co., Inc.
1350 Ave. of the Americas (APD)
New York, NY 10019
212-261-6500

"Complete Book of Children's Allergies, The"
B.R. Feldman, MD
David Carroll
Times Books
Available from:
Asthma & Allergy Foundation of
America
1125 15th St. N.W. #502 (APD)
Washington, DC 20005
202-466-7643
Fax 202-466-8940
and:
Asthma Outreach Library

37 Pillsbury Rd. (APD)
Sandown, NH 03873
603-329-5301
and:
Priorities®
70 Walnut St. (APD)
Wellesley, MA 02181
800-553-5398
and:
Random House, Inc.
201 E. 50th St. 31st Flr. (APD)
New York, NY 10022
212-751-2600
Orders 800-733-3000
Inquiries 800-726-0600

"Emergency Room: An ABC Tour"
Available from:
Pediatric Projects, Inc.
PO Box 1880 (APD)
Santa Monica, CA 90406

"Furry"
Holly Keller
Available from:
Asthma & Allergy Foundation of
America
1125 15th St. N.W. #502 (APD)
Washington, DC 20005
202-466-7643 l
Fax 202-466-8940

"Going to the Hospital"
Available from:
Assn. for Care of Children's Health
7910 Woodmont Ave. #300 (APD)
Bethesda, MD 20814-3015
301-654-6549
Fax 301-986-4553

"Hospital Game, The"
E. Crocker
Available from:
Assn. for Care of Children's Health
7910 Woodmont Ave. #300 (APD)
Bethesda, MD 20814-3015
301-654-6549
Fax 301-986-4553

Controlling Your Environment

Information In Print

"Hospital Journal"
Available from:
Assn. for Care of Children's Health
7910 Woodmont Ave. #300 (APD)
Bethesda, MD 20814-3015
301-654-6549
Fax 301-986-4553

"Hospital Story, A"
Available from:
Assn. for Care of Children's Health
7910 Woodmont Ave. #300 (APD)
Bethesda, MD 20814-3015
301-654-6549
Fax 301-986-4553

"Hospital Story: A Book for Children and Parents Together"
Available from:
Pediatric Projects, Inc.
PO Box 1880 (APD)
Santa Monica, CA 90406

IN PRINT FOR TEENS

"For Teenagers: Your Stay in the Hospital"
Available from:
Assn. for Care of Children's Health
7910 Woodmont Ave. #300 (APD)
Bethesda, MD 20814-3015
301-654-6549
Fax 301-986-4553

"Teens Face to Face with Chronic Illness"
Suzanne LeVert
Available from:
Asthma & Allergy Foundation of America
1125 15th St. N.W. #502 (APD)
Washington, DC 20005
202-466-7643
Fax 202-466-8940

OF RELATED INTEREST

"About Your Medicines"
(Available through doctors)
Available from:
U.S. Pharmacopeia, Inc.
12601 Twinbrook Pkwy (APD)
Rockville, MD 20852
800-227-8772
301-881-0666
Fax 301-816-8299

"Advice for the Patient: Drug Information in Lay Language"
USP DI®
Available from:
U.S. Pharmacopeia, Inc.
12601 Twinbrook Pkwy (APD)
Rockville, MD 20852
800-227-8772
301-881-0666
Fax 301-816-8299

"Air Cleaners for Allergy Relief"
Available from:
Research Products Corp.
1015 E. Washington Ave. (APD)
PO Box 1467 (APD)
Madison, WI 53701-1467
800-545-2219
608-257-8801
Fax 608-257-4357

"Air Cleaning Facts"
Available from:
Research Products Corp.
1015 E. Washington Ave. (APD)
PO Box 1467 (APD)
Madison, WI 53701-1467
800-545-2219
608-257-8801
Fax 608-257-4357

Air Pollution
Series of leaflets:
"Air Pollution and Exercise"
"Air Pollution and Your Health"
"Air Pollution Fact Sheet: Ozone Air Pollution"
"Air Pollution in Your Home"

Controlling Your Environment

Information In Print

"Air Pollution Primer"
"Air Pollution Tips for Exercisers"
Available from:
American Lung Assn.
800-LUNG-USA (5864-872)
Refers to local ALA for information

"Allergy Environment Control"
Judy Lee Bachman, PhD
Available from:
Health Services Consultants
2670 Del Mar Heights Rd. #194 (APD)
Del Mar, CA 92014

"Allergy Environment Guidebook"
Judy Lee Bachman, PhD
Available from:
Health Services Consultants
2670 Del Mar Heights Rd. #194 (APD)
Del Mar, CA 92014

"Allergy Free Garden"
Available from:
Asthma Foundation of Southern
Arizona
National Foundation for Asthma
PO Box 30069 (APD)
Tucson, AZ 85751-0069
520-323-6046

"Allergy Plants"
Mary Jelks, MD
Available from:
Allergy Asthma Technology
4151 N. Kedzie (APD)
PO Box 18398 (APD)
Chicago, IL 60618
800-621-5545
312-465-8020
Fax 312-465-7619
and:
World-Wide Publications
611 E. Wells St. (APD)
PO Box 24339 (APD)
Tampa, FL 33623

"Anaphylaxis Part 1"
Available from:
American Allergy Assn.
1259 El Camino #254 (APD)

Menlo Park, CA 94025
415-322-1663
Internet AllergyAid@aol.com

"Anaphylaxis Part 2"
Available from:
American Allergy Assn.
1259 El Camino #254 (APD)
Menlo Park, CA 94025
415-322-1663
Internet AllergyAid@aol.com

"Caring for Your Child in the Emergency Room"
Available from:
Assn. for Care of Children's Health
7910 Woodmont Ave. #300 (APD)
Bethesda, MD 20814-3015
301-654-6549
Fax 301-986-4553

"Clearing the Air at Work"
Available from:
Americans for Nonsmokers' Rights
2530 San Pablo Ave. #J (APD)
Berkeley, CA 94702
PO Box 668 (APD)
Berkeley, CA 94704
510-841-3032

"Consumer Drug Digest"
Available from:
American Soc. of Hospital Pharmacists
(ASHP)
7272 Wisconsin Ave. (APD)
Bethesda, MD 20814
202-289-1700

"Consumer Guide to Product Information"
Medication information, precautions
Available from:
Thrift Drug Co.
615 Alpha Dr. (APD)
Pittsburgh, PA 15238
412-782-8730

"Consumer Health & Nutrition Index"
Available from:

Controlling Your Environment

Information In Print

S. Karger, AG
26 W. Avon Rd. (APD)
Box 529 (APD)
Farmington, CT 06085
203-675-7834

"Consumer Health Information Source Book"
Available from:
S. Karger, AG
26 W. Avon Rd. (APD)
Box 529 (APD)
Farmington, CT 06085
203-675-7834

"Drug Information for the Health Care Provider"
Available from:
U.S. Pharmacopeia, Inc.
12601 Twinbrook Pkwy (APD)
Rockville, MD 20852
800-227-8772
301-881-0666
Fax 301-816-8299

"Drug Interactions"
FDA
Available from:
American Allergy Assn.
1259 El Camino #254 (APD)
Menlo Park, CA 94025
415-322-1663
Internet AllergyAid@aol.com

"Educational Plannning for Students with Chronic Health" Conditions: Information for Parents, Educators, and Health Care Providers"
Ellie Goldberg, MEd
79 Elmore St. (APD)
Newton, MA 02159

"Environmental Controls"
Available from:
National Allergy Supply, Inc.
4400 Georgia Hwy. 120 (APD)
PO Box 1658 (APD)
Duluth, GA 30136
800-522-1448

In Atlanta 404-623-8077
Fax 404-623-5568

"Evaporative Coolers: A Fact Sheet on Cooler Care"
Available from:
Pollution Probe
12 Madison Ave. (APD)
Toronto, ON M5R 2S1
Canada

"Exotic Pets"
Available from:
People Drug Stores, Inc.
6315 Bren Mar Dr. (APD)
Alexandria, VA 22312
703-750-6710

"Fly Control Handbook"
Available from:
Beneficial BioSystems
PO Box 8461 (APD)
Emeryville, CA 94662

"Guide To Accredited Camps"
Available from:
American Camping Assn.
Bradford Woods
5000 State Rd. 67 North (APD)
Martinsville, IN 46151-7902

"Guide to Prescription and Over-the-Counter Drugs"
Available from:
Delta Delacorte
Div. of Bantam Doubleday Dell
666th Ave. (APD)
New York, NY 10103
800-221-4676
212-765-6500

"Hay Fever Facts"
Available from:
American Lung Assn.
800-LUNG-USA (5864-872)
Refers to local ALA for information

"Hay Fever"
Available from:

Controlling Your Environment

Information In Print

American Council on Science and Health
47 Maple St. (APD)
Summit, NJ 07901

"Health Effects of Smoking on Children"
Available from:
American Lung Assn.
800-LUNG-USA (5864-872)
Refers to local ALA for information

"Health Information for International Travel"
Superintendent of Documents
Government Printing Office
Washington, DC 20402

"Health Insurance Fact and Answer Book, The"
Geri Harrington
Available from:
Harper & Row, Publishers, Inc.
10 E. 53rd St.
New York, NY 10022
212-207-7000
800-242-7737

"Help for Children: Hotlines, Helplines, and Other Resources"
Miriam J. Williams Wilson, RN
Available from:
Rocky River Publishers
PO Box 1679 (APD)
Shepherdstown, WV 25443
304-876-2711

"Help Your Health - You Can; We Can"
Available from:
People Drug Stores, Inc.
6315 Bren Mar Dr. (APD)
Alexandria, VA 22312
703-750-6710

"Helping Children Cope"
Joan Fassler
Available from:
Assn. for Care of Children's Health
7910 Woodmont Ave. #300 (APD)

Bethesda, MD 20814-3015
301-654-6549
Fax 301-986-4553

"Here Are Some Things You Should Know about Prescription Drugs"
Item No. 537W
Available from
Consumer Information Center
Pueblo, CO 81009

"Hospital Checklist"
Available from:
Assn. for Care of Children's Health
7910 Woodmont Ave. #300 (APD)
Bethesda, MD 20814-3015
301-654-6549
Fax 301-986-4553

"How the Immune System Works"
FDA
Available from:
American Allergy Assn.
1259 El Camino #254 (APD)
Menlo Park, CA 94025
415-322-1663
Internet AllergyAid@aol.com

"How to Choose a Humidifier"
Available from:
Research Products Corp.
1015 E. Washington Ave. (APD)
PO Box 1467 (APD)
Madison, WI 53701-1467
800-545-2219
608-257-8801
Fax 608-257-4357

"How to Organize a Self-Help Group"
Available from:
National Self-Help Clearinghouse
25 W. 43rd St. Rm. 620 (APD)
New York, NY 10036
212-642-2944
NY City Referrals 212-586-5770
Fax 212-719-2488

Controlling Your Environment

Information In Print

"How to Prevent Drug Interactions"
Available from:
Nonprescription Drug Manufacturers
Assn.
NDMA
1150 Connecticut Ave. NW (APD)
Washington, DC 20036
202-429-9260
Fax 202-223-6835

"Humidification Facts"
Available from:
Research Products Corp.
1015 E. Washington Ave. (APD)
PO Box 1467 (APD)
Madison, WI 53701-1467
800-545-2219
608-257-8801
Fax 608-257-4357

"Ideas for Activities with Hospitalized Children"
Available from:
Assn. for Care of Children's Health
7910 Woodmont Ave. #300 (APD)
Bethesda, MD 20814-3015
301-654-6549
Fax 301-986-4553

"Inactive Ingredient Labeling"
Available from:
American Allergy Assn.
1259 El Camino #254 (APD)
Menlo Park, CA 94025
415-322-1663
Internet AllergyAid@aol.com

"Insurance: What do you Need? How Much is Enough?"
David W. Kennedy
Available from:
Knight-Ridder Press
PO Box 5367 (APD)
Tucson, AZ 53517

"International Travel Health Guide"
Stuart R. Rose, MD
Available from:
Travel Medicine, Inc.
351 Pleasant St. #312 (APD)
Northampton, MA 01060
413-584-0381

"Knowing Your Rights: Check out the Facts Before You Check into the Hospital"
Available from:
American Assn. of Retired Persons
(AARP)
1909 K St. N.W. (APD)
Washington, DC 20049
202-728-4451

"Living with Chronic Illness"
Cheri Register
Collier Macmillan
Available from:
MacMillan Publishing Co.
866 Third Ave. (APD)
New York, NY 10022
NY 212-702-2000
800-257-5755

"Making Your Own Household Cleaners"
Available from:
Pollution Probe
12 Madison Ave. (APD)
Toronto, ON M5R 2S1
Canada

"Medicine Labels and You"
Available from:
Nonprescription Drug Manufacturers
Assn.
NDMA
1150 Connecticut Ave. NW (APD)
Washington, DC 20036
202-429-9260
Fax 202-223-6835

"Molds"
FDA
Available from:
American Allergy Assn.
1259 El Camino #254 (APD)
Menlo Park, CA 94025
415-322-1663

Controlling Your Environment

Information In Print

Internet AllergyAid@aol.com

"Moulds and Health: Who is at Risk?"
Yousef Al-Doory, PhD
with Shirley Ramsey, PhD
Available from:
Charles C Thomas, Publisher
2600 S. First St. (APD)
Springfield, IL 62794-9265

"Nasal Allergy and Orthodontics"
Stanley M. Sokolow, DDS
Available from:
American Allergy Assn.
1259 El Camino #254 (APD)
Menlo Park, CA 94025
415-322-1663
Internet AllergyAid@aol.com

"New Dimensions in Self-Help"
Available from:
National Self-Help Clearinghouse
25 W. 43rd St. Rm. 620 (APD)
New York, NY 10036
212-642-2944
NY City Referrals 212-586-5770
Fax 212-719-2488

"No Smoking: Lungs at Work"
Available from:
American Lung Assn.
800-LUNG-USA (5864-872)
Refers to local ALA for information

"Nonprescription Drugs"
Available from:
American Allergy Assn.
1259 El Camino #254 (APD)
Menlo Park, CA 94025
415-322-1663
Internet AllergyAid@aol.com

"Organizing a Self-Help Clearinghouse"
Available from:
National Self-Help Clearinghouse
25 W. 43rd St. Rm. 620 (APD)
New York, NY 10036
212-642-2944

NY City Referrals 212-586-5770
Fax 212-719-2488

"Ozone, UV & Your Skin"
Available from:
ICS Books, Inc
1370 E 86th Pl. (APD)
Merrillville, IN 46410
PO Box 10767 (APD)
Merrillville, IN 46410-0767
219-769-0585
Fax 210-769-6085
In Canada
Vanwel Publishing
800-661-6138
Fax 416-937-1760

"Parenting Plus: Raising Children with Special Health Needs"
Peggy Finston, MD
Dutton, NY

"Patient Guide to Prescription Information"
Available from:
Pharmex, Div. of
Automatic Business Products Co, Inc
PO Box 57 (APD)
Willimantic, CT 06226
800-243-8192
203-456-4255

"Poison Oak and Poison Ivy"
Available from:
Bio-Integral Resource Center, The
PO Box 7414 (APD)
Berkeley, CA 94707
510-524-2567
Fax 510-524-1758

"Preparing Your Child for the Hospital: A Checklist"
Available from:
Assn. for Care of Children's Health
7910 Woodmont Ave. #300 (APD)
Bethesda, MD 20814-3015
301-654-6549
Fax 301-986-4553

Controlling Your Environment

Information In Print

"Preventing Mildew"
FDA
Available from:
American Allergy Assn.
1259 El Camino #254 (APD)
Menlo Park, CA 94025
415-322-1663
Internet AllergyAid@aol.com

"Read the Label and Use Medicines Safely"
Available from:
Giant Food, Inc.
PO Box 1804 (APD)
Washington, DC 20013
301-341-4365

"Removing Mildew"
FDA
Available from:
American Allergy Assn.
1259 El Camino #254 (APD)
Menlo Park, CA 94025
415-322-1663
Internet AllergyAid@aol.com

"Self-Help Organizations and Professional Practice"
T.J. Powell
Available from:
National Assn. of Social Workers
7981 Eastern Ave. (APD)
Silver Spring, MD 20910

"Self-Help Reporter"
Quarterly
Available from:
National Self-Help Clearinghouse
25 W. 43rd St. Rm. 620 (APD)
New York, NY 10036
212-642-2944
NY City Referrals 212-586-5770
Fax 212-719-2488

"Smog and Air Pollution"
Available from:
American Allergy Assn.
1259 El Camino #254 (APD)
Menlo Park, CA 94025
415-322-1663

Internet AllergyAid@aol.com

"Sneezeless Landscaping"
Call your local American Lung Assn. for availability

"Starting and Operating Support Groups"
Available from:
National Resource Center for
for Family Support Programs
Family Resource Coalition
200 S. Michigan Ave. #1520 (APD)
Chicago, IL 60604

"Story of Humidity, The"
Available from:
Research Products Corp.
1015 E. Washington Ave. (APD)
PO Box 1467 (APD)
Madison, WI 53701-1467
800-545-2219
608-257-8801
Fax 608-257-4357

"Sun and Your Skin, The"
Dr. J.L.M. Hawk
Available from:
American Allergy Assn.
1259 El Camino #254 (APD)
Menlo Park, CA 94025
415-322-1663
Internet AllergyAid@aol.com

"Take Care with Over-the-Counter Allergy Medicine"
Available from:
Nonprescription Drug Manufacturers Assn.
NDMA
1150 Connecticut Ave. NW (APD)
Washington, DC 20036
202-429-9260
Fax 202-223-6835

"Take Charge of Your Health"
Stephen Astor, MD
Available from:
Two A's Industries, Inc.
285 South Dr. (APD)

Controlling Your Environment

Information In Print

Mountain View, CA 94040-4318
415-968-3111

"TMC's Allergy Free Garden: A Guide to Allergy Free Landscaping"
Available from:
Tucson Medical Center
Chest and Allergy Clinic
PO Box 42195 (APD)
Tucson, AZ 85733
520-324-5110

"Tracking the Skin's Reactions to Drugs"
Available from:
American Allergy Assn.
1259 El Camino #254 (APD)
Menlo Park, CA 94025
415-322-1663
Internet AllergyAid@aol.com

"Travelers' Medical Resource"
Available from:
ICS Books, Inc
1370 E 86th Pl. (APD)
Merrillville, IN 46410
PO Box 10767 (APD)
Merrillville, IN 46410-0767
219-769-0585
Fax 210-769-6085
In Canada
Vanwel Publishing
800-661-6138
Fax 416-937-1760

"Understanding Calcium and Osteoporosis"
Staff of the American Allergy Assn.
Irene T. McPherrin, MD
Available from:
Allergy Publications
PO Box 640 (APD)
Menlo Park, CA 94025
415-322-1663

"USAN & USP Dictionary of Drug Names"
Available from:
U.S. Pharmacopeia, Inc.

12601 Twinbrook Pkwy (APD)
Rockville, MD 20852
800-227-8772
301-881-0666
Fax 301-816-8299

"Using Medicines Wisely"
Available from:
American Lung Assn.
800-LUNG-USA (5864-872)
Refers to local ALA for information

"Vacation Time"
Available from:
American Allergy Assn.
1259 El Camino #254 (APD)
Menlo Park, CA 94025
415-322-1663
Internet AllergyAid@aol.com

"Weeds 'n' Things"
(Allergens in southern Arizona)
Linda Alpert, RN, BSN
Available from:
Asthma Foundation of Southern Arizona
National Foundation for Asthma
PO Box 30069 (APD)
Tucson, AZ 85751-0069
520-323-6046

"Your Hospital: Meeting the Special Needs of Children"
Available from:
Assn. for Care of Children's Health
7910 Woodmont Ave. #300 (APD)
Bethesda, MD 20814-3015
301-654-6549
Fax 301-986-4553

IN PRINT FOR PROFESSIONALS

"Adverse Reactions to Cosmetics"
Anton C. De Grott, MD
Gordon L. Lackie, Editor
Available from:
Scholium Int'l, Inc.

Controlling Your Environment

Information In Print

99 Seaview Blvd. (APD)
Port Washington, NY 11050-4610
516-484-3290

"Allergic and Vasomotor Rhinitis: Clinical Aspect"
Niels Mygind
Bent Weeke
Available from:
Coronet Books
311 Bainbridge St. (APD)
Philadelphia, PA 19147
215-925-5083

"Allergic Diseases from Infancy to Adulthood"
C. Warren Bierman
David S. Pearlman
Available from:
W.B. Saunders Co.
Subs. of Harcourt/Brace/Jovanovich, Inc.
Curtis Center
Independence Square W (APD)
Philadelphia, PA 19106
800-545-2322
PA 215-238-7800

"Allergic Diseases"
Roy Patterson, MD
Lippincott Medical
Available from:
Harper & Row, Publishers, Inc.
10 E. 53rd St.
New York, NY 10022
212-207-7000
800-242-7737

"Allergic Diseases: Diagnosis & Management"
Roy Patterson, MD
Available from:
Periger Books
Imprint of Putnam Publishing Group
200 Madison Ave. (APD)
New York, NY 10016
800-631-8571
212-951-8400

"Allergies: Complete Guide to Diagnosis, Treatment, & Daily Management"
Young, MD
Available from:
Anderson Continuing Education
for Nursing Professionals
3268 Ramos Cir. (APD)
PO Box 276297 (APD)
Sacramento, CA 95827
800-532-2332
and:
Consumers Union
256 Washington St. (APD)
Mt. Vernon, NY 10553

"Allergy and Inflammation"
A.B. Kay, MD
Available from:
Academic Press, Inc.
Subs. of Harcourt Brace Jovanovich, Inc.
465 S. Lincoln Dr. (APD)
Troy, MI 63379
619-231-6616
800-346-8648

"Allergy"
Allen P. Kaplan, MD, Editor
Available from:
Churchill Livingstone, Inc.
650 Ave. of the Americas (APD)
New York, NY 10011
800-553-5462
212-206-5000
Fax 212-727-7808
Customer Service 800-503-5426
and
Churchill Livingstone, Inc.
128 Long Acre (APD)
London, WC25 9AN
United Kingdom
011-44-71836-5852

"Allergy: Principles & Practice"
Middleton, et al.
Available from:
C.V. Mosby Co.
Subs. of Times Mirror Co.
11830 Westline Industrial Dr. (APD)

Controlling Your Environment

Information In Print

PO Box 46908 (APD)
St. Louis, MO 63146-9988
800-325-4177
MO 314-872-8370
Orders 800-426-4545

"Allergy: Theory & Practice"
Philip Korenblat, MD
James H. Wedner, MD
Available from:
W.B. Saunders Co.
Subs. of Harcourt/Brace/Jovanovich, Inc.
Curtis Center
Independence Square W (APD)
Philadelphia, PA 19106
800-545-2322
PA 215-238-7800

"Allergy Products Directory"
Controlling Your Environment
Allergy/Asthma Finding Help
Asthma Resources Directory
Protecting Your Skin
Foods Resources Directory
Available from:
Allergy Publications
PO Box 640 (APD)
Menlo Park, CA 94025
415-322-1663

American Hospital Formulary Service Comprehensive: current drug monographs; quarterly updates
Available from:
American Soc. of Hospital Pharmacists (ASHP)
7272 Wisconsin Ave. (APD)
Bethesda, MD 20814
202-289-1700

American Lung Assn. Reprints
Call your local ALA branch for reprints of the following articles:
"A Randomized Trial of A.C.T. (Asthma Care Training) for Kids"
C.E. Lewis, MD et. al.
"A School Health Education Program for Children with Asthma Aged 8-11 Years"
D. Evans, et. al.
"Asthma Education: A National Strategy" (NHLBI & NIAID)
S.R. Parker, et. al.
"Asthma Self-Management Education Research and Implications for Clinical Practice
N.M. Clark, et. al.
"Asthma Self-Management Programs: Premises not Promises
E.L. Klingelhofer, et. al.
"Collaborative Asthma Self-Management Evaluation Designs"
M.C. Hindi-Alexander, et. al.
"Living with Asthma: Replications and Extensions"
T.L. Creer
"Making Childhood Asthma Management Education Happen in the Community: Translating Health Behavioral Research into Local Programs"
C.B. Krutzsch
"Managing Better: Children, Parents, and Asthma"
N.M. Clark, et. al.
"Self-Management Education of Children with Asthma: Air Wise"
W.L. McNabb, et. al.
"The Impact of Health Education on Frequency and Cost of Health Care Used by Low Income Children with Asthma"
N.M. Clark, et. al.
"The Role of Patient Education in the Management of Childhood Asthma"
S.R. Wilson-Pessano
"Workshop on Asthma Self-Management, Summary of Workshop Discussion"
S.R. Wilson-Pessano, et. al.
Available from:
American Lung Assn.
800-LUNG-USA (5864-872)
Refers to local ALA for information

"Asthma & Allergy in Pregnancy & Early Infancy"
Michael Schatz, MD, Editor
Robert S. Zeiger, MD, Editor

Controlling Your Environment

Information In Print

Available from:
Marcel Dekker, Inc.
270 Madison Ave. (APD)
800-228-1160
NY 212-696-9000

"Color Atlas of Allergy, A"
William F. Jackson, MA, MB, BChir, MRCP
Rino Cerio, BSc, MB, BS, MRCP
Available from:
C.V. Mosby Co.
Subs. of Times Mirror Co.
11830 Westline Industrial Dr. (APD)
PO Box 46908 (APD)
St. Louis, MO 63146-9988
800-325-4177
MO 314-872-8370
Orders 800-426-4545

"Consumer Guide for Room Air Cleaners"
Available from:
Assn. of Home Appliance Manufacturers
AHAM
20 N. Wacker Dr. (APD)
Chicago, IL 60606
312-984-5800

"Current Perspectives in Immunodermatology"
Rona M. Mackie, Editor
Available from:
Churchill Livingstone, Inc.
650 Ave. of the Americas (APD)
New York, NY 10011
800-553-5462
212-206-5000
Fax 212-727-7808
Customer Service 800-503-5426
and
Churchill Livingstone, Inc.
128 Long Acre (APD)
London, WC25 9AN
United Kingdom
011-44-71836-5852

"Current Therapy in Allergy, Immunology & Rheumatology"
Lichtenstein & Fauci
Available from:
C.V. Mosby Co.
Subs. of Times Mirror Co.
11830 Westline Industrial Dr. (APD)
PO Box 46908 (APD)
St. Louis, MO 63146-9988
800-325-4177
Orders 800-426-4545

"Drug Information for the Health Care Provider"
Available from:
U.S. Pharmacopeia, Inc.
12601 Twinbrook Pkwy (APD)
Rockville, MD 20852
800-227-8772
301-881-0666
Fax 301-816-8299

"Eosinophils in Asthma & Allergy"
A.B. Kay, MD
Available from:
Blackwell Scientific Pubns., Inc.
238 Main St. (APD)
Cambridge, MA 02142
800-445-6638
617-225-0430

"Essential Immunology"
I. M. Roitt, MA, DSc,
Available from:
C.V. Mosby Co.
Subs. of Times Mirror Co.
11830 Westline Industrial Dr. (APD)
PO Box 46908 (APD)
St. Louis, MO 63146-9988
800-325-4177
Orders 800-426-4545

"Evaluation and Management of Allergic and Asthmatic Disorders"
Eric Gershwin
Stephen M. Nagy, Editor
Available from:
Grune & Stratton

Controlling Your Environment

Information In Print

Subs. of Harcourt Brace Jovanovich, Inc.
111 Fifth Ave. (APD)
New York, NY 10003
212-741-4888

"Guide to Atmospheric Pollen Counting and Differentiation A"
Available from:
Center Laboratories
35 Channel Dr. (APD)
PO Box 70 (APD)
Port Washington, NY 11050
Customer service 800-223-6837

"Key Facts in Immunology"
David S. Scott
Jeffrey R. Dawson
Available from:
Churchill Livingstone, Inc.
650 Ave. of the Americas (APD)
New York, NY 10011
800-553-5462
212-206-5000
Fax 212-727-7808
Customer Service 800-503-5426
and
Churchill Livingstone, Inc.
128 Long Acre (APD)
London, WC25 9AN
United Kingdom
011-44-71836-5852

"Late Phase Allergic Reactions"
Walter Dorsch
Available from:
CRC Press, Inc.
Subs of Times Mirror Co.
2000 Corporation Blvd. N.W. (APD)
Boca Raton, FL 33431
800-272-7737
407-994-0555

"Manual of Clinical Problems in Asthma, Allergy & Related Disorders, A"
Don A. Bukstein
Robert C. Strunk
Available from:
Little, Brown & Co.

Div. of Time, Inc.
34 Beacon St. (APD)
Boston, MA 02108
800-343-9204
MA 617-227-0730

"Medication Teaching Manual: A Guide for Patient Counseling"
Available from:
American Soc. of Hospital Pharmacists (ASHP)
7272 Wisconsin Ave. (APD)
Bethesda, MD 20814
202-289-1700

"New Developments in the Therapy of Allergic Disorders & Asthma"
S.A. Langer, MD
Available from:
S. Karger, AG
26 W. Avon Rd. (APD)
Box 529 (APD)
Farmington, CT 06085
203-675-7834

"Primer on Allergic & Immunologic Diseases"
Richard Lockey, MD, Editor
　　English, Spanish
Available from:
American Academy Allergy/Imm.
611 E. Wells St. 4th Flr. (APD)
Milwaukee, WI 53202-3816
800-822-ASMA (2762)
414-272-6071
Fax 414-276-3349

"Problem Buildings: Building-Associated Illness and the Sick Building Syndrome"
J. Cone, MD, MPH, Editor
M. Hodgson, MD, MPH, Editor
Available from:
Hanley & Belfus, Inc.
Dist. by C.V. Mosby Co.
210 S. 13th St. (APD)
Philadelphia, PA 19107
215-546-7293

Controlling Your Environment

Information In Print

"Progress in Allergy"
P. Kallos, MD
Available from:
S. Karger, AG
26 W. Avon Rd. (APD)
Box 529 (APD)
Farmington, CT 06085
203-675-7834

"Respiratory Allergy"
Gaetano Melillo, MD
Gianni Marone, MD
Philip S. Norman, MD
Available from:
C.V. Mosby Co.
Subs. of Times Mirror Co.
11830 Westline Industrial Dr. (APD)
PO Box 46908 (APD)
St. Louis, MO 63146-9988
800-325-4177
MO 314-872-8370
Orders 800-426-4545

"Rhinitis and Asthma: Similarities and Differences"
Niels Mygind, MD
Ronald Dahl, MD
Ulf Pipkorn, MD
Available from:
C.V. Mosby Co.
Subs. of Times Mirror Co.
11830 Westline Industrial Dr. (APD)
PO Box 46908 (APD)
St. Louis, MO 63146-9988
800-325-4177
MO 314-872-8370
Orders 800-426-4545

"The Manual of Allergy and Immunology"
Glenn Lawlor, MD, Editor
Thomas Fischer, MD, Editor

Available from:
Little, Brown & Co.
Div. of Time, Inc.
34 Beacon St. (APD)
Boston, MA 02108
800-343-9204
MA 617-227-0730

"Theoretical and Clinical Aspects of Allergic Diseases"
H. Bostrom, Editor
N. Ljungstedt. Editor
Available from:
Coronet Books
311 Bainbridge St. (APD)
Philadelphia, PA 19147
215-925-5083

"Understanding Allergy Sensitivity & Immunity: A Comprehensive Guide"
Janice Vickerstaff Joneja, PhD
Leonard Bielory, MD
Available from:
Rutgers Univ. Press
109 Church St. (APD)
New Brunswick, NJ 08901
800-446-9323
908-932-7764

INTERAX
Microfiche of prescribed medications
Available from:
Pharmex, Div. of
Automatic Business Products Co, Inc
PO Box 57 (APD)
Willimantic, CT 06226
800-243-8192
203-456-4255

INDEX

Controlling Your Environment

Index

Index

Our thanks to the

non-profit organizations

and the companies in the pages following

for their interest in this project

Controlling Your Environment

Asthma and Allergy Foundation of America (AAFA)

America's leading organization for people with asthma and allergies

- Provides up-to-date, practical and timely articles in our newsletter,
- Sponsors a nationwide network of local chapters,
- Offers peer support through 145 local, affiliated support groups,
- Funds important medical research,
- Maintains a large clearinghouse of current and affordable educational materials,
- Advocates on behalf of the 50 million Americans with asthma and allergies,
- Offers special services to physicians and allied health professionals.

Call or write:

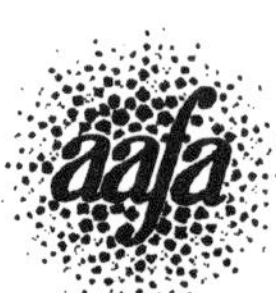 Asthma and Allergy Foundation of America
1125 15th Street, NW Suite 502
Washington, DC 20005
(202) 466-7643 or (800) 7-ASTHMA
(202) 466-8940 FAX 

The Allergy and Asthma Network•Mothers of Asthmatics, Inc. (AAN•MA), is a nonprofit health education organization dedicated to assisting 50 million people with allergies and asthma and their families. Individual and professional memberships include the following benefits:

- A subscription to AAN•MA's monthly newsletter, *The MA Report*.

- A **10 percent discount** on AAN•MA publications, videos, peak flow meters, nebulizer accessories.

- Membership to the **AAN Pharmacy Program** offering discounts on medications.

- Toll-free **hotline** staff support.

- **Marketplace** - offering discounts on allergy and asthma products.

- Special medical **updates and bulletins**.

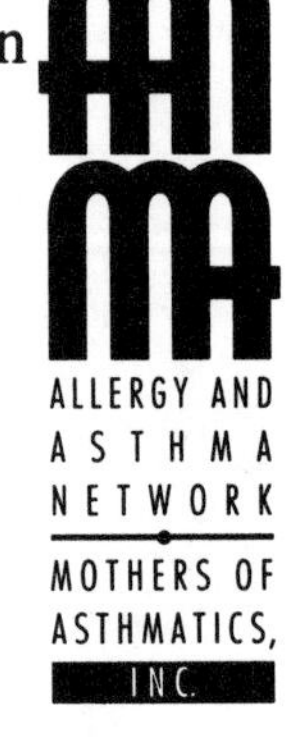

Controlling Your Environment

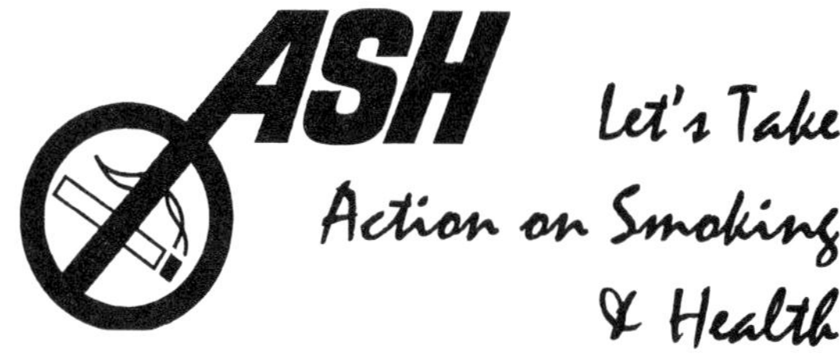

99.98% of Americans smoke, whether they like it or not! We are forced to inhale other people's tobacco smoke—as a condition of holding a job, dining in a restaurant, shopping in a mall, or flying internationally.

Action on Smoking & Health is a national, nonprofit charitable organization that is supported entirely by tax-deductible contributions from individuals and private foundations. Using the tremendous power of the law to represent nonsmokers in courts and legislative bodies and before regulatory agencies, ASH has been successfully fighting for the rights of nonsmokers for over a quarter-century! ASH is responsible for cigarette commercial-free radio and television, smokefree flights and bus rides, and many other victories.

Yes! I want to support the work of ASH with a contribution of: ☐ $100 ☐ $50 ☐ $15✻ ☐ Other ______

☐ **SPECIAL OFFER:** we'll send the informative booklet "Taking Action to Protect You and Your Family From Passive Smoke" for an additional $3.50 (postpaid) — a 25% discount for Allergy Products Directory readers!

Name ____

Address ____

City, State, Zip ____

Your contribution to ASH is tax-deductible. Please make your check payable to ASH and send it to 2013 H St. NW, Washington, DC 20006   ✻ If you contribute a minimum of $15, we'll send you our bi-monthly newsletter.

Asthma.
It doesn't have to restrict your life.

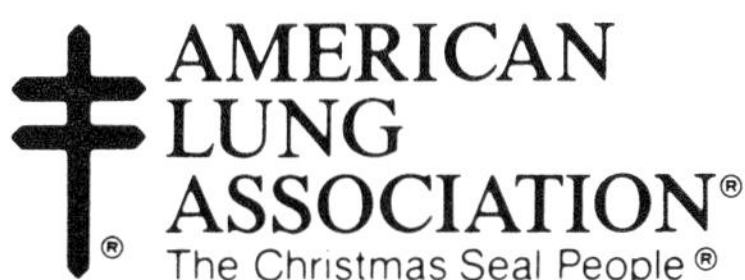

AMERICAN LUNG ASSOCIATION®
The Christmas Seal People ®

Controlling Your Environment

SEND FOR
AMERICAN ALLERGY ASSOCIATION'S
PUBLICATION'S LIST

1259 El Camino #254
Menlo Park, CA 94025

Enclose a self-addressed envelope
and two stamps

➤ "Your Office Environment"

AAA Info Sheets help you recognize trouble areas, causes and symptoms.
Help you tackle the problems at work in a more knowledgeable manner.
Request Office Environment and enclose: $8

➤ "Allergy Alerts from Living with Allergies"

American Allergy Association recognizes the special problems that you face in your daily life. *Allergy Alerts* gives you the facts you need to evaluate advertising that may mislead or misinform.

These alerts cover a wide range of areas from dyes in medications to medication interactions, food additives like sulfites, new foods like spelt, situations that could trigger asthma, problems with collagen, contact lens solutions, latex, even fabric softeners.

Be armed with the information you need to protect yourself and your family from misinformation or new products that may pose allergy problems.
When the news is too good to be true, you need the facts.
Request Allergy Alerts and enclose $11

➤ "Pollen Times — By State, By Month"

Don't let your travel plans be ruined.
Don't compromise your business effectiveness.
Plan your business trip   Plan your vacation` Avoid pollen problems.
*Know **when** grasses, weeds, or trees are likely to be pollinating.
*Know **where** grasses, weeds, or trees are likely to be pollinating.
Request Pollen Times and enclose $7

➤ "10 Steps toward Allergy Relief"

There are many things that you can do when you seek relief from allergies and these Information Sheets take you through the steps, helping you to make the decisions necessary for your medical health and well being.
Request 10 Steps and enclose $2 plus self-addressed, stamped envelope.

➤ "Guide to Gluten-Free Diets"

Safe substitutes for baking and cooking
Differentiates celiac disease from wheat allergy
Sources of gluten in the diet. Warnings on when to check with the manufacturer
Buying guide for foods and ingredients — Plus a list of recipe books.
Request Gluten-free Diets and enclose $11

Allergy Publications
1259 El Camino #254 ●Menlo Park, CA 94025

➤ "Eating Without. . .Packet"

12 Information Sheets describe the most common food allergens
Specific problems with common foods and supplements
The facts on milk ingredient labeling, milk allergy and milk sensitivity
PLUS: 16-page handbook selected by Harvard Health Newsletter as a resource:
Understanding Calcium and Osteoporosis
Request Eating Without and enclose $11

➤ "The New Labels"

Terms defined. What do all these new label words mean?
How to more easily understand what the labels are telling you
What are the meanings of the words that are used on the labels?
Exceptions, Omissions, and Problems.
What labels do not tell you. How the labels can mislead you
Health Claims. What is allowed and what is not.
Ingredient Labeling. Learn what must be listed and how.
Request Labels and enclose $6 plus self-addressed, stamped envelope

➤ "Infant Formulas for Allergic Infants and Dietetic Concerns for Toddlers"

How those differences affect testing, symptoms, and diet
Misleading food labels — Reliable food labels
What's in milk?
When substitutes are suitable and when they are not
Other formulas: Neocate, Whey or Casein or Protein Hydrolysates or meat-based formula
Evaluating infant formulas
Is protection possible for your child?
What about elemental diets
Other drinks: goat's milk, soy milk
FDA labeling requirements under the new law
Children under two — Children under four
Request Toddlers and enclose $11

Allergy Publications
1259 El Camino #254 ●Menlo Park, CA 94025

————AMERICAN ALLERGY ASSOCIATION————
1259 El Camino #254, Menlo Park, CA 94025

FOR YOUR HEALTH CONCERNS

American Allergy Association is a non-profit, educational organization, formed in 1979 to reach those suffering from asthma and allergies due to pollen, molds, dust, danders, foods, irritants. We offer. . .

● **DATASearch** of our extensive data base of allergy and asthma products, services, resources, help sources, and publications.

● *Living with Allergies* our hand book of in-depth articles on allergy, foods, book reviews, product information, allergy alerts, reports from journals.

● **Allergy/Asthma ResourceLink** for on-line information at hooked.net

● **Allergen-free recipe books** for cakes, cookies, muffins, breads, soups, salads, main courses and desserts. Write and tell us which foods you must avoid.

● **Directories** for asthma, environmental control, household care, personal needs, dust, pollen, mildew, cosmetics. Write for our publications list.

● **Allergy Information Series** of handbooks based on the thousands of questions AAA has answered over the years from patients, from nurses, from doctors, from dietitians, and from reference libraries. This series addressed the problem of "What do people want to know and how can we best meet that need.?"

When writing, please enclose a self-addressed envelope with two stamps.

Comments and Suggestions

Allergy Publications is always looking for ways to improve its publications. Please take a moment to send us your opinion to the address above.

1.   What did you like or dislike about the organization of the directory:

2.   Are there any products, services, or publications you think should be included in the next edition? (We need the product or service name, the company, and if possible, the address and telephone number or the title and author.)

3.   Comments. (We like to hear good things, too.)